T0348411

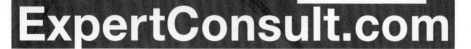

Rapid Response Events in the Critically Ill

Rapid Response Events in the Critically Ill

A Case-Based Approach to Inpatient Medical Emergencies

SYED ARSALAN AKHTER ZAIDI, MD, MCR
Clinical Assistant Professor of Medicine
Internal Medicine
University of Pittsburgh Medical Center
Pittsburgh, PA

KAINAT SALEEM, MD, MCR
Clinical Assistant Professor of Medicine
Internal Medicine
University of Pittsburgh Medical Center
Pittsburgh, PA

ELSEVIER

Elsevier
1600 John F. Kennedy Blvd.
Ste 1800
Philadelphia, PA 19103-2899

RAPID RESPONSE EVENTS IN THE CRITICALLY ILL: ISBN: 978-0-323-87239-3
A Case-Based Approach to Inpatient Medical Emergencies

Content Strategist: Michael Houston
Content Development Specialist: Shilpa
Publishing Services Manager: Shereen Jameel
Project Manager: Beula Christopher
Design Direction: Patrick C. Ferguson

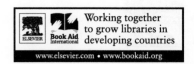

Working together
to grow libraries in
developing countries

www.elsevier.com • www.bookaid.org

Last digit is the print number: 9 8 7 6 5 4 3 2 1

*I would like to thank and **dedicate** this work to **my wife** and co-editor, Kainat, for providing me the impetus to write this book – an often talked about aspiration of mine that became a reality – and **my parents** for their continued support and belief in me; I would not have been who I am without their blessings.*

Syed

*I've always believed that achieving success depends on motivation, dedication, confidence, and most of all, the desire and dedication to succeed. I would like to dedicate this work to **my husband** and co-editor, Arsalan, who believed in me to be able to take on this task and supported me along the way. I also want to dedicate this book to my **parents**, who motivated me and always believed in me, contributing to my confidence.*

Kainat

The idea for this book evolved over several years while I served as a supervising physician at a leading tertiary care academic center. My role as a "code leader" for over 500 rapid response events in 2 years led me to learn about many common scenarios that can be dealt with more effectively with a suitable knowledge base. Many textbooks provide detailed information on managing critically ill patients and inpatient emergencies, but a textbook focused on dealing with just rapid response events in a case-based format was lacking. Our efforts in this text are mainly to provide an easy-to-read guide for medical students, residents, fellows, and hospitalists who routinely deal with inpatient medical emergencies. This book is compiled using the most up-to-date information at the time of writing, but as we know that medical science is in the process of constant evolution, readers should seek updated guidelines as needed. Providers are requested to make their clinical decisions based on their clinical judgment at the bedside, as all patients and clinical scenarios are unique.

A rapid response team (RRT) or a medical emergency team (MET) consists of nurses and other health care professionals/paramedical staff (respiratory therapists, pharmacists, emergency department personnel, and others) who bring critical care expertise to the bedside. The concept behind a well-run rapid response is to stabilize a critical patient and introduce the necessary interventions to prevent further clinical deterioration. An RRT is equipped to provide ICU-level care at any location in the hospital while the patient is stabilized for transport to ICU if needed.

This book consists of five main sections: Cardiology, Respiratory, Gastrointestinal, Endocrinology, and miscellaneous. Each section contains a case-based approach to an inpatient emergency related to that system. Each chapter consists of a simple case presentation, including pertinent patient history, investigations, and interventions based on a provisional diagnosis. The cases and patient information are made-up by the authors, and any similarity to a real patient will be purely coincidental. The case is followed by a comprehensive discussion about the diagnosis in that case. The discussion includes clinical features, diagnostic criteria, and a stepwise approach to managing the diagnosis in a code event. Since all codes are based on the rapid response principles of "Airway, Breathing, Circulation", these management steps are common in various chapters. Therefore, starting each rapid response with "Airway, Breathing, and Circulation" allows the readers to get a comprehensive overview of the management of each case without having to refer to other chapters.

To aid the readers, we have tried to follow a consistent format in the content presentation so that information can be readily located. This format has been adopted to support critical thinking as the readers read through the initial presentation, history, physical examination, and vital signs and make a presumptive diagnosis. However, some chapters could not be structured so due to their content. We hope that our organization of this text will be helpful for all the readers.

ACKNOWLEDGMENTS

We want to express our sincere appreciation for the assistance and support provided by all the contributors in developing this book. The journey from just a concept to an actual content-rich textbook involved hundreds of hours of work which would not have been possible without all who contributed.

Particular mention goes to Dr. Firas Abdulmajeed and Dr. Muhammad Adrish, who took time out of their hectic schedules to review the book's content and suggest valuable additions and edits. Their expertise and knowledge of critical care medicine helped enhance this textbook immensely. I also want to thank Dr. Muhammad Saad, who shared his expert opinion in Cardiology and helped make this text as up-to-date as possible with the latest guidelines. Last but not least, I thank Dr. Bushra Zaidi, my sister and my closest friend, for her valuable time in reviewing the final content and providing support during the proofreading process.

Firas Abdulmajeed, MD, ChB
Assistant Professor of Critical Care
   Medicine and Neurology
Director of Medical ICU
University of Pittsburgh Medical Center
   Mercy Hospital
Pittsburgh, PA

Abdelrhman M. Abo-zed, MD
Resident Physician
Internal Medicine
University of Pittsburgh Medical Center
   Mercy Hospital
Pittsburgh, PA

Mohammad Adrish, MD, MBA
Associate Professor
Medicine – Pulmonary, Critical Care and
   Sleep Medicine
Baylor College of Medicine
Houston, TX

Rahul R. Bollam, MD
Resident Physician
Internal Medicine
University of Pittsburgh Medical Center
   Mercy Hospital
Pittsburgh, PA

Waliul Chowdhury, MD
Resident Physician
Internal Medicine
University of Pittsburgh Medical Center
   Mercy Hospital
Pittsburgh, PA

Melissa Chrites, DO
Attending Physician
USAFR
Coraopolis, PA

Michael Heslin, DO
Resident Physician
Physical Medicine and Rehabilitation
University of Pittsburgh Medical Center
   Mercy Hospital
Pittsburgh, PA

Kainat Saleem, MD, MCR
Clinical Assistant Professor of Medicine
Internal Medicine
University of Pittsburgh Medical Center
Pittsburgh, PA

Ali Uddin, MD
Resident Physician
Internal Medicine
University of Pittsburgh Medical Center
   Mercy Hospital
Pittsburgh, PA

Syed Arsalan Akhter Zaidi, MD, MCR
Clinical Assistant Professor of Medicine
Internal Medicine
University of Pittsburgh Medical Center
Pittsburgh, PA

CONTENTS

PART 4   Cases With Gastrointestinal Pathologies

Cases With Cardiovascular Pathologies

CHAPTER 1

Chest Pain in a Patient With Coronary Artery Disease – I

Waliul Chowdhury ▪ Syed Arsalan Akhter Zaidi ▪ Firas Abdulmajeed
▪ Mohammad Adrish

Case Study

A rapid response event was initiated by the bedside nurse for acute onset hypotension. On prompt arrival of the rapid response team, it was noted that the patient was a 66-year-old female with a known history of ST-elevation myocardial infarction (STEMI) status post coronary artery bypass grafting a year ago, hypertension, and type 2 diabetes. She initially presented to the hospital for right flank pain and was being treated for a urinary tract infection. Upon further questioning at the bedside, the patient mentioned that she had been having substernal chest pain for the past 1 h. Her chest pain had continued to worsen, and she now had associated diaphoresis and tachypnea.

VITALS SIGNS

Temperature: 37.4 °F, axillary
Blood Pressure: 90/40 mmHg
Pulse: 105 beats per min (bpm), sinus tachycardia on telemetry (see Fig. 1.1)
Respiratory Rate: 22 breaths per min
Pulse Oximetry: 99% on room air

FOCUSED PHYSICAL EXAMINATION

The patient was an elderly female who was in moderate distress, holding her chest and appeared diaphoretic. She responded briefly to her name but swiftly stopped responding to further commands. She was moving all her limbs spontaneously. The heart rate was 105-110 bpm, with a regular rhythm and no murmurs. The abdominal exam did not elicit any tenderness, and the rest of her physical exam was benign.

INTERVENTIONS

The patient was given a 1 L fluid bolus which increased her blood pressure to 120/70 mmHg. A complete metabolic panel, troponin level, and magnesium levels were ordered. An EKG was done, which showed sinus tachycardia, with no acute ischemic findings. Chest X-ray at bedside showed no evidence of pneumothorax, consolidation, widened mediastinum, or enlarged aortic knob and no evidence of fluid overload. The pretest probability of PE was low, so a d-dimer test was ordered, which was normal. The patient was given one dose of 0.3 mg sublingual nitroglycerin (NTG), which improved her chest pain. Based on her cardiac history and current presentation, she was loaded with 325 mg of aspirin and 600 mg of clopidogrel and started on a therapeutic dose of enoxaparin after consultation with cardiology.

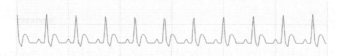

Fig. 1.1   Telemetry strip showing lead ii with a heart rate of 105 bpm, and sinus rhythm

TABLE 1.1 ■ **Differential diagnosis of chest pain**

Life-threatening	Non-life-threatening
Acute coronary syndrome	Lung infection
Acute aortic dissection	Pericarditis
Pulmonary embolism	Gastroesophageal reflux disease
Tension pneumothorax	Costochondritis
Pericardial tamponade	Panic attack
Esophageal rupture	Aortic stenosis

FINAL DIAGNOSIS: UNSTABLE ANGINA

Generalized Approach to Acute Severe Chest Pain

There is a wide range of causes of chest pain in a rapid response setting, but the differential can be narrowed down with an organized history, physical, and appropriate workup. Chest pain is the second most common presenting complaint in the United States, with 7.6 million emergency department visits yearly. Prompt recognition and exclusion of the life-threatening differentials of chest pain are of paramount importance. However, it can be tricky at times as patients may appear deceptively well (Table 1.1). This emphasizes the importance of appropriate workup.

ACUTE CORONARY SYNDROME (ACS)

ACS results either from rupture of atherosclerotic plaques or formation of intramural thrombus, which reduces blood flow to the myocardium causing ischemia via mismatch in the oxygen supply vs. demand. If this mismatch is reversible and not significant enough to cause myocardial necrosis, it is called unstable angina. If the myocardial ischemia is irreversible with associated myocardial injury, it is called a myocardial infarction (STEMI vs. non-STEMI, discussed in detail in later chapters). EKG is the diagnostic investigation of choice, aided by elevated cardiac enzymes in the appropriate setting.

ACUTE AORTIC DISSECTION

Aortic dissection begins with a tear in the inner layer (tunica intima) of the aortic wall. This causes blood to travel between the intimal and medial layers of the vessel. The pulsatile blood flow causes the dissection to spread and subsequently causes obstruction of the branch arteries leading to end-organ ischemia. The type of chest pain is typically stabbing chest pain radiating to the back. Computed tomography (CT) angiogram is the diagnostic investigation of choice.

PULMONARY EMBOLISM (PE)

PE occurs when a distal deep venous clot gets dislodged, travels through the right side of the heart, and gets lodged at the branch point in the main pulmonary artery (saddle embolus) or one of its distal branches (segmental or sub-segmental clots). This occlusion can cause acute pulmonary hypertension, dysfunction of the right ventricle leading to right-sided heart failure, a mismatch in gas exchange, and possibly infarction of lung parenchyma. CT angiogram is the diagnostic investigation of choice.

PNEUMOTHORAX

Pneumothorax is the presence of air in the pleural space. It typically occurs because of an abnormal connection between the pulmonary parenchyma and pleural space. Tension pneumothorax is a life-threatening form of pneumothorax that occurs because of a one-way valve opening into the pleural space that allows air to enter this space but does not allow it to move back into the lung. This leads to increased pressure within the pleural space that can displace mediastinal structures and cause hemodynamic compromise. Primary spontaneous pneumothorax occurs typically in younger males that are thin and tall. Secondary spontaneous pneumothorax typically occurs in patients with chronic obstructive lung disease, cystic fibrosis, and asthma. Chest X-ray is the diagnostic investigation of choice.

MEDIASTINITIS

Mediastinitis is either inflammation or infection of the mediastinal space. Common causes include esophageal perforation (Boerhaave's syndrome), odontogenic infections, and iatrogenic causes secondary to cardiac, upper gastrointestinal, or airway procedures. The mortality rate is high, ranging from 14% to 42%, despite surgical or medical management, and delays in diagnosis can further increase mortality. Chest CT is the diagnostic investigation of choice.

PERICARDIAL TAMPONADE

Pericardial tamponade occurs when fluid around the heart accumulates under pressure, causing impaired filling of the heart. Severely compromised cardiac filling presents as cardiogenic shock and requires an immediate reduction in pericardial pressure via pericardiocentesis. Causes of tamponade can include aortic dissection, thoracic trauma, ventricular free wall rupture after myocardial infarction (refer to Chapter 13 for further reading), or as a complication of acute pericarditis secondary to an infection, malignancy, or uremia. An EKG is the diagnostic investigation of choice.

Suggested Approach to Chest Pain in a Rapid Response Setting

The following protocol can be used for immediate risk assessment and management in inpatient scenarios where chest pain is being evaluated. This stepwise approach can be used to evaluate emergency room patients. The usual sequence of history taking, physical exam, investigations, and resuscitative interventions is rarely followed during a rapid response. Instead, these measures often run parallel to each other in a code situation. The following components of the rapid response are discussed in the traditional sequence only to ease understanding. For a flowchart of evaluation and management of chest pain, see Figs. 1.2 and 1.3.

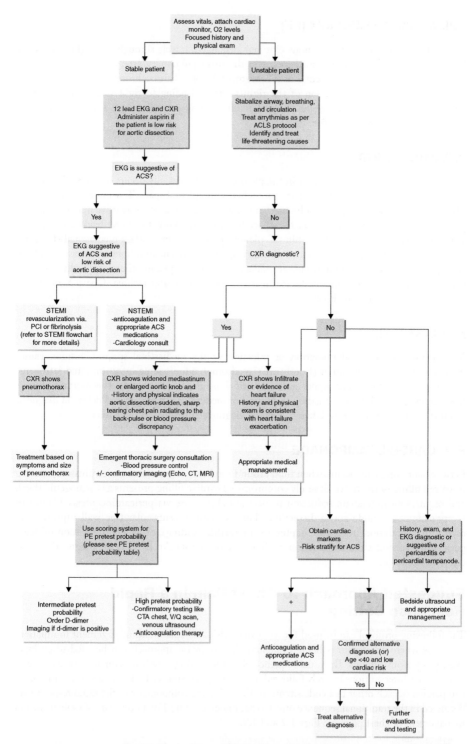

Fig. 1.2 Evaluating a patient with acute chest pain

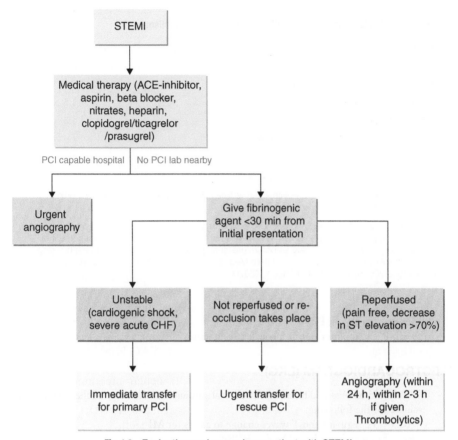

Fig. 1.3 Evaluating and managing a patient with STEMI

FOCUSED HISTORY AND PHYSICAL

- The acuity of signs and symptoms
- A detailed description of chest pain (location, quality, intensity, radiation, timing, setting, alleviating/aggravating factors – particularly improvement with nitrates, associated symptoms – fever or cough, prior similar symptoms)
- Prior cardiac history
- Prior history of malignancy, PE, or deep venous thrombosis. Quick WELLS Score can be calculated for the likelihood of PE (Table 1.2; refer to Chapter 19 for additional details)
- History of recent use of aspirin, beta-blockers, statins, or anticoagulants
- Physical exam should begin with an assessment of the airway, breathing, and circulation. Assess for hypoxia (oxygen saturation <90%), breath sounds (absence of breath sounds might suggest pneumothorax), bradycardia, tachycardia, or a new cardiac murmur

LABS

- BMP/CMP, magnesium – looking for electrolyte abnormalities
- Lactate – an early sign of occult shock
- Troponin – looking for signs of necrosis of cardiac myocytes. Troponins can take up to 6 h from the onset of ischemia to become positive in a blood test

TABLE 1.2 ▣ **WELLS score for the likelihood of pulmonary embolism**

Criteria	Points
Clinical signs and symptoms of deep vein thrombosis	3
PE is the most likely diagnosis	3
Tachycardia (pulse >100)	1.5
Immobilization/surgery in the last four weeks	1.5
Prior deep vein thrombosis/pulmonary embolism	1.5
Hemoptysis	1
Active malignancy, treated within the past six months	1

Score interpretation: Low risk = <2 points; Intermediate risk = 2-6 points; High risk = >6 points
PE unlikely = <4 points; PE likely = >4 points

Wells PS, Anderson DR, Rodger M, Stiell I, Dreyer JF, Barnes D, Forgie M, Kovacs G, Ward J, Kovacs MJ. Excluding pulmonary embolism at the bedside without diagnostic imaging: management of patients with suspected pulmonary embolism presenting to the emergency department by using a simple clinical model and d-dimer. Ann Intern Med. 2001 Jul 17;135(2):98-107. doi: 10.7326/0003-4819-135-2-200107170-00010. PMID: 11453709.

- d-dimer – to rule out PE
- Pro-BNP – to look for right ventricular dysfunction

ELECTROCARDIOGRAM (EKG)

- EKG should be obtained based on the clinical suspicion of the cause of chest pain and can evaluate for the following:
  - ACS – ST segment and T waves change to assess for MI
  - PE – Sinus tachycardia, $S_I Q_{III} T_{III}$, RBBB
  - Pericardial tamponade – Low voltage QRS complexes, electrical alternans
  - Acute pericarditis – Widespread ST elevations, PR depressions

IMAGING

- Chest X-ray to rule out consolidation, widening of the mediastinum, pneumothorax, and pleural effusion.
- CT angiogram chest to evaluate for PE vs. aortic dissection

INTERVENTIONS

We recommend that all patients be assessed for airway, breathing, circulation based on the advanced cardiac life support algorithm. IV fluid boluses should be considered for hypotension based on the overall clinical scenario. Balanced fluids (e.g., plasmalyte) should be used where available; otherwise, normal saline can be utilized. Vasopressors should be appropriate in patients not responding to fluids. For persistent chest pain in appropriate clinical situations, sublingual NTG should be tried to alleviate the pain. 0.3 mg sublingual (S/L) NTG is usually effective for cardiac pain; this dose can be repeated up to three times at 5 min intervals. If pain persists, IV morphine can be considered per institutional guidelines. Morphine has the dual effect of an analgesic and an anxiolytic. Anxiety from chest pain can worsen tachycardia, which increases the myocardium's oxygen demand, which would then worsen the ischemia and pain. Morphine can interrupt this vicious circle. Low doses of lorazepam can also be considered per institutional guidelines in appropriate clinical scenarios, e.g., if a patient has a known history of anxiety, is hyperventilating, or showing other signs of anxiety. It is paramount to ensure the hemodynamic stability of the patient before attempting sedation of any kind.

Suggested Reading

Barstow C, Rice M, McDivitt JD. Acute coronary syndrome: diagnostic evaluation. *Am Fam Physician.* 2017;95(3):170–177.

Hollander JE, Chase M. Evaluation of the adult with chest pain in the emergency department. https://www.uptodate.com/contents/evaluation-of-the-adult-with-chest-pain-in-the-emergency-department.

Kelly CR, Kirtane AJ, Stant J, et al. An updated protocol for evaluating chest pain and managing acute coronary syndromes. *Crit Pathw Cardiol.* 2017;16(1):7–14. doi:10.1029/2001JB000884.

Reamy BV, Williams PM, Odom MR. Pleuritic chest pain: sorting through the differential diagnosis. *Am Fam Physician.* 2017;96(5):306–312.

Chest Pain in a Patient With Coronary Artery Disease – II

Waliul Chowdhury ▧ Syed Arsalan Akhter Zaidi ▧ Firas Abdulmajeed ▧ Mohammad Adrish

Case Study

A rapid response event was initiated by the bedside nurse for sudden onset chest pain. On prompt arrival of the rapid response team (RRT), it was noted that the patient was a 59-year-old male with a known history of bronchial asthma, coronary artery disease who had a coronary artery bypass graft eight years ago, and coronary stent placement five years ago. The patient was admitted to the hospital two days ago for an asthma exacerbation. A few minutes before this RRT event, the patient complained of acute onset, severe, substernal, crushing chest pain that was ten out of ten in intensity, and was radiating to his left shoulder. He was also diaphoretic and was feeling nauseated but did not vomit.

VITAL SIGNS

Temperature: 98.4 °F, axillary
Blood Pressure: 170/90 mmHg
Pulse: 110 beats per min (bpm) – sinus tachycardia on telemetry
Respiratory Rate: 14 breaths per min
Pulse Oximetry: 97% on room air

FOCUSED PHYSICAL EXAM

The patient was a middle-aged diaphoretic male in moderate distress because of chest pain. Appropriate personal protective equipment was established, and the patient was examined. His cardiovascular exam was notable for tachycardia with normal heart sounds; no murmurs, rubs, or gallops were heard. No jugular venous distension or pedal edema was noted. There was no chest wall or epigastric tenderness. A change in position or movement of his upper extremities did not have any effect on the chest pain. His lungs were clear on auscultation. The remainder of the physical exam was unremarkable.

INTERVENTIONS

A stat 12-lead electrocardiogram (EKG) was obtained, which showed ST-segment elevations in lead V1-V4, I, and aVL (see Fig. 2.1A for ST-segment morphologies in acute coronary syndrome [ACS], and Fig. 2.1B for EKG tracing of anterior wall ST-elevation myocardial infarction [STEMI]). These changes were new compared to patient's EKG at admission. Sublingual nitroglycerin was administered. Stat troponin I level, basic metabolic panel (BMP), brain natriuretic peptide (BNP), and magnesium levels were obtained and were all normal. A stat cardiology consult was arranged, the diagnosis of STEMI was confirmed, and the cardiac catheterization lab was

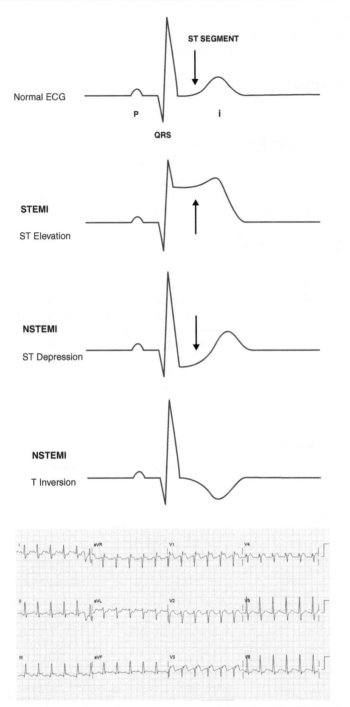

Fig. 2.1   **A,** EKG tracings showing different morphologies of ST-segment in different forms of ACS. **B,** EKG tracing showing ST-segment elevations in V1-V4, and ST depressions in leads I, aVL.

activated. The patient was given a loading dose of 324 mg chewable aspirin and 300 mg of clopidogrel. A heparin drip was started, and the patient was taken to the lab for a successful percutaneous coronary intervention and was subsequently admitted to the coronary care unit.

FINAL DIAGNOSIS

Acute anterior wall STEMI

Acute Coronary Syndrome

The blood supply of the myocardium is derived from the right and left coronaries arteries which arise from the root of the aorta (Table 2.1). As the coronary blood supply is composed of end-arteries with minimal collateral supply, occlusion of any of the left or right coronary artery branches can produce ischemia in a distinct part of the heart that can be identified EKG strip.

DEFINITION AND DIAGNOSIS

The three presentations encompassing ACS include unstable angina, non-ST-segment elevation MI, and ST-segment elevation MI (see Table 2.2 for features of these presentations of ACS).

History and a physical examination are of paramount importance; evaluation for signs and symptoms such as positional chest pain, reproducible chest pain, sharp chest pain radiating to the back, and burning epigastric pain, productive cough, fever, and sick contacts can point toward alternate diagnoses such as acute pericarditis, costochondritis, aortic dissection, gastroesophageal reflux, and pneumonia, respectively. HEART score can be a quick bedside tool for use in ambiguous cases where it is difficult to differentiate between ACS and other causes of chest pain. The HEART score helps calculate the likelihood of ACS-related death, MI, or urgent revascularization in the next two weeks (see Table 2.3).

TABLE 2.1 ■ Coronary anatomy and corresponding EKG leads

Coronary artery	Myocardial supply	Representative EKG leads
Left coronary artery	Left ventricle, left atrium	V1-V6 (anterior) anteroseptal (V1-V4), anterolateral (V3-V4)]
Left anterior descending artery	Right ventricle, left ventricle, interventricular septum	V1-V4 (anteroseptal)
Left circumflex artery	Left atrium, left ventricle	I, aVL (lateral) V5, V6 (apical) II, III, aVF (inferior)
Left marginal artery	Left ventricle	I, aVL (lateral limb) V5, V6 (apical)
Right coronary artery	Right atrium, right ventricle	aVR, V1 (Basal) II, III, aVF (inferior) V5-V6 (apical)
Posterior descending artery	Right ventricle, left ventricle, interventricular septum	I, aVL (lateral) V5, V6 (apical) II, III, aVF (inferior)
Right marginal artery	Right ventricle, apex	V5-V6 (apical) II, III, aVF (inferior)

TABLE 2.2 ■ **Diagnostic criteria for acute coronary syndrome**

ACS type	Features
Unstable angina	• Substernal crushing chest pain at rest • May have signs of ischemia or infarction on EKG, e.g., depressed ST wave or new T-wave inversion. • No elevation in cardiac enzymes
Non-ST-elevation myocardial infarction (NSTEMI)	• Substernal crushing chest pain at rest • May have signs of ischemia or infarction on EKG, e.g., depressed ST wave or new T-wave inversion. • Elevation in cardiac enzymes
ST-elevation myocardial infarction (STEMI)	• Substernal crushing chest pain at rest • New ST-elevation in two contiguous leads >0.1 mV in all leads except for leads V2-V3. Cutoffs for leads V2-V3: $\geq$0.2 mV for males over 40 years, $\geq$0.25 mV for males less than 40 years, $\geq$0.15 mV in all females. • May or may not have elevation in cardiac enzymes

TABLE 2.3 ■ **HEART score for calculating the risk of major cardiovascular adverse events**

HEART Score[†]	
Element	Points
History	
• Highly suspicious	2
• Moderately suspicious	1
• Slightly or non-suspicious	0
EKG findings	
• Significant ST changes	2
• Non-specific repolarization changes	1
• Normal	0
Age (years)	
• $\geq$65	2
• 45-65	1
• $\leq$45	0
Risk factors	
• $\geq$Three risk factors* or history of atherosclerotic disease	2
• One or two risk factors	1
• No known risk factors	0
Troponin	
• $\geq$ Three times the normal limit	2
• >One to <three times the normal limit	1
• $\leq$ Normal limit	0

*Risk factors: hypertension, hypercholesterolemia, diabetes mellitus, family history of premature coronary artery disease, current smoking or quit smoking <1 month ago, obesity (BMI $\geq$30 kg/m^2) Score interpretation:0-3 points = low (0.6%-1.7%) risk of major cardiac adverse events 4-6 points = intermediate (16.6%) risk of major cardiac adverse events7-10 points = high (50.1%) risk of major cardiac adverse events
[†]Six AJ, Backus BE, Kelder JC. Chest pain in the emergency room: value of the HEART score. Neth Heart J. 2008;16(6):191-196. doi:10.1007/BF03086144

Suggested Approach to a Patient With Suspected ACS

For inpatient scenarios where ACS is considered the primary cause of acute symptoms, the following approach can be used for rapid evaluation and management. This approach is based on a thorough literature search and updated guidelines and can also be applied to emergency room scenarios, as the management is universal. See Fig. 2.2 for a basic flowchart of the evaluation and management of ACS.

FOCUSED HISTORY AND PHYSICAL EXAMINATION

- The acuity of signs and symptoms
- A detailed description of the chest pain (location, quality, intensity, radiation, timing, setting, alleviating/aggravating factors, associated symptoms, prior similar symptoms)
- History of atherosclerotic disease (including cerebrovascular or peripheral vascular disease) or risk factors for atherosclerotic disease as mentioned in Table 2.3
- History of recent use of aspirin, beta-blockers, statins, anticoagulation
- Physical exam should begin with an assessment of the airway, breathing, and circulation. Assess for hypoxia (oxygen saturation <90%), bradycardia, tachycardia, or a new cardiac murmur.

LABORATORY TESTS

- Cardiac biomarkers-troponin I (which can take up to 6 h to be detectable in the blood), CK-MB, and myoglobin as the markers of myocardial injury
- BNP to evaluate for acute heart failure
- BMP and magnesium level for the assessment of electrolyte derangements that can be arrhythmogenic.

EKG

- Cardiac rhythm monitoring should be established on an emergent basis, ideally with an external defibrillator to assess for devolution into malignant arrhythmias.
- Screening 12-lead EKG should be obtained on an emergent basis which can show the changes mentioned in Table 2.1. Short interval follow-up EKG (within 15 min) should be obtained to assess for evolving changes.

IMAGING STUDIES

- Chest X-ray can be obtained if the patient develops a new oxygen requirement or a new murmur to evaluate for acute onset pulmonary edema from heart failure. However, this should not delay other necessary investigations.

THERAPEUTIC INTERVENTIONS

ACS is a medical emergency. We recommend that all patients be assessed for airway, breathing, and circulation. The airway should be secured, intubated if necessary, especially when new-onset respiratory failure is present. This would ensure adequate oxygen supply to the myocardium. The patient should be placed on a cardiac monitor, and pacer pads should be attached immediately. Ensure adequate blood pressure and peripheral perfusion. Hypotension should be corrected to allow for adequate myocardial blood flow in the setting of infarcted/stunted myocardium. Vasopressors should be used if indicated. Tachy- or bradyarrhythmias should be treated per the

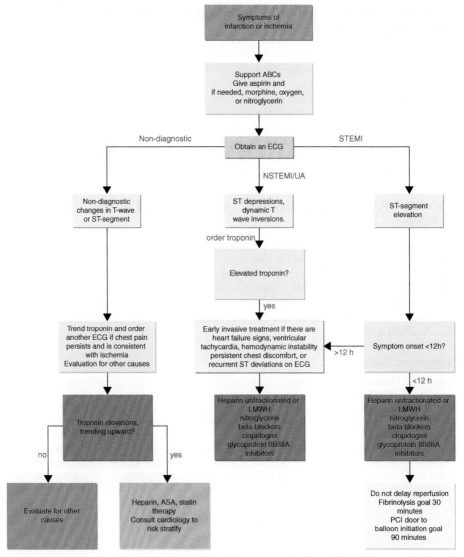

Fig. 2.2 Basic flowchart for the assessment and management of a patient with suspected acute coronary syndrome.

advanced cardiac life support (ACLS) protocol, and 325 mg chewable aspirin should be administered immediately. This can be given rectally in patients who cannot take it orally. Sublingual or transdermal nitroglycerin is used to alleviate pain. Care should be taken in hypotensive patients or those with suspected right ventricular infarct. Intravenous morphine can also be used to relieve pain and dyspnea associated with ACS. Once airway and hemodynamics are secured and EKG is obtained, immediate cardiology consultation should be obtained to activate the cardiac catheterization lab for percutaneous coronary intervention if warranted. The patient should be transferred to the cardiac intensive care unit for further management if warranted.

Summary of the Stepwise Approach for a Patient With Suspected ACS

Step 1: Patient with signs and symptoms of ACS on focused history and physical?

Step 2: Assess for airway and hemodynamic status, and proceed with intubation if indicated. Correct hypotension.

Step 3: Establish cardiac rhythm monitoring and obtain screening 12-lead EKG. Obtain lab work. Obtaining lab work should not delay EKG.

Step 4: Administer aspirin. Administer nitroglycerin and morphine as indicated. Consider clopidogrel vs other antiplatelet agents and anticoagulants per institutional guidelines.

Step 6: Obtain immediate cardiological consultation and activation of cardiac catheterization lab if appropriate.

CODING A PATIENT WITH CARDIAC ARREST FROM ACUTE CORONARY SYNDROME

If a patient with suspected ACS has a cardiac arrest, we suggest following the ACLS protocol to ensure proper securement of the airway and treatment of any arrhythmias per guidelines. Particular attention should be paid to correct hypoxia, and intubation should be done early if indicated. VTach/VFib patients will require defibrillation, while bradycardic patients will require atropine, epinephrine, and maybe artificial transcutaneous pacing. We recommend scheduling a stat consult with cardiology and transferring such patients to a cardiac intensive care unit once hemodynamics are secured.

Suggested Reading

Anderson JL, Morrow DA. Acute myocardial infarction. *N Engl J Med.* 2017;376(21):2053–2064. https://doi. org/10.1056/NEJMra1606915.

Barstow C. Acute coronary syndrome: presentation and diagnostic evaluation. *FP Essent.* 2020;490:11–19.

Barstow C, Rice M, McDivitt JD. Acute coronary syndrome: diagnostic evaluation. *Am Fam Physician.* 2017;95(3):170–177.

Hollander JE, Chase M. Evaluation of the adult with chest pain in the emergency department. https://www. uptodate.com/contents/evaluation-of-the-adult-with-chest-pain-in-the-emergency-department.

Kelly CR, Kirtane AJ, Stant J, et al. An updated protocol for evaluating chest pain and managing acute coronary syndromes. *Crit Pathw Cardiol.* 2017;16(1):7–14. https://doi.org/10.1097/HPC.0000000000000098.

CHAPTER 3

Chest Pain in a Patient With Hypertensive Emergency

Waliul Chowdhury ▦ Kainat Saleem ▦ Firas Abdulmajeed ▦ Mohammad Adrish

Case Study

A rapid response event was initiated by the bedside nurse for new-onset, severe chest pain. Upon prompt arrival of the rapid response team, it was found that the patient was a 47-year-old male with a known history of insulin-dependent diabetes mellitus, hypertension, and substance abuse. He was admitted a few hours earlier for altered mental status and bizarre behavior, and a urine toxicology screen was found to be positive for cocaine and methamphetamines. The patient had developed acute onset, sub-sternal, 10/10 chest pain 10 min before the rapid response event was initiated. The pain was stabbing and radiating to his back. He was nauseous but denied any other symptoms.

VITAL SIGNS

Temperature: 100°F, axillary
Blood pressure: 240/135 mmHg
Pulse: 145 beats per min (bpm) – narrow complex tachycardia on telemetry
Respiratory rate: 32 breaths per min
Pulse oximetry: 97% oxygen saturation on room air

FOCUSED PHYSICAL EXAM

The patient was a middle-aged male sitting up in bed in severe distress. His respiratory exam showed tachypnea and labored breathing, but the lungs were clear to auscultation. A cardiac exam showed tachycardia with a regular rhythm; no murmurs were identified. No edema was present. The abdominal exam was benign.

INTERVENTIONS

A cardiac monitor was attached. A stat electrocardiogram (EKG) was obtained, which showed sinus tachycardia; no ST changes related to acute ischemia were present. The patient was given 2 mg IV morphine for pain. He was also given 10 mg IV labetalol for elevated blood pressure, and a stat bedside chest X-ray was obtained. Chest X-ray showed a widened mediastinum indicating aortic dissection. The patient was started on esmolol infusion, and a stat computed tomography (CT) angiogram of chest and abdomen per dissection protocol was ordered. Imaging was consistent with dissection of the descending thoracic aorta (Fig. 3.1). An emergent consult was called to thoracic surgery, and the patient was transferred to the intensive care unit for further management.

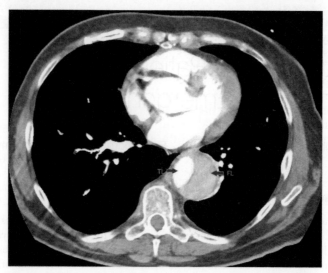

Fig. 3.1   CT angiogram of the chest showing an intimal tear in the descending thoracic aorta and formation of false lumen separated from the true lumen by an intimal flap.

TABLE 3.1 ■ **Anatomical classification of aortic dissection**

Classification system	Subtypes
Daily (Stanford) classification system	Type A – Dissection involving the ascending aorta and/or arch of the aorta, regardless of distal extent Type B – Dissections distal to the arch of the aorta
DeBakey classification system	Type 1 – Intimal tear originating in the ascending aorta and involvement of aortic arch or beyond Type 2 – Intimal tear originating in the ascending aorta, dissection confined to the ascending aorta Type 3 – Intimal tear originating in the descending aorta and involvement of the aorta only beyond the origin of the left sub-clavian artery

FINAL DIAGNOSIS : ACUTE AORTIC DISSECTION SECONDARY TO HYPERTENSIVE EMERGENCY

Acute Aortic Dissection

Aortic dissection is a life-threatening, catastrophic illness caused by a tear in the tunica intima of the aorta; this leads to the entry of blood into the wall of the aorta under pressure, creating a false lumen that creates a separation between the aortic wall layers. Aortic dissection can be classified anatomically based on the location of the pathologic condition. Two classification systems are used, as shown in Table 3.1.

Aortic dissection can be classified clinically based on the duration from symptom onset to presentation: hyperacute (<24 h), acute (1-14 days), subacute (15-90 days), and chronic (>90 days). The dissection can also be classified as complicated vs. uncomplicated, based on the presence of complications such as proximal or distal malperfusion, rapid expansion, impending rupture or

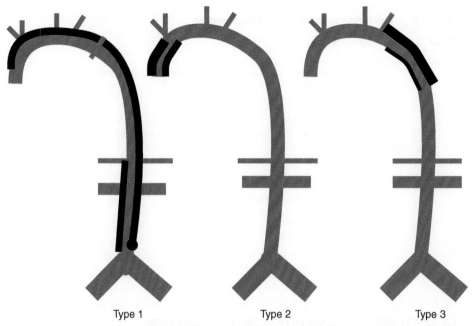

Type 1   Type 2   Type 3

Fig. 3.2   Schematic diagram of the Debakey classification system. Type I and II Debakey dissections are classified as type A dissections under the Daily system. Type 3 Debakey dissection would correspond to type B dissection under the Daily system.

frank rupture of the aortic wall, hypertension refractory to three or more classes of maximum doses of anti-hypertensives, or uncontrolled pain. The dissection can also be classified according to location (Fig. 3.2).

Aortic dissection is more common in males than females and is more commonly seen in people older than 65 years. Various risk factors contribute to the development of aortic dissection (Table 3.2).

Prompt identification of aortic dissection is of critical importance. Without intervention, the mortality rate of ascending aortic dissection approaches 1%-2% per hour after symptom onset. Propagation of the false lumen proximally can lead to hemopericardium and cardiac tamponade, acute aortic valve insufficiency, and myocardial infarction from compression of coronary artery lumens. Neurological complications can occur if dissection compromises the carotid blood flow. Distal propagation of the false lumen can cause vascular compromise to kidneys, bowel, and lower extremities. A frank rupture can cause immediate death by exsanguination.

Suggested Approach to a Patient With Suspected Aortic Dissection

For inpatient scenarios where acute aortic dissection is being considered, the following approach can be used for rapid evaluation and management. This approach is based on a thorough literature search and updated guidelines and can also be applied to emergency room scenarios. See Fig. 3.3 for a flowchart of the evaluation and management of suspected aortic dissection.

TABLE 3.2 ■ Risk factors associated with aortic dissection

Class	Examples
Medical	• Hypertension – most common risk factor • Substance abuse – cocaine and methamphetamines, which are associated with hypertensive crises • Atherosclerosis • Vasculitis • Pregnancy and delivery • Prior thoracic aortic aneurysm • Prior cardiac surgery • Prior aortic surgery
Genetic/ congenital	• Connective tissue disorders • Marfan syndrome • Vascular type Ehlers-Danlos syndrome • Turner syndrome • Loey-Dietz syndrome • Bicuspid aortic valve
Iatrogenic/ traumatic	• Intra-aortic balloon pump • Motor vehicle accident – especially with rapid deceleration

FOCUSED HISTORY AND PHYSICAL EXAMINATION

- The acuity of signs and symptoms
- A detailed description of chest pain (location, quality, intensity, radiation, timing, setting, alleviating/aggravating factors, associated symptoms, prior similar symptoms)
- History of risk factors and associations mentioned in Table 3.2
- History of recent use of antiplatelet agents or anticoagulation
- Physical exam should begin with an assessment of airway, breathing, and circulation. Blood pressure in both arms should be measured
- Assessment of distal pulses should be done, including carotids
- Evaluation for signs of aortic insufficiency (a murmur might not be audible in severe aortic regurgitation), new-onset heart failure (jugular venous distension), and cardiac tamponade (pulsus paradoxus) should be done

LABORATORY TESTS

- Cardiac biomarkers such as troponins – to evaluate for myocardial infarction, which is a major differential as well as a complication of aortic dissection
- CBC – to evaluate for any signs of acute hemorrhage
- Electrolytes, lactate level – to evaluate for end-organ damage
- d-dimer – although a non-specific test, values below 500 ng/dL have good negative predictive value in aortic dissection
- Type and screen – in preparation for possible upcoming interventions

ELECTROCARDIOGRAM

- Screening 12-lead EKG should be obtained on an emergent basis to rule out coronary ischemia, as acute coronary syndrome is a major differential and a known complication of aortic dissection.

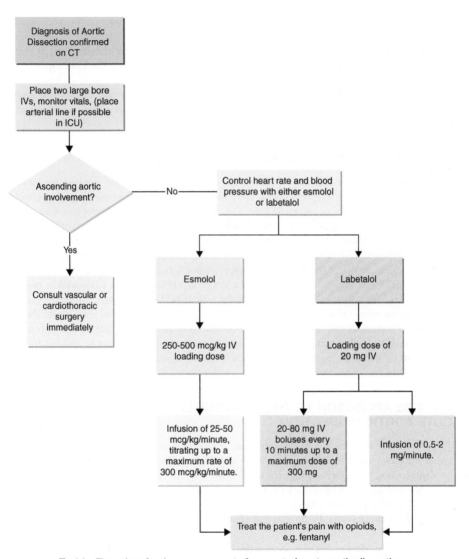

Fig. 3.3 Flow chart for the management of suspected acute aortic dissection.

IMAGING STUDIES

- Chest X-ray – should be obtained at the bedside. A widened mediastinum can point toward dissection. The presence of a new unilateral pleural effusion or a change in the cardiac contour can also point toward dissection in some scenarios.
- CT angiogram of chest and abdomen – should be obtained emergently in all hemodynamically stable patients suspected of having aortic dissection. The entirety of the aorta should be imaged, not just the portion confined to the chest
- MR angiography – MRA has a higher sensitivity and specificity for the diagnosis of aortic dissection; however, it is rarely used in rapid response settings given the time required for the study and inaccessibility to the patient.
- Transesophageal echocardiogram – rarely used in rapid response setting. However, it would be the imaging of choice in unstable patients because of portability, high sensitivity, and high specificity.

THERAPEUTIC INTERVENTIONS

Aortic dissection is a life-threatening emergency. All patients should be assessed for airway, breathing, and circulation. Hypotension is an ominous sign, and prompt investigations should be initiated to evaluate for acute aortic valve insufficiency, cardiac tamponade, and frank rupture. Emergent surgical consultation should be obtained in this case. The presence of neurological compromise should also trigger an emergent surgical consult. In stable patients, pain control should be addressed with opioids. Anxiety is also a concomitant factor and can be addressed with short-acting benzodiazepines. IV anti-hypertensive infusions should be initiated. Beta-blockers like esmolol and labetalol remain the drugs of choice even in cases with a history of cocaine use. Medications are titrated to a heart rate of 60 beats per min. Given the risk of rebound hypertension from alpha stimulation, other beta-blockers such as metoprolol should be avoided. Intravenous calcium channel blockers and nitrates can be added for added control. Type A dissection is a surgical emergency. Surgical intervention should not be delayed for the management of stroke or myocardial infarction. Patients should be managed in the intensive care unit.

STEPWISE APPROACH TO THE MANAGEMENT OF SUSPECTED ACUTE AORTIC DISSECTION

Step 1: Assess for airway and hemodynamic status. Hypotension is an ominous sign; cardiothoracic and vascular surgical consult should be called immediately in a patient with hypotension secondary to suspected aortic dissection. An emergent bedside transesophageal echocardiogram can be obtained at the discretion of the surgical team.

Step 2: In stable patients, EKG should be obtained to evaluate for myocardial ischemia.

Step 3: Pain control with IV opioids and anxiety control with IV benzodiazepines should be initiated.

Step 4: Highly selective beta-blockers such as esmolol or non-selective beta-blockers such as labetalol should be initiated. Once the heart rate is controlled, vasodilators are initiated.

Step 5: CT angiogram of the chest and abdomen should be obtained to evaluate the extent of dissection.

Step 6: Thoracic surgery and vascular consults should be obtained immediately, and the patient should be transferred to the intensive care unit for further management.

Suggested Reading

Fukui T. Management of acute aortic dissection and thoracic aortic rupture. *J Intensive Care*. 2018;6(1):1–8. https://doi.org/10.1186/s40560-018-0287-7.

Black JH III, Burke CR. Management of acute aortic dissection. https://www.uptodate.com/contents/management-of-acute-aortic-dissection?search=aortic dissection&source=search_result&selectedTitle=2~150 &usage_type=default&display_rank=2.

Nienaber CA, Clough RE, Sakalihasan N, et al. Aortic dissection. *Nat Rev Dis Prim*. 2016;2(1):16053. https://doi.org/10.1038/nrdp.2016.53.

CHAPTER 4

Tachycardia in a Patient With Atrial Fibrillation

Waliul Chowdhury ▪ Syed Arsalan Akhter Zaidi ▪ Firas Abdulmajeed ▪ Mohammad Adrish

Case Study

A rapid response event was initiated by the bedside nurse for sudden onset palpitations. Upon the prompt arrival of the rapid response team, the patient was found to be a 56-year-old male with a known history of hemorrhagic stroke status post-tissue plasminogen activator (t-PA) a month prior with residual right-sided neurological deficits and tobacco abuse disorder. The patient was admitted to the hospital two days prior for management of infected decubitus ulcers. His symptoms had started 15 min before the rapid response was called, and he complained about palpitations and dizziness.

VITAL SIGNS

Temperature: 98 °F, axillary
Blood Pressure: 159/89 mmHg
Pulse: 160 beats per min (bpm)–narrow complex, irregular rhythm on telemetry (Fig. 4.1)
Respiratory Rate: 22 breaths per min
Pulse Oximetry: 95% oxygen saturation on room air

FOCUSED PHYSICAL EXAM

The patient was a middle-aged male in mild distress. Appropriate personal protective equipment was established, and the patient was examined. The patient was alert and oriented. He reported having an uncomfortable, fluttery feeling in his chest. He also complained of dizziness even while lying flat. However, he denied any overt chest pain. His cardiac exam showed tachycardia with an irregular rhythm. Jugular venous distension was not appreciated, and no peripheral edema was present. Lung and abdominal exams were benign.

INTERVENTIONS

A cardiac monitor and pads were attached immediately. The monitor showed narrow complex tachycardia with irregularly spaced complexes and a rate variability between 140 and 180 bpm. Stat electrocardiogram (EKG) was obtained, which was notable for the absence of P waves. The patient was given 5 mg intravenous (IV) metoprolol push which did not decrease the heart rate. The patient's blood pressure fell to 110/83 mmHg, and a 500 cc fluid bolus was initiated. He was given another 5 mg of IV metoprolol which again did not affect the heart rate. Then, 10 mg IV of diltiazem was given, which decreased the heart to a range of 120-130 bpm. The patient was started on a continuous diltiazem drip and moved to the stepdown unit. Stat electrolyte panel,

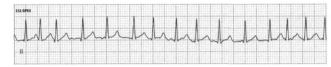

Fig. 4.1 Telemetry strip showing a narrow complex tachycardia with a heart rate of ~150 beats per min. No P waves can be seen, and the R-R interval is variable.

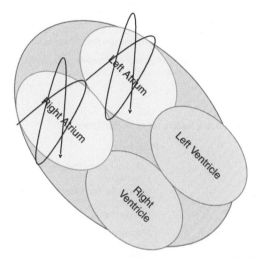

Fig. 4.2 Schematic representation of chaotic conduction seen in atrial fibrillation.

magnesium level, troponin level, and complete blood count were ordered, which were unremarkable. Given his recent history of hemorrhagic stroke, anticoagulation was not initiated.

FINAL DIAGNOSIS

Atrial fibrillation with rapid ventricular response.

Atrial Fibrillation

Atrial fibrillation is the most common cardiac arrhythmia, which causes greater than 450,000 hospitalizations every year in the United States. It has also been associated with an estimated 158,000 deaths each year. It is a rapid, irregular heart rhythm produced by the rapid firing of a single focus in the atria, most commonly in the pulmonary veins. The short duration of action potential in the atrial muscle fibers and their short refractory period play a key role in sustaining the extremely fast conduction rate seen in atrial fibrillation, which can cause atrial contraction rates as high as 400/min. This leads to the replacement of the coordinated conduction and contraction of the atria (represented by P waves on EKG) by the rapid, chaotic "fibrillation" of atrial musculature (seen as a wavy undulation of isoelectric axis or F waves – see Fig. 4.2). Atrial fibrillation is often classified based on the frequency and duration of arrhythmic episodes (Table 4.1).

Despite the rapid firing of atria, the ventricular rate usually does not exceed 200 bpm because of the "slow response" nature of atrioventricular (AV) nodal fibers, which serves as the rate-limiting step in cardiac conduction. The broad range of heart rate in rapid ventricular response lies between 90 and 170 bpm unless special circumstances such as an accessory conduction pathway,

TABLE 4.1 ■ Classifications of atrial fibrillation

Category	Features
Paroxysmal/intermittent atrial fibrillation	• Terminates spontaneously or with intervention within seven days of onset • Returns at a variable frequency
Persistent atrial fibrillation	• Fails to terminate within seven days • Can have subsequent episodes of paroxysmal atrial fibrillation
Long-standing persistent atrial fibrillation	• It lasts longer than 12 months
Permanent atrial fibrillation	• Persistent atrial fibrillation where rhythm control is no longer being pursued
"Lone" atrial fibrillation	• Any category of atrial fibrillation without underlying structural heart disease • Less commonly used term these days

TABLE 4.2 ■ Associations and risk factors for atrial fibrillation

Class	Factors
Cardiac diseases	• Coronary artery disease • Heart failure • Congenital heart disease – atrial septal defect • Hypertrophic cardiomyopathy • Congenital QT or P wave duration abnormalities
Non-cardiac diseases	• Hypertension • Venous thromboembolism • Obstructive sleep apnea • Hypomagnesemia • Obesity • Diabetes mellitus • Chronic kidney disease
Environmental/lifestyle	• Age • Male sex • Family history • Genetics • Birth weight • Smoking • Alcohol • Caffeine

catecholamine access, or hyperthyroidism are present. The most common presenting symptoms include palpitations, dizziness, lightheadedness, weakness, and fatigue. Symptoms of cardiac ischemia such as chest pain and dyspnea and symptoms of hemodynamic compromise such as syncope can present occasionally. However, patients with atrial fibrillation can be asymptomatic from an arrhythmia standpoint. This "occult" atrial fibrillation is usually discovered during the work-up of consequences of atrial fibrillation such as stroke and transient ischemic attack, where it is found to be the cause of cerebrovascular accident in about a quarter of the patients.

Table 4.2 lists the different associations and risk factors of atrial fibrillation. Atrial fibrillation has been associated with an increased risk of stroke, myocardial infarction, heart failure, systemic embolism, venous thromboembolism, and dementia. Systemic anticoagulation is initiated based on the patient's risk of systemic embolism. The CHA_2DS_2-VASc score is often used to calculate this risk of systemic embolism (Table 4.3).

TABLE 4.3 ■ CHA$_2$DS$_2$-VASc* score for anticoagulation in atrial fibrillation

Risk factors	Assigned score
Congestive heart failure, signs of heart failure, or evidence of reduced ejection fraction	+1
Hypertension	+1
Age 65-74 years	+1
Age 75 years or more	+2
Diabetes	+1
Female sex	+1
Previous stroke, transient ischemic attack, or thromboembolism	+2
Vascular disease, aortic plaque, myocardial infarction, or peripheral arterial disease	+1
Maximum score	9

Interpretation of score:
0 = No anticoagulation (can be considered in individual cases)
1 = Anticoagulation based on clinical judgment and individual risk
2 or higher = Anticoagulation recommended
*Lip GY, Nieuwlaat R, Pisters R, Lane DA, Crijns HJ. Refining clinical risk stratification for predicting stroke and thromboembolism in atrial fibrillation using a novel risk factor-based approach: the euro heart survey on atrial fibrillation. Chest. 2010 Feb;137(2):263–272. doi: 10.1378/chest.09-1584. Epub 2009 Sep 17. PMID: 19762550.

Rate control vs. rhythm control strategy is considered equivalent for the treatment of atrial fibrillation. Some recent studies have shown a potential reduction in mortality and stroke with rhythm control compared to rate control in high-risk patients. However, strong recommendations are lacking. Long-term management of atrial fibrillation is outside the scope of this chapter.

For the management of rapid ventricular response episodes, beta-blockers and calcium channel blockers remain the first-line therapy. Digoxin can be used in complex cases per institutional guidelines and clinician preference. Antiarrhythmics such as amiodarone are reserved for refractory cases and patients who do not tolerate beta-blockers and calcium channel blockers. Other antiarrhythmic agents such as sotalol or dofetilide are rarely used in the rapid response setting, and expert consultation should be obtained before considering these agents in an emergency. Electrical cardioversion is reserved for patients with hemodynamic instability. It should be noted that chemical or electrical cardioversion in atrial fibrillation of >48 h duration without preceding anticoagulation is associated with a 5%-7% risk of stroke. It is essential to weigh the risks and benefits of cardioversion in all cases of atrial fibrillation with a rapid ventricular response.

Suggested Approach to a Patient With Atrial Fibrillation and Rapid Ventricular Response in a Rapid Response Setting

The following approach can be used to evaluate and manage patients with atrial fibrillation and rapid ventricular response event. These steps are based on a thorough review of the literature and can also be used in an emergency department setting as the management is similar (see Fig. 4.3 for a flowchart of management of atrial fibrillation with rapid ventricular response). The usual sequence of history taking, physical exam, investigations, and resuscitative interventions are often not followed during a rapid response; these measures often run parallel to each other in a

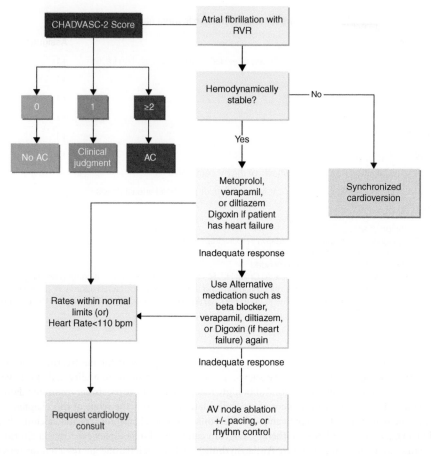

Fig. 4.3   Flowchart of evaluation and management of atrial fibrillation with rapid ventricular response.

code situation. The following components of the rapid response are discussed in the traditional sequence only to ease understanding.

FOCUSED HISTORY AND PHYSICAL EXAMINATION

- The acuity of signs and symptoms, prior history of arrhythmias
- Medication history, including AV nodal medications that are being held or have been discontinued recently and anticoagulation agents
- History of high-risk medical comorbidities that can precipitate atrial fibrillation such as heart failure, hyperthyroidism, myocardial ischemia, sepsis, volume depletion, hypoxia
- Physical exam should begin with an evaluation of airway, breathing, and circulation
- Volume status should be assessed, can include pulmonary auscultation for crackles, the cardiovascular exam for jugular venous distension, peripheral perfusion, and peripheral edema

EKG

- EKG should be obtained in all patients on an emergent basis to confirm the diagnosis of atrial fibrillation with rapid ventricular response

LABORATORY TESTS

- Basal metabolic panel and magnesium level – to assess for significant electrolyte abnormalities as a trigger
- Troponin level – to evaluate for myocardial ischemia
- Thyroid-stimulating hormone – to assess for hypo- or hyperthyroidism as a trigger

IMAGING

- Imaging is not required for the diagnosis of atrial fibrillation. However, the following studies can be obtained to evaluate for effects of rapid ventricular response:
  - Chest X-ray can be obtained if there is suspicion of pulmonary edema

THERAPEUTIC INTERVENTIONS

Atrial fibrillation with rapid ventricular response can be a medical emergency if it is associated with hemodynamic instability. We recommend that all patients be assessed for airway, breathing, and circulation. The airway should be secured as necessary. In hemodynamically unstable patients, emergent, electrical cardioversion is indicated per the advanced cardiac life support algorithm. Institutional guidelines should be considered for borderline cases. In hemodynamically stable patients, irregularly irregular rhythm should be confirmed with an EKG. Beta-blockers or calcium channel blockers should be used for rate control. Digoxin can be used in complex cases based on institutional guidelines. Rhythm control with amiodarone can be used in refractory cases or earlier, depending on clinical judgment and institutional guidelines. Sotalol and dofetilide are rarely used in a rapid response situation and should be attempted only after expert consultation with cardiology. The risk of thromboembolism associated with atrial fibrillation of >48 h duration should be considered when attempting chemical or electrical cardioversion. The assessment of volume status is vital as both volume overload and volume depletion can precipitate atrial fibrillation. The overall clinical picture will help determine whether fluid resuscitation vs. diuresis should be attempted to correct the underlying cause.

STEPWISE APPROACH TO THE MANAGEMENT OF A PATIENT WITH VENTRICULAR TACHYCARDIA

Step 1: Assess for airway and hemodynamic status. Attach cardiac monitor and place pacer pads. Secure airway if indicated.

Step 2: Synchronized cardioversion should be attempted if the patient is unstable hemodynamically.

Step 3: In stable patients, obtain stat EKG to confirm the irregularly irregular rhythm.

Step 4: Use beta-blockers vs. calcium channel blockers to control heart rate.

Step 4B: If first-line therapies are ineffective, digoxin can be considered per institutional practice.

Step 5: Amiodarone can be used in refractory cases for rhythm control. The risk of thromboembolism in patients without adequate anticoagulation, with atrial fibrillation of >48 h duration, should be kept in mind while attempting electrical or chemical cardioversion.

Step 6: Diuretics vs. IV fluids should be used based on the patient's volume status and clinical judgment.

Suggested Reading

Amin A, Houmsse A, Ishola A, Tyler J, Houmsse M. The current approach of atrial fibrillation management. *Avicenna J Med*. 2016;6(1):8–16. https://doi.org/10.4103/2231-0770.173580.

Michaud GF, Stevenson WG. Atrial fibrillation. *N Engl J Med*. 2021;384(4):353–361. https://doi.org/10.1056/NEJMcp2023658.

Staerk L, Sherer JA, Ko D, Benjamin EJ, Helm RH. Atrial fibrillation: epidemiology, pathophysiology, clinical outcomes. *Circ Res*. 2017;120(9):1501–1517. https://doi.org/10.1161/CIRCRESAHA.117.309732.

Xu J, Luc JGY, Phan K. Atrial fibrillation: review of current treatment strategies. *J Thorac Dis*. 2016;8(9):E886–E900. https://doi.org/10.21037/jtd.2016.09.13.

CHAPTER 5

Tachycardia in a Patient With Ischemic Cardiomyopathy

Waliul Chowdhury ▪ Syed Zaidi ▪ Mohammad Adrish ▪ Firas Abdulmajeed

Case Study

A rapid response event was initiated by the bedside nurse for a patient who had sudden onset palpitations, followed by a pre-syncope event as the patient was walking to the restroom. Upon prompt arrival of the rapid response team, it was noted that the patient was a 45-year-old male with a history of ischemic cardiomyopathy and substance use disorder who was admitted earlier in the day after acute alcohol intoxication. At the time of admission, the patient's drug screen was positive for cocaine, methamphetamines, and opiates.

VITAL SIGNS

Temperature: 98.3 °F, axillary
Blood Pressure: 156/85 mmHg
Pulse: 208 beats per min (bpm) – wide complex tachycardia on telemetry (see Fig. 5.1)
Respiratory Rate: 22 breaths per min
Pulse Oximetry: 93% oxygen saturation on room air

FOCUSED PHYSICAL EXAMINATION

The patient was a middle-aged man lying in bed in mild distress. Appropriate personal protective equipment was established, and the patient was examined. The patient was alert and oriented. He reported having an uncomfortable feeling in his chest. However, he denied any dizziness or overt chest pain. His cardiac examination showed regular tachycardia. Jugular venous distension was not appreciated, and no peripheral edema was present. His lung and abdominal exams were benign.

INTERVENTIONS

Cardiac defibrillator pads were attached immediately. The monitor showed wide complex tachycardia indicating possible ventricular tachycardia (VT) vs. atrial fibrillation with aberrancy. Then, 500 cc normal saline bolus was started. Stat dose of 6 mg adenosine IV was administered without any change in heart rate. Then, 12 mg IV adenosine was administered again without any effect. Stat electrocardiogram (EKG) was obtained, which showed monomorphic wide complexes consistent with VT. As next step, 150 mg IV amiodarone was administered over 10 min, which failed to terminate the malignant rhythm. A second bolus of 150 mg IV amiodarone was administered, leading to successful cardioversion to normal sinus rhythm. EKG obtained after chemical cardioversion showed a normal QRS complex without any underlying bundle branch block. Stat troponin, electrolyte panel, including magnesium level, were obtained during the event, which

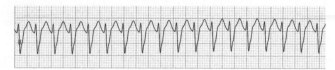

Fig. 5.1   Telemetry strip showing wide complex, monomorphic tachycardia.

TABLE 5.1 ▪ **Morphologies of ventricular tachycardia**

Monomorphic	Polymorphic
• Regular wide complex tachycardia with uniform consecutive beats with similar morphology • Commonly associated with structural heart disease, e.g., ischemic heart disease (especially prior MI), cardiomyopathies (dilated, infiltrative, hypertrophic), LV non-compaction	• Regular wide complex tachycardia with a frequent variation of QRS morphology and/or QRS axis • Commonly associated with QT prolongation: congenital vs. acquired (discussed in detail in Chapter 16)

were all within normal limits. A 24 h IV infusion of amiodarone was initiated, and the patient was moved to the step-down unit.

FINAL DIAGNOSIS

Ventricular tachycardia

Ventricular Tachycardia

The sino-atrial node is the pacemaker of the heart. The details of the cardiac conduction system are discussed in Chapter 9. Based on the hierarchy in the electrical conduction pathway, ventricular myocytes have the slowest firing rate (20-40 bpm), which is overridden by the much faster impulse generation of all the higher pacemakers. The impulse generated by a ventricular focus produces the classic wide QRS complex ($\geq$120 ms), and the two ventricles are not depolarizing simultaneously. This widened QRS complex can also be seen in the presence of a bundle branch block which also means that the two ventricles are not depolarizing simultaneously.

Definition and diagnosis: Tachycardia is defined as a resting heart rate >100 bpm. Tachycardia arising from a ventricular focus is called VT. VT can be non-sustained (lasting <30 s) or sustained (lasting $\geq$30 s or causing hemodynamic compromise before reaching the 30 s mark). VT can be monomorphic or polymorphic (Table 5.1).

Suggested Approach to a Patient With Suspected Sustained VT

For inpatient scenarios where sustained VT is considered the primary diagnosis, the following approach can be used for rapid evaluation and management of the patient. This approach is based on a thorough literature search and updated guidelines and can be expanded and used in emergency room situations. See Fig. 5.2 for a flowchart of management of sustained VT.

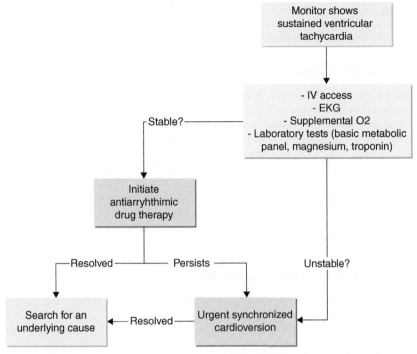

Fig. 5.2 Flowchart for the management of sustained ventricular tachycardia.

FOCUSED HISTORY AND PHYSICAL EXAMINATION

- Vital signs, looking for signs of hemodynamic instability like low blood pressure and hypoxia. This will help decide whether defibrillation is required.
- Mental status and oxygen requirement, assessing the need for intubation.
- Signs and symptoms of ongoing cardiac ischemia.
- History of ischemic heart disease, use of arrhythmogenic medications.
- Native cardiac rhythm (review prior EKGs if available) if hemodynamics allow.

LABORATORY TESTS

- Electrolyte panel including magnesium and potassium levels since hypokalemia and hypo-magnesemia can both precipitate torsades de pointes (TdP).
- Troponin level to assess for myocyte ischemia.
- Arterial blood gas if suspicion of hypoxia or severe acidosis.
- TSH, free T3, and T4, since thyroid dysfunction can be a potential risk factor.

ELECTROCARDIOGRAM

- EKG should be obtained in all cases. The following features are characteristic:
  - Wide QRS complex ($\geq$120 ms).
  - Uniform regularly spaced QRS complexes.

IMAGING

- Imaging has no specific role in the evaluation of a patient with VT.

THERAPEUTIC INTERVENTIONS

Sustained VT is a medical emergency. We recommend that all patients be assessed for airway, breathing, and circulation. In patients without a pulse, synchronized electrical cardioversion is the most critical step in resuscitation, followed by cardiopulmonary resuscitation (CPR) per the advanced cardiac life support (ACLS) protocol and institutional guidelines. Adenosine can be considered in patients with a pulse, which can help differentiate between a ventricular focus and a supraventricular focus with aberrancy. Chemical cardioversion with 150 mg IV amiodarone is generally considered the next appropriate step. Procainamide and sotalol are part of the ACLS algorithm. However, we recommend their use per institutional guidelines and expert consultation. Electrical cardioversion should be considered for refractory cases and in worsening hemodynamics. Evaluation for underlying cardiac ischemia should be done by consulting with cardiology as appropriate. See Table 5.2 for some key points to remember for stable vs. unstable VT patients.

SUMMARY OF A STEPWISE APPROACH TO A PATIENT WITH VT

Step 1: Assess for airway and hemodynamic status. Attach cardiac monitor and place pacer pads. Secure airway if indicated.

Step 2: Obtain stat EKG to evaluate underlying rhythm. Compare to the native rhythm on prior EKGs, if hemodynamics allow.

Step 3: Use IV adenosine to differentiate between VT and supraventricular tachycardia with aberrancy.

Step 4: Prompt synchronized cardioversion should be done in unstable patients.

Step 5: In hemodynamically stable patients, chemical cardioversion should be attempted with amiodarone vs. other antiarrhythmic agents based on ACLS protocol and institutional guidelines.

CODING A PATIENT WITH VT

If a patient with VT has a cardiac arrest, we suggest following the ACLS protocol to secure the airway and early synchronized cardioversion followed by effective CPR per guidelines.

TABLE 5.2 ■ Key points to remember in patients who are stable vs. unstable in VT

Unstable	Stable
Urgent cardioversion is recommended in pulseless VT	Therapy should be prompt to avoid deterioration
Antiarrhythmic drugs are not recommended as first-line therapy	Treatment is mainly pharmacologic
Managed via ACLS and high energy counter-shock	Begin with an intravenous antiarrhythmic agent and reserve electrical cardioversion for refractory patients or for those who become unstable
Subsequent shocks should be given with defibrillator if persistent	If not terminated, external cardioversion may be needed with pharmacologic agents

Antiarrhythmic agents such as IV amiodarone should be given early in the process. IV lidocaine should be considered based on institutional guidelines. Patients should be evaluated for ongoing cardiac ischemia and myocardial infarction, and emergent cardiac consultation should be obtained for coronary revascularization if myocardial infarction is suspected.

Suggested Reading

AlKalbani A, AlRawahi N. Management of monomorphic ventricular tachycardia electrical storm in structural heart disease. *J Saudi Hear Assoc.* 2019;31(3):135–144. https://doi.org/10.1016/j.jsha.2019.05.001.

Killu AM, Stevenson WG. Ventricular tachycardia in the absence of structural heart disease. *Heart.* 2019;105(8):645LP–656LP. https://doi.org/10.1136/heartjnl-2017-311590.

Koplan BA, Stevenson WG. Ventricular tachycardia and sudden cardiac death. *Mayo Clin Proc.* 2009;84(3): 289–297. https://doi.org/10.1016/S0025-6196(11)61149-X.

Roberts-Thomson KC, Lau DH, Sanders P. The diagnosis and management of ventricular arrhythmias. *Nat Rev Cardiol.* 2011;8(6):311–321. https://doi.org/10.1038/nrcardio.2011.15.

Senaratne JM, Sandhu R, Barnett CF, Grunau B, Wong GC, van Diepen S. Approach to ventricular arrhythmias in the intensive care unit. *J Intensive Care Med.* 2020;36(7):731–748. https://doi.org/10.1177/088506 6620912701.

Tang PT, Do DH, Li A, Boyle NG. Team management of the ventricular tachycardia patient. *Arrhythmia Electrophysiol Rev.* 2018;7(4):238–246. https://doi.org/10.15420/aer.2018.37.2.

CHAPTER 6

Tachycardia in a Patient With Alcohol Withdrawal

Rahul R. Bollam ▪ Kainat Saleem ▪ Mohammad Adrish ▪ Firas Abdulmajeed

Case Study

A rapid response event was initiated by the bedside nurse for a patient who developed persistent tachycardia on telemetry. On arrival of the rapid response team, the patient was lying in bed, diaphoretic and uncomfortable. The patient was a 32-year-old male with a history of alcohol abuse, admitted to the hospital three days prior requesting alcohol detox. The patient was on a phenobarbital taper and as-needed diazepam for alcohol withdrawal symptoms. An alcohol withdrawal assessment score (Clinical Institute Withdrawal Assessment Alcohol (CIWA) score) was administered 15 min before the code was called and was 21.

VITAL SIGNS

Temperature: 98.4 °F, axillary
Blood Pressure: 150/90 mmHg
Pulse: 179 beats per min (bpm) (Fig. 6.1)
Respiratory Rate: 18 breaths per min
Pulse Oximetry: 99% oxygen saturation on room air

FOCUSED PHYSICAL EXAMINATION

The patient was a young male who appeared diaphoretic and visibly uncomfortable. He was alert, oriented, and responding to questions appropriately. Coarse tremors were present on the extension of the upper extremities. He denied difficulty breathing, palpitations, and pain. His cardiac exam showed tachycardia with normal heart sounds and no murmurs. His lung and abdominal exams were benign.

INTERVENTIONS

A cardiac monitor was attached with telemetry showing narrow complex tachycardia. The patient was given lorazepam 2 mg IV because of concern for worsening alcohol withdrawal, given the elevated CIWA score. A stat 12-lead EKG was obtained, and it showed regular, narrow complex tachycardia; P waves could not be appreciated given a heart rate >150 bpm. The patient appeared to be in supraventricular tachycardia with an unknown underlying rhythm. He was asked to blow in a 10 cc syringe for 15 seconds, while simultaneously lowering his head and raising his legs. This maneuver was repeated without success. Then, 6 mg of IV adenosine followed by a 20 cc normal saline flush was given, which successfully converted the patient's cardiac rhythm to normal sinus rhythm. Post-conversion EKG was obtained, which showed sinus rhythm at 110 bpm. Stat troponin and electrolyte levels were obtained, and potassium and magnesium were repleted

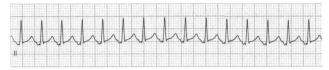

Fig. 6.1 Telemetry strip showing tachycardia at 179 bpm.

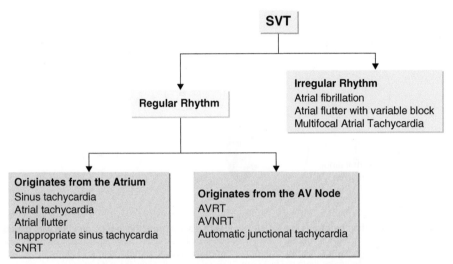

Fig. 6.2 Classification of SVT based on the location of arrhythmic focus.

intravenously. The patient was reloaded with phenobarbital, started on scheduled lorazepam doses, and remained on the medical ward with continuous telemetry monitoring.

FINAL DIAGNOSIS

Supraventricular tachycardia

Supraventricular Tachycardia

DEFINITION AND DIAGNOSIS

Tachycardia is defined as a resting heart rate >100 bpm. Supraventricular tachycardia (SVT) is a tachyarrhythmia that originates from the atrial or atrioventricular (AV) nodal tissues. It is the most common dysrhythmia in children and young, otherwise healthy patients. SVT can be classified based on the site of origin (atrium or AV node) or regularity (irregular or regular; Fig. 6.2).

Usually, patients are asymptomatic between episodes of tachycardia. Arrhythmia-related symptoms include palpitations, fatigue, lightheadedness, chest pain, dyspnea, anxiety, presyncope, or syncope. Gradual onset and gradual termination of episodes suggest sinus tachycardia. Sudden onset and abrupt termination are considered characteristics of paroxysmal arrhythmias. Most SVTs are produced through a re-entry mechanism and can be classified based on the location of re-entry.

AV Nodal Re-entry Tachycardia (AVNRT)

This is the most common form of SVT, and the re-entry circuit lies within the AV node. These are typically paroxysmal and occur spontaneously or provoked with exertion/physiologic stress, caffeine, alcohol, beta-agonists, or sympathomimetics. EKG typically shows regular, narrow complex (QRS <120 ms) tachycardia at 140-280 bpm. P waves are absent. Pseudo R waves may be seen in V1, V2, or pseudo-S waves in leads II, III, and aVF. These pseudo waves signify P waves buried in the QRS complex (Figs. 6.3 and 6.4).

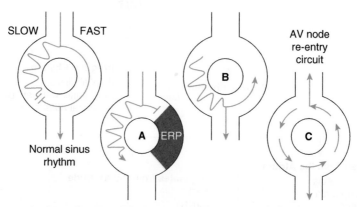

Fig. 6.3 Two conduction pathways in AV node; slow with a short refractory period and fast with a long **refractory period.** Normal sinus impulse travels down both paths simultaneously, leading to faster conduction in the faster pathway, which then turns refractory while conduction is ongoing in the slow pathway. If a pre-mature atrial impulse arrives while the fast pathway is refractory, the impulse is directed toward the slow pathway (A). The impulse then runs around and runs up the fast pathway, no longer refractory (B). This creates the re-entry circuit leading to rapid heart rate (C).

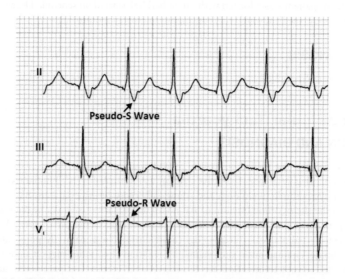

Fig. 6.4   EKG findings in AVNRT. Pseudo R waves and pseudo S waves are prominent.

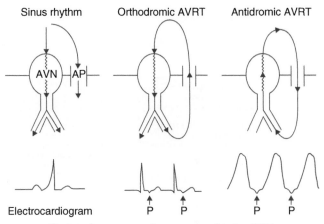

Fig. 6.5 Accessory pathway responsible for AVRT.

AV Re-entrant Tachycardia (AVRT)

The re-entry circuit is formed by the normal conduction system and an accessory pathway. Pre-mature atrial or ventricular beats often trigger AVRT. These can be divided into the following based on the direction of re-entry conduction and EKG morphology (Fig. 6.5).

- **Orthodromic Conduction:** Anterograde conduction occurs via the AV node, with retrograde conduction occurring via the accessory pathway. QRS complexes are usually <120 ms with P waves buried in the QRS complex or retrograde.
- **Antidromic Conduction:** Anterograde conduction occurs via the accessory pathway with retrograde conduction via the AV node. QRS complexes are wide because of abnormal ventricular depolarization via the accessory pathway.

Atrial Tachycardia

Impulse originates within the atria but outside the sinus node. Both atrial flutter and multi-focal atrial tachycardia are specific types of atrial tachycardia.

Other

Rare types of SVT are inappropriate sinus tachycardia, focal junctional tachycardia, non-paroxysmal junctional tachycardia, sinoatrial node re-entry tachycardia.

Suggested Approach to a Patient With Suspected SVT

For a patient who develops SVT while in the hospital, the following approach can be used to evaluate and treat the acute event. This can be expanded and used in emergency room situations, as these suggestions are based on thorough literature research and updated guidelines for the management of SVT. The usual sequence of history taking, physical exam, investigations, and resuscitative interventions are often not followed during a rapid response; these measures often run parallel to each other in a code situation. The following components of the rapid response are discussed in the traditional sequence only to ease understanding. See Fig. 6.6 for a basic flowchart for the evaluation and management of a patient with SVT.

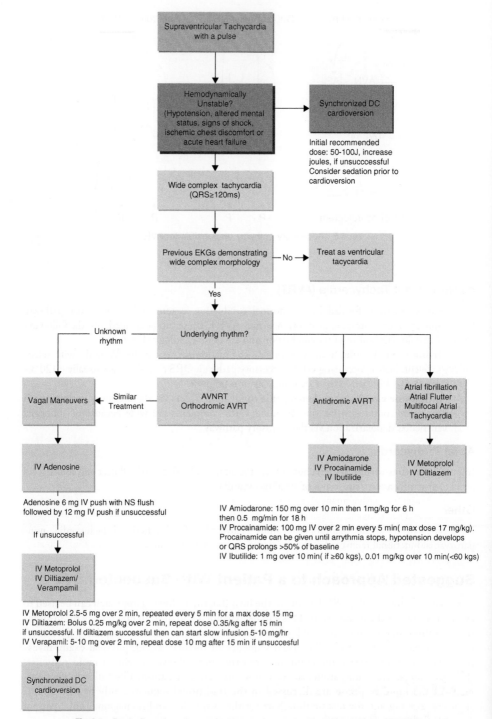

Fig. 6.6 Basic flowchart for evaluation and management of a patient with SVT.

FOCUSED HISTORY AND PHYSICAL EXAMINATION

- The acuity of signs and symptoms.
- Native cardiac rhythm (review prior EKGs if available).
- History of structural heart disease or pre-excitation syndromes.
- Physical exam should begin with an assessment of airway, breathing, and circulation. Assess for signs of shock and decreased end-organ perfusion.
- Assess for pain, fever, and volume depletion.

EKG

- 12-lead EKG should be done in all patients with tachycardia. The following features are characteristic of SVTs.
  - Regularly spaced QRS complexes.
  - Narrow QRS complex ($\leq$120 ms) unless there is an underlying bundle branch block. If the history of wide complex morphology cannot be determined, assume it is ventricular tachycardia.

LABORATORY TESTS AND IMAGING STUDIES

- Labs are usually not indicated for the acute management of SVT.
- Ancillary testing can rule out secondary causes of SVT, such as cardiac ischemia, venous thromboembolism, infection, or hyperthyroidism.

THERAPEUTIC MANAGEMENT

SVT can become a medical emergency. In a pulseless patient or a patient with hemodynamic compromise, we recommend following the advanced cardiac life support (ACLS) protocol for synchronized cardioversion and cardiopulmonary resuscitation (CPR). For a hemodynamically stable patient, vagal maneuvers can be used to abort the SVT. Patients can be asked to exhale into a 10 mL syringe with force sufficient to move the plunger for 15 s, followed by passive leg raise for 15 s. Carotid sinus massage should be used with extreme caution in the elderly and those with a known atherosclerotic disease at risk of stroke. 6 mg IV adenosine can be used to abort the rhythm in cases refractory to vagal maneuvers. The dose of adenosine can be escalated based on the ACLS algorithm while keeping the risk of sinus arrest in mind. Beta-blockers and calcium channel blockers can be used in cases not responsive to adenosine. Antiarrhythmic agents such as IV amiodarone can be used based on the patient's hemodynamics, ACLS protocol, and institutional guidelines.

SUMMARY OF A STEPWISE APPROACH TO A PATIENT WITH SUPRAVENTRICULAR TACHYCARDIA

Step 1: Assess for airway and hemodynamic status. Attach cardiac monitor and place pacer pads. Secure airway if indicated.

Step 2: Obtain stat EKG to evaluate underlying rhythm. Compare to the native rhythm on prior EKGs, if hemodynamics allow.

Step 3: If hemodynamically stable, attempt vagal maneuvers to abort re-entry.

Step 4: Administer adenosine, beta-blockers, calcium channel blockers, and/or amiodarone per ACLS protocol and institutional guidelines.

Step 5: In hemodynamically unstable patients, attempt electrical vs. chemical cardioversion based on ACLS protocol and institutional guidelines.

Step 6: Use IV fluids and pressors as indicated.

CODING A PATIENT WITH SUPRAVENTRICULAR TACHYCARDIA

If a patient with SVT has a cardiac arrest, we suggest following the pulseless electrical activity arrest ACLS protocol to ensure securement of proper airway and initiation of effective CPR, per guidelines. Once the pulse is obtained, if SVT is persistent, synchronized cardioversion should be done. Post-cardiac arrest care should be initiated once the return of spontaneous circulation (ROSC) is achieved. Electrical or chemical cardioversion should be attempted based on ACLS protocol and institutional guidelines in hemodynamically unstable patients with a pulse. Sedatives or analgesics can be used prior to cardioversion.

Suggested Reading

Bibas L, Levi M, Essebag V. Diagnosis and management of supraventricular tachycardias. *CMAJ*. 2016; 188(17-18):E466–E473. https://doi.org/10.1503/cmaj.160079.

Kotadia ID, Williams SE, O'Neill M. Supraventricular tachycardia: an overview of diagnosis and management. *Clin Med*. 2020;20(1):43–47. https://doi.org/10.7861/clinmed.cme.20.1.3.

Lerman BB, Markowitz SM, Cheung JW, Liu CF, Thomas G, Ip JE. Supraventricular tachycardia: mechanistic insights deduced from adenosine. *Circ Arrhythm Electrophysiol*. 2018;11(12):e006953. https://doi.org/10.1161/CIRCEP.118.006953.

Levine GN. Supraventricular tachycardia. *Cardiol Secrets Fourth Ed*. 2013:267–272. https://doi.org/10.1016/B978-1-4557-4815-0.00035-0.

CHAPTER 7

Tachycardia in a Patient With Severe Pain

Rahul R. Bollam ▪ Kainat Saleem ▪ Syed Arsalan Akhter Zaidi

Case Study

A rapid response code was activated for a patient who developed persistent tachycardia on continuous telemetry. Upon the arrival of the condition team, the patient was noted to be a 60-year-old male with a past medical history of peptic ulcer disease and alcohol use, admitted two days prior for severe abdominal pain. The patient had undergone an esophagogastroduodenoscopy (EGD) a few hours before the condition was called. EGD had shown evidence of gastritis. The patient had been started on proton pump inhibitors.

VITAL SIGNS

Temperature: 97.6 °F, axillary
Blood Pressure: 170/90 mmHg
Heart Rate: 160 beats per min (bpm) (Fig. 7.1)
Respiratory Rate: 30 breaths per min
Oxygen Saturation: 99% oxygen saturation on room air

FOCUSED PHYSICAL EXAMINATION

The patient was a middle-aged male who appeared diaphoretic and visibly uncomfortable. He was awake, oriented, and responding to questions. His abdominal examination showed epigastric tenderness but no distension or guarding. The remainder of his examination was unremarkable.

INTERVENTIONS

A cardiac monitor and pads were attached immediately, with telemetry showing narrow complex, regular tachycardia. The patient was given 2 mg intravenous (IV) morphine immediately for pain relief. Electrocardiogram (EKG) was obtained, which showed sinus tachycardia. Complete blood count (CBC), electrolytes, lactate, amylase, and troponin level were ordered. The patient's history of peptic ulcers and recent findings of EGD were noted. The patient was given a dose of antacid medication and sucralfate. An additional dose of 4 mg IV morphine was given for unresolved pain, and a chest/abdominal X-ray was obtained at the bedside, which was unremarkable. Stat computed tomography (CT) for abdomen and pelvis were ordered, which showed findings consistent with acute pancreatitis. The patient was started on treatment for pancreatitis with adequate fluid hydration and a pain control regimen.

FINAL DIAGNOSIS

Sinus tachycardia in the setting of severe pain caused by acute pancreatitis.

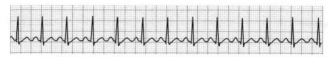

Fig. 7.1 Telemetry strip showing regular, narrow complex tachycardia with identifiable P waves consistent with sinus tachycardia.

TABLE 7.1 ■ **Features of normal and primary sinus tachycardia**

	Features/subtypes
Normal sinus tachycardia	Appropriate increase in heart rate in response to physiological, pathological, or pharmacological stimuli

	• Physiological causes
	  ■ emotion, anxiety, panic attack, physical exertion, pain
	• Pathological causes
	  ■ Disease-related: heart failure, myocardial infarction, valvulopathies, pericarditis, pulmonary embolism, pneumothorax, asthma, pneumonia, pulmonary edema, thyrotoxicosis, hypoglycemia, pheochromocytoma, anemia, hypovolemia, fever, infection, shock
	  ■ Medications/drugs: norepinephrine, dopamine, dobutamine, salbutamol, atropine, methylxanthines, chemotherapeutic agents such as doxorubicin and daunorubicin, albuterol, amphetamines, ecstasy, cannabis, cocaine, lysergic acid diethylamide
	  ■ Withdrawal: beta-blockers, illicit substances, alcohol
	  ■ Dietary exposures: caffeine, chocolate, and alcohol

Primary sinus tachycardia	Increase in heart rate that is not appropriate for the degree of physiological, pharmacological, or pathological stress

	• Inappropriate sinus tachycardia
	  ■ Persistently high (>100 bpm) resting heart rate in the absence of a precipitating cause
	  ■ Usually associated with palpitations
	• Postural orthostatic tachycardia syndrome
	  ■ Inappropriate sinus tachycardia triggered by orthostatic stress, relieved by lying down in the absence of orthostatic hypotension and autonomic dysfunction
	• Sinus node reentry tachycardia
	  ■ Sudden onset, paroxysmal, non-sustained sinus tachycardia

Sinus Tachycardia

Sinus tachycardia is a heart rate greater than 100 bpm generated from the sinus node. It can be classified clinically into normal or physiologic (appropriate sinus tachycardia) and primary sinus tachycardia (Table 7.1). Sinus tachycardia is the most common rhythm disturbance.

It is essential to differentiate between sinus tachycardia and other atrial tachyarrhythmias forms. On EKG, sinus tachycardia presents as a regular narrow complex tachycardia (Fig. 7.2). Other rhythms that can present as a narrow complex tachycardia are atrial tachycardia or atrial flutter. Atrial tachycardia will usually have an atrial rate >100 bpm with an unusual P wave axis (Fig. 7.3). Atrial flutter will most commonly present with inverted flutter waves in the lead II, III, and aVF with positive flutter waves in V1 (Fig. 7.4). Timing of the onset of tachycardia can also help differentiate between sinus tachycardia and other types of atrial tachyarrhythmias. Abrupt onset of tachycardia would point toward a non-sinus tachyarrhythmia.

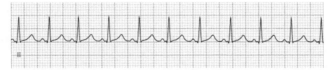

Fig. 7.2 Sinus tachycardia at a rate of 130 bpm, normal morphology of P waves, and regular rhythm with a QRS complex followed by each P wave.

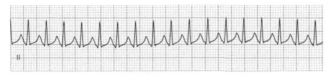

Fig. 7.3 Atrial tachycardia at a rate of 220 bpm.

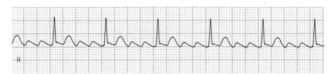

Fig. 7.4 Atrial flutter at an atrial rate of 300 bpm and a ventricular rate of 75 bpm.

Suggested Approach to a Patient With Suspected Sinus Tachycardia

For inpatient scenarios where sinus tachycardia is suspected, the following approach can be used to evaluate and manage the patient acutely. The ultimate management decisions are based on the treating clinician's discretion, expertise, and institutional guidelines.

HISTORY AND PHYSICAL EXAMINATION

- Assess for the presence of symptoms and the acuity of signs and symptoms.
- Prior history of similar occurrences.
- Baseline heart rate and rhythm.
- History of arrhythmias, medication use, triggers including fever and pain.
- Physical exam should assess for diseases and pathologies that can trigger sinus tachycardia.

LABS

- Laboratory tests can be done to evaluate the underlying cause of tachycardia.
- CBC – can be done to evaluate for anemia.
- Electrolyte panel – can be done to evaluate for volume depletion.
- Thyroid-stimulating hormone (TSH) – can be done to assess for thyroid disturbances.
- Troponin – can be done if there is suspicion of myocardial ischemia.

EKG

- EKG should be obtained to distinguish from other atrial arrhythmias.
  - Normal sinus demonstrates upright P waves in the leads I, II, aVL, and negative P wave in lead aVR. Sinus tachycardia is heart rate >100 with a normal P wave axis.
  - Atrial flutter and atrial tachycardia would have features described earlier in the chapter.
- ST changes would point toward a cardiac pathologic condition based on the clinical scenario.

IMAGING

- Imaging is not necessary for the diagnosis of sinus tachycardia. However, it can be pursued to evaluate for triggers.
  - A chest X-ray can be obtained to rule out pneumonia, effusion, pneumothorax, pulmonary edema.
  - CT angiogram of the chest can be pursued if there is clinical suspicion of pulmonary embolism.

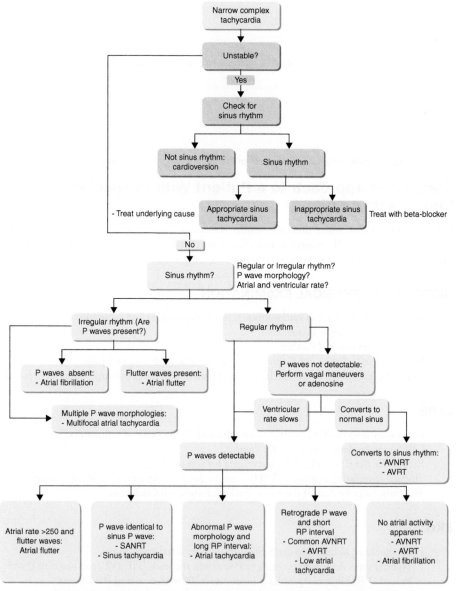

Fig. 7.5 Flowchart for the assessment and management of sinus tachycardia.

THERAPEUTIC INTERVENTIONS

Treatment of sinus tachycardia is usually dependent on identifying the underlying cause. Rate control should not be instituted in acute settings in patients with sinus tachycardia. The focus should be on determining and treating the underlying cause. This rhythm generally does not cause hemodynamic instability. If hemodynamic instability is present, other arrhythmias should be considered higher on the differential list. This chapter will focus on therapeutic interventions directed toward general (physiologic) causes of sinus tachycardia. For the management of specific pathologies, please refer to their respective chapters.

In patients with severe pain, management should be guided by routine pain assessment and a stepwise approach (see flowchart for management in Fig. 7.5). IV opioid analgesics such as hydromorphone, fentanyl, morphine, and IV non-steroidal anti-inflammatory drugs such as ketorolac are the most common pain control agents used in a rapid response setting because of their quick onset of action. IV acetaminophen is less effective as a pain control agent. However, it could be the preferred drug if fever is present as well. Acute severe panic attacks and anxiety can be treated with benzodiazepines or hydroxyzine based on clinician judgment and institutional guidelines. Alcohol withdrawal and withdrawal from illicit drugs should be treated per the institutional protocols. IV benzodiazepines are commonly used in the scenario. The agent of choice is dependent on clinical preference and institutional guidelines. Blood loss and volume depletion should be treated with blood transfusions and IV fluids, respectively.

SUMMARY OF A STEPWISE APPROACH TO A PATIENT WITH SINUS TACHYCARDIA

Step 1: Assess for airway and hemodynamic status. Attach cardiac monitor and place pacer pads. Secure airway if indicated.

Step 2: Obtain stat EKG to evaluate rhythm.

Step 3: Once the diagnosis of sinus tachycardia is established, the focus should be switched to determining and treating the underlying cause using lab testing and imaging as needed.

Step 4: Rate control should not be instituted as sinus tachycardia is generally not the primary pathologic condition and is a response to some other issue.

Suggested Reading

Buttà C, Tuttolomondo A, Giarrusso L, Pinto A. Electrocardiographic diagnosis of atrial tachycardia: classification, P-wave morphology, and differential diagnosis with other supraventricular tachycardias. *Ann Noninvasive Electrocardiol Off J Int Soc Holter Noninvasive Electrocardiol*. 2015;20(4):314–327. https://doi.org/10.1111/anec.12246.

Kotadia ID, Williams SE, O'Neill M. Supraventricular tachycardia: an overview of diagnosis and management. *Clin Med*. 2020;20(1):43–47. https://doi.org/10.7861/clinmed.cme.20.1.3.

Markowitz SM, Thomas G, Liu CF, Cheung JW, Ip JE, Lerman BB. Atrial tachycardias and atypical atrial flutters: mechanisms and approaches to ablation. *Arrhythm Electrophysiol Rev*. 2019;8(2):131–137. https://doi.org/10.15420/aer.2019.17.2.

Patel A, Markowitz SM. Atrial tachycardia: mechanisms and management. *Expert Rev Cardiovasc Ther*. 2008;6(6):811–822. https://doi.org/10.1586/14779072.6.6.811.

Yusuf S, Camm AJ. The sinus tachycardias. *Nat Clin Pract Cardiovasc Med*. 2005;2(1):44–52. https://doi.org/10.1038/ncpcardio0068.

CHAPTER 8

Tachycardia and Hypotension in a Patient on Anticoagulation

Rahul R. Bollam ■ Mohammad Adrish ■ Firas Abdulmajeed

Case Study

A rapid response code was activated for a patient who developed decreased responsiveness along with tachycardia and hypotension. On arrival of the condition team, the patient was lying in bed, minimally responsive to painful stimuli. The patient was a 72-year-old female with a history of diabetes and coronary artery disease who was admitted to the hospital one day prior with unstable angina and was started on therapeutic dosing of enoxaparin (at 1 mg/kg twice a day). Her pain improved, and the plan was to continue her anticoagulation for a total of three days and to get a cardiac cath within one week in the outpatient setting. Overnight, the patient's condition deteriorated, she became increasingly hypotensive, and the blood pressure had been unresponsive to 2 L of IV fluid boluses.

VITAL SIGNS

Temperature: 98.9 °F, axillary
Blood Pressure: 80/50 mmHg
Heart Rate: 120 beats per min, sinus tachycardia on telemonitor
Respiratory Rate: 20 breaths per min
Pulse Oximetry: 99% oxygen saturation on room air

FOCUSED PHYSICAL EXAMINATION

The patient was an elderly female who was poorly responsive to verbal stimuli, but was moving her extremities in response to pain. Her respiratory and cardiovascular examination was otherwise unremarkable. A neurological exam was non-focal. No apparent signs of overt bleeding were identified. No excessive or unusual bruising was visible. Her extremities were cool to touch, with distal pulses weakly palpable.

INTERVENTIONS

A cardiac monitor and pacer pads were attached to the patient. Then, 1 L of IV fluid (Plasma-Lyte) bolus was initiated. Stat complete blood count (CBC) and lactate level were obtained. The patient's blood pressure failed to respond to the rapid fluid bolus, and norepinephrine infusion was initiated. Her mean arterial pressure showed improvement with these measures. The patient's mental status improved with improvement in blood pressure. CBC was reported in the meanwhile and showed a drop of 3 g/dL in her hemoglobin level. Type and screen were sent stat, and two units of packed red cells were ordered. Non-contrast computed tomography (CT) of the abdomen pelvis was ordered (results shown in Fig. 8.1). A CT angiogram was deferred at the time because

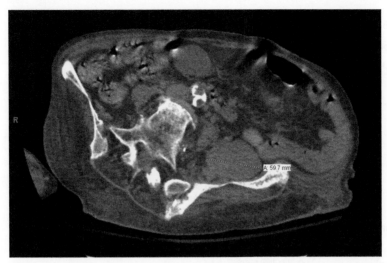

Fig. 8.1 Non-contrast CT of the abdomen and pelvis showing a left-sided retroperitoneal hemorrhage.

of the patient's tenuous hemodynamic status. The order for her next doses of enoxaparin was discontinued, and she was transferred to the intensive care unit (ICU) for further management of hemorrhagic shock due to retroperitoneal bleed.

FINAL DIAGNOSIS

Hemorrhagic shock due to retroperitoneal bleed

Shock

Shock is a state of circulatory failure characterized by hypoxia at tissue and cellular levels because of reduced oxygen delivery, increased oxygen consumption, or inability to utilize the delivered oxygen adequately. Shock is classified into four etiologies based on the underlying pathophysiology: *distributive, cardiogenic, hypovolemic, and obstructive*. Undifferentiated shock is the presence of shock without a clearly defined underlying mechanism. This chapter will focus on the management of shock caused by reduced circulating volume, namely hypovolemic and distributive shock. Management of shock because of "pump failure" can be found in Chapter 12.

Hypovolemic shock is caused purely by the loss of intravascular volume. In contrast, *distributive shock* is caused by a reduction in systemic vascular resistance leading to a drop in diastolic blood pressure and mean arterial pressure. The common etiologies of each are discussed in Table 8.1.

The signs and symptoms of hypovolemic and distributive shock can be similar; tachycardia, hypotension, and weak peripheral pulses are common to both types of shock. Hypovolemic shock is characterized by cool extremities and prolonged capillary refill. However, distributive shock is classically described as warm extremities with flushed skin.

A comprehensive history and physical examination are critical in the management of shock. For patients suspected of having hypovolemic shock, determining the source of volume loss is essential as management hinges on the replacement of volume and limiting/stopping volume loss. A history of recent trauma, surgery, or other interventional procedures should raise a flag for occult bleeding. Large volume upper and lower gastrointestinal (GI) bleeds usually manifest

TABLE 8.1 ■ **Common causes of hypovolemic and distributive shock**

Category	Causes and Examples
Hypovolemic shock	Hemorrhagic causes • Blunt/penetrating trauma • Upper GI bleed • Operative/post-procedural • Aneurysmal rupture • Post-partum Non-hemorrhagic causes • Volume loss through GI tract–diarrhea, vomiting, high output nasogastric tube/colostomy drainage • Volume loss through the skin–heat stroke • Volume loss through the kidney–diuretic use, post-obstructive diuresis • Volume loss in third spaces–pancreatitis, cirrhosis, post-operative
Distributive shock	Infective causes • Sepsis Non-infective causes • SIRS–pancreatitis, burns • Toxic shock syndrome • Anaphylaxis

TABLE 8.2 ■ **Composition of intravenous fluids compared to plasma**

Fluid	Sodium	Potassium	Chloride	Lactate
Plasma	135-145 mEq/L	3.5-5 mEq/L	94-111 mEq/L	1-2 mEq/L
Normal Saline (0.9% NS)	154 mEq/L	-	154 mEq/L	-
Lactated Ringer	130 mEq/L	4.0 mEq/L	109 mEq/L	28 mEq/L
Plasma-Lyte	140 mEq/L	5 mEq/L	98 mEq/L	-

themselves; management of these specific etiologies can be found in Chapters 51 and 52. Patients with septic shock generally have a focus of infection that can be found through a detailed history, physical exam, and appropriate investigations. Patients with anaphylaxis typically have a history of exposure to an agent followed by abrupt precipitation of hypotension and shock.

The management of shock focuses on the restoration of adequate circulation. Volume replacement forms the basis of management. The choice of replacement fluid depends on the cause of hypovolemia and shock. In cases of non-hemorrhagic shock, crystalloid solutions can be used as the first-line resuscitation fluid. Crystalloids are preferred over colloid solutions. Among crystalloids, normal saline is the most used and the most inexpensive resuscitation fluid available. However, the use of normal saline for large volume resuscitation has been associated with hyperchloremic metabolic acidosis. Balanced fluids, such as Plasma-Lyte, are the preferred fluid of choice for large volume resuscitations. The composition of various intravenous fluids is given in Table 8.2.

Colloid solutions are rarely used as the first-line resuscitative fluid for the management of hypovolemia. Intravenous albumin can expand the intravascular volume but is expensive. Hyperoncotic albumin has been used in individuals with intravascular volume depletion but total body volume overload, such as cirrhotic patients. However, studies have not shown any added benefit of this approach.

In patients with hemorrhagic shock, replacement of lost volume with blood products is the mainstay of therapy. Typed and cross-matched packed red blood cells (PRBC) are the first blood product to be transfused. However, patients with hemorrhage lose whole blood and require the replacement of other blood products as well. The protocols for plasma and platelet transfusion will be discussed later in this chapter. In the absence of typed and screened packed red cells, unmatched type O Rh–blood type can be used in emergencies per institutional protocol. In patients with religious restrictions on blood transfusions, such as *Jehovah's witnesses*, hemoglobin-based oxygen carriers have been used in emergency settings. However, there is insufficient data regarding their safety and efficacy in patients with hemorrhagic shock.

Massive transfusion protocol refers to the transfusion of a large volume of blood products within a short period of time. It is usually defined by transfusion of ≥10 units PRBC within 24 h or > 4 units PRBC in 1 h. It is commonly utilized in motor vehicle accidents and penetrating trauma. However, it may be required in non-trauma cases such as massive GI bleed, ruptured aortic aneurysm, obstetric hemorrhage, or post-/peri-operative bleed. Packed red cells, platelets, and plasma are transfused in a predetermined ratio of 1:1:1; however, the institution's massive transfusion protocol should be followed. Massive transfusions are associated with unique complications such as metabolic alkalosis, hypocalcemia, hyperkalemia, and hypothermia. These complications are best monitored in a critical care setting.

In patients where adequate volume resuscitation has been unable to raise the mean arterial pressure above 65 mmHg, or in any patients with profound, life-threatening hypotension, vasopressors should be initiated. The choice of vasopressors is dependent on the availability of appropriate venous access. However, a central venous or intraosseous access can be obtained emergently in a rapid response setting. A brief review of various vasopressors is available in Table 8.3.

Patients on anticoagulation with massive bleeding may require reversal of anticoagulation. A brief review of reversal agents is given in Table 8.4.

Severe hemorrhage can occur in patients who have acutely received tissue plasminogen activator (tPA). Although tPA has a short half-life and dissipates from the blood within minutes, the levels of clotting factors may stay low for a significant duration after tPA has been eliminated from

TABLE 8.3 ■ **Characteristics of various vasopressors**

Drug	Dose range	Target receptors	Effect on cardiac output	Effect on systemic vascular resistance
Norepinephrine	0.01-3.3 mcg/kg/min	*Major*–alpha-adrenergic *Minor*–beta-adrenergic	↑	↑↑↑
Epinephrine	0.01-2 mcg/kg/min	*Major*–beta-adrenergic *Minor*–alpha-adrenergic	↑↑↑	↑
Dopamine	1-20 mcg/kg/min	Dose-dependent	Dose-dependent	Dose-dependent
Vasopressin	0.03 U/min	V1 and V2	↓	↑↑↑
Phenylephrine	0.5-6 mcg/kg/min	Alpha-adrenergic	↓	↑↑↑

TABLE 8.4 ■ **Commonly used anticoagulation agents and reversal agents**

Anticoagulant	Reversal Agent	Caveat
Intravenous unfractionated heparin (half-life 60-90 min)	• Discontinuation of heparin would be sufficient because of the short half-life in most cases. • If urgent/emergent reversal is required, then protamine sulfate can be used (1 mg per 90-100 U of heparin given in the past 2-3 h)	Protamine is a protein derived from fish sperm and carries the risk of anaphylaxis in those previously exposed, including diabetes who have received protamine containing insulin (NPH, PZI) and individuals with fish allergy
Low molecular weight heparin (LMWH) (half-life 3-6 h)	• No specific reversal agent is present for LMWH. • Protamine sulfate can be used (1 mg per 1 mg LMWH, can be given up to 50 mg if the dose was given within 8 h)	Rapid administration of protamine can cause hypotension and bradycardia
Fondaparinux (half-life 17-21 h)	• No Food and Drug Administration (FDA) approved reversal agents available • Prothrombin complex concentrate (PCC) or recombinant factor VIIa can be used	Fondaparinux may be dialyzable
Intravenous direct thrombin inhibitors–Argatroban (half-life 45 min), Bivalirudin (half-life 25 min)	• No reversal agents for these agents • Discontinuation would be sufficient in most cases because of a short half-life	Argatroban and Bivalirudin are dialyzable drugs
Warfarin (half-life 36 h)	• Intravenous vitamin K (5-10 mg) and four-factor PCC can be given (dose of PCC is based on INR)	If four-factor PCC is not available, FFP can be used
Factor Xa inhibitors–Apixaban (half-life 11-13 h), Rivaroxaban (half-life 5-9 h), apixaban)	• Andexanet alfa is available as a reversal agent • Limited evidence is present to support the use of four-factor PCC. However, it can be used if a reversal agent is not available or non-emergent bleed	PCC works for ~6-8 h; therefore, direct oral anticoagulants may outlast its effect, resulting in rebound coagulopathy
Oral direct thrombin inhibitor–Dabigatran (half-life 14-17 h)	• Idarucizumab is available as a reversal agent • Hemodialysis can be done if reversal agent is not present or non-emergent bleed	

the bloodstream. Cryoprecipitate, fresh frozen plasma (FFP), and tranexamic acid can be given to these patients. In patients on antiplatelet agents or those with platelet dysfunction because of uremia, desmopressin can be given to improve platelet function. Platelet transfusion can also be given; however, evidence does not support its use. Consultation with cardiology or neurology is strongly recommended prior to administering antidotes in patients who have acutely received tPA or antiplatelet agents for stroke or after percutaneous intervention or coronary artery bypass.

An *anaphylactic shock* is a unique form of shock with variable and unpredictable outcomes. Most patients present with cutaneous signs and symptoms such as urticaria, angioedema, flushing, and pruritis before progressing to respiratory and hemodynamic compromise. However, 10%-20% of the patients do not have cutaneous signs and symptoms. Early recognition of anaphylaxis and administration of intramuscular epinephrine is critical to prevent life-threatening consequences. Intravenous epinephrine can be used in refractory cases. Aggressive fluid resuscitation is generally required to counter massive volume shifts that characterize this form of shock. Corticosteroids and antihistamines are used as adjunctive therapy.

Suggested Approach to a Patient With Non-Cardiogenic Shock

In patients suspected of having hypovolemic or distributive origin shock, we suggest the following approach to management. The usual sequence of history taking, physical exam, investigations, and resuscitative interventions is often not followed during a rapid response; these measures often run parallel to each other in a code situation. The following components of the rapid response are discussed in the traditional sequence only to ease understanding.

HISTORY AND PHYSICAL EXAMINATION

- Duration of onset and timing of symptoms.
- History of causes such as trauma, GI bleed, infection, previous episodes of anaphylaxis.
- Medication history should include antiplatelet agents, anticoagulants, any potential trigger for anaphylaxis.
- In case of suspected hemorrhagic shock, history should be obtained regarding contraindications/considerations to transfusion (Jehovah witness, immunosuppressed/transplant recipient, presence of antibodies).
- Physical exam should begin with an assessment of airway, breathing, and circulation.
- Assess for active bleeding in appropriate cases such as hematemesis, melena, hematochezia, or hematoma.

LABORATORY TESTING

- The following lab work should be obtained in all forms of shock:
  - CBC—elevated white count would point toward infection; acute drop in hemoglobin would point toward an occult bleed; low platelet count would identify a blood component that might need replacement in appropriate cases.
  - Lactate level—can serve as an indirect marker of tissue perfusion and severity of shock.
  - Basic metabolic panel (BMP)—to assess the degree of acidosis.
- For hemorrhagic shock, the following labs should be obtained in addition:
  - Type and cross-match of blood—should be obtained in anticipation of blood transfusion.
  - Coagulation studies—prothrombin time, activated partial thromboplastin time (aPTT), international normalized ratio (INR), and fibrinogen level to guide resuscitation and anticoagulation reversal in appropriate cases.
- For septic shock, the following labs should be obtained in addition to the standard blood work:
  - Blood cultures—should ideally be obtained before the initiation of antibiotic therapy.
  - Urinalysis and culture—should be obtained in appropriate patients for source identification.
- No specific blood work is required for the assessment of anaphylactic shock.

IMAGING STUDIES

- In patients suspected of hemorrhagic shock with overt bleeding, imaging might not be necessary. However, in patients where an occult bleed is suspected, non-contrast CT imaging can be done as a first step to identify the side of bleeding. Cause-specific imaging such as CT angiogram for GI bleeds should be obtained based on the clinical scenario and clinician judgment. Please refer to Chapters 51 and 52 for investigations specific to GI bleeding.

- In patients with suspected septic shock, imaging can be delayed until the patient is stabilized further in a critical care setting. Imaging should be obtained for the identification of the source of sepsis.

THERAPEUTIC INTERVENTIONS

Management of shock should begin with an assessment of the airway, breathing, and circulation as per the advanced cardiac life support protocol. The airway should be secured in patients who cannot maintain adequate oxygenation and ventilation. Endotracheal intubation should be pursued where indicated. Two large-bore peripheral IVs should be placed. Central venous access or intraosseous access should be obtained in appropriate cases. IV fluid resuscitation should be initiated. In patients with hemorrhagic shock because of trauma, the role of IV fluid resuscitation is less established. In these patients, volume resuscitation should ideally be done with blood products. However, it takes some time to arrange blood products, and IV fluids should be used in the interim. Vasopressors should be initiated in appropriate cases to maintain adequate circulation.

Further management is dependent on the cause of shock. In patients with hemorrhagic shock and external bleeding, e.g., bleeding dialysis fistula, the compressibility of the site should be assessed. Direct pressure vs. tourniquet should be considered as indicated. Angiography and interventional radiology interventions might be necessary for patients with occult internal bleeding. GI bleed might require endoscopic management. In bleeding patients on anticoagulation, reversal agents should be considered. Blood products should be transfused as indicated. In patients with septic shock, antibiotics should be initiated as soon as possible. Patients with anaphylaxis require intramuscular vs. intravenous epinephrine. Patients on beta-blockers might require glucagon because of muted response to epinephrine. H1 antihistamines, H2 antihistamines, and corticosteroids should be administered. All patients with shock should be managed in an ICU.

Suggested Reading

Doerschug KC, Schmidt GA. Shock: Diagnosis and Management. In: Oropello JM, Pastores SM, Kvetan V, eds. *Critical Care*. McGraw-Hill Education; 1AD. http://accessmedicine.mhmedical.com/content.aspx?aid=1136413997.

Kislitsina ON, Rich JD, Wilcox JE, et al. Shock – classification and pathophysiological principles of therapeutics. *Curr Cardiol Rev*. 2019;15(2):102–113. https://doi.org/10.2174/1573403X15666181212125024.

Soong JTY, Soni N. Circulatory shock. *Medicine (United Kingdom)*. 2013;41(2):64–69. https://doi.org/10.1016/j.mpmed.2012.11.012.

CHAPTER 9

Bradycardia in a Patient With Atrial Fibrillation

Rahul R. Bollam ▓ Syed Arsalan Akhter Zaidi ▓ Firas Abdulmajeed
▓ Mohammad Adrish

Case Study

A rapid response event was initiated by the bedside nurse for new-onset hypotension and brady-cardia. On prompt arrival of the rapid response team, it was noted that the patient was a 65-year-old male with a known history of atrial fibrillation treated with oral metoprolol, who was admitted to the hospital two days before for evaluation and management of uncontrolled tachycardia. The patient had been treated initially with a diltiazem infusion which was later transitioned to oral extended-release formulation earlier in the day. The patient continued to receive his home meto-prolol during this hospitalization.

VITAL SIGNS

Temperature: 99.6 °F, axillary
Blood Pressure: 70 mmHg palpable systolic, diastolic not obtainable
Heart Rate: 47 beats per min (bpm) – sinus bradycardia on telemetry (Fig. 9.1)
Respiratory Rate: 22 breaths per min
Pulse Oximetry: 97% oxygen saturation on room air

FOCUSED PHYSICAL EXAMINATION

The patient was a middle-aged man lying in bed in no apparent distress. Appropriate personal protective equipment was established, and the patient was examined. The patient was lethargic and would not respond to any verbal commands. However, he would move all four extremities to painful stimuli. His carotid pulse was weak but palpable. His focused cardiac exam showed inaudible heart sounds. Jugular venous distension was not appreciated. His lung and abdominal exams were benign.

INTERVENTIONS

A cardiac monitor with transcutaneous pacer pads was attached immediately. The monitor showed sinus bradycardia. A 1000 mL bolus of normal saline was started. A stat dose of 0.5 mg atropine was administered without any improvement in heart rate. Two more doses of 0.5 mg atropine were administered without any response. Stat dose of 2 g IV calcium chloride was administered with resultant improvement in heart rate to 50 bpm. Repeat blood pressure check showed improve-ment to 84/58 mmHg. Stat electrocardiogram (EKG) was obtained, which showed sinus bra-dycardia without any ST changes suspicious of acute ischemia. The patient's mental status also improved with these interventions. Stat labs, including complete blood count, basic metabolic

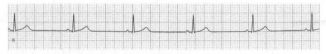

Fig. 9.1   Telemetry strip showing sinus bradycardia (rate of 47 bpm).

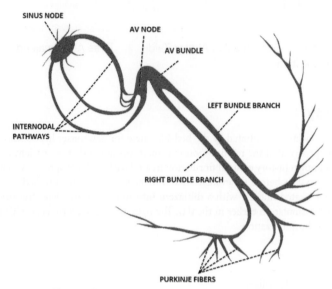

Fig. 9.2   Electrical conduction pathway in the heart.

panel, magnesium, troponin, and lactate level, were sent and were all within normal limits. The patient was started on a calcium infusion and transferred to the intensive care unit (ICU) for further management.

FINAL DIAGNOSIS

Bradycardia because of significant atrioventricular (AV) nodal blockade

Bradycardia

Cardiac rhythm is initiated and maintained by the sinoatrial (SA) node, and the electrical impulse generated here passes through the atria to the AV node. AV node is the rate-limiting step in the cardiac conduction pathway and is the major physiological and pharmacological rate control site. The impulse passes from the AV node to the Bundle of His, which lies in the interventricular septum. The electrical pathway splits into right and left bundles that depolarize the two ventricles simultaneously (Fig. 9.2). All the foci in the cardiac conduction pathway can serve as pacemakers for the heart; however, the rate at which they generate the electrical impulses differs. The intrinsic firing rate of the SA node is 60-100 bpm which overrides the much slower atrial foci (60-80 bpm), junctional foci (40-60 bpm), and the ventricular foci (20-40 bpm). Defects in the SA node will allow the next pacemaker with the highest firing rate to take over.

DEFINITION AND DIAGNOSIS

Bradycardia is defined as a resting heart rate of <60 bpm in adults. Moreover, 49% of symptomatic bradycardia is caused by disturbances of automaticity/conduction, with the remaining caused by reversible causes. See Table 9.1 for various etiologies of bradycardia.

The morphology of the QRS complex seen on an EKG helps determine the approximate site of the cardiac pacemaker. See Fig. 9.3 for narrow complex vs. wide complex bradycardia and the respective etiologies. See Fig. 9.4 for an example of QRS complex in sinus bradycardia and Fig. 9.5 for an example of a rhythm strip of complete heart block with junctional escape rhythm.

In most patients, bradycardia does not directly cause symptoms, although comorbid conditions might be exacerbated by reduced cardiac output (angina, heart failure). Symptoms of slow heart rate include lightheadedness, pre-syncope or syncope, worsening angina or heart failure, cognitive slowing, and exercise intolerance. Bradycardia minimally increases the diastolic filling, which increases stroke volume. However, if this compensatory factor cannot compensate adequately for the decreased heart rate, it can potentially lead to cardiogenic shock.

Suggested Approach to a Patient With Sinus Bradycardia

For inpatient scenarios where sinus bradycardia is suspected, the following approach can be used to evaluate and manage the patient acutely. The ultimate management decisions are based on the treating clinician's discretion, expertise, and institutional guidelines. The usual sequence of history taking, physical exam, investigations, and resuscitative interventions are often not followed during

TABLE 9.1 ■ Etiology of bradycardia

Etiology of bradycardia	
Physiologic	• Sleep • Endurance in athletes • Related to aging
Pathologic	***Non-Pharmacological*** • Vagal stimulation (pain, carotid sinus hypersensitivity) • Inferior wall myocardial infarction, myocarditis • Sinus node disease/dysfunction • Hypothermia • Anorexia nervosa • Hyperkalemia, hypermagnesemia • Hypothyroidism • Brainstem herniation (Cushing reflex) • Infections such as Lyme disease, syphilis, aortic valve endocarditis with ring abscess ***Pharmacological*** • Beta-blockers • Calcium channel blockers • Digoxin • Central alpha-2 agonists (clonidine and dexmedetomidine) • Amiodarone • Opioids • GABA agonists (barbiturates, benzodiazepines, baclofen) • Organophosphates

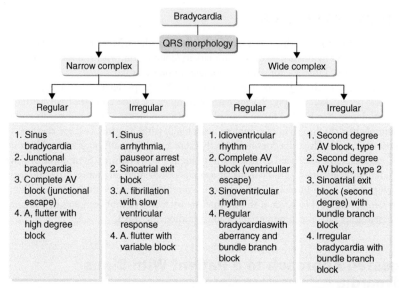

Fig. 9.3 Identification of a cardiac pacemaker and underlying cause of bradycardia based on QRS morphology.

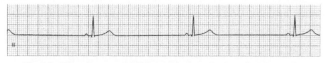

Fig. 9.4 Waveform and QRS morphology in sinus bradycardia.

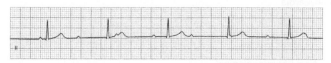

Fig. 9.5 Waveform and QRS morphology in complete AV nodal block with junctional escape.

a rapid response; these measures often run parallel to each other in a code situation. The following components of the rapid response are discussed in the traditional sequence only to ease understanding. See Fig. 9.6 for a basic flowchart to assess and manage a patient with acute onset bradycardia.

FOCUSED HISTORY AND PHYSICAL EXAMINATION

- Check for hypothermia
- The acuity of signs and symptoms
- Native cardiac rhythm (review prior EKGs if available)
- History of recent use of AV nodal blocking agents
- Physical exam should begin with an assessment of airway, breathing, and circulation
- Assess for signs of shock and decreased end-organ perfusion

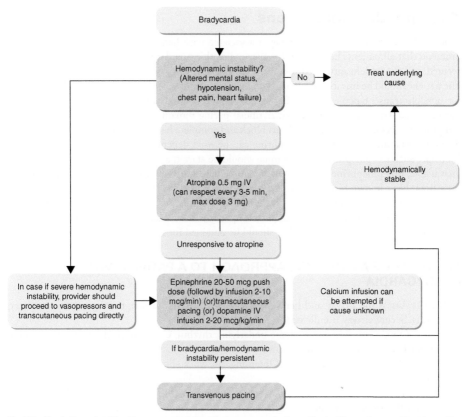

Fig. 9.6 Basic flowchart for the assessment and management of a patient with acute onset bradycardia.

LABORATORY TESTS

- Troponin level to evaluate for cardiac ischemia
- Electrolyte panel including glucose level to evaluate for severe electrolyte derangements
- Arterial blood gas with lactate to evaluate for acidemia
- A coagulation profile can be obtained in anticipation of any further interventions
- Thyroid-stimulating hormone and free T4 level to evaluate for severe hypothyroidism
- Digoxin level can be considered if there is a history of use of this medication

ELECTROCARDIOGRAM

- EKG should be obtained in all cases for the following reasons:
  - To identify the site of pacemaker based on QRS morphology (sinus bradycardia vs. high-grade AV block vs. junctional escape vs. ventricular escape)
  - To evaluate for inferior wall myocardial infarction (ST changes in leads II, III, aVF)

IMAGING STUDIES

- There is no specific role of imaging in the acute evaluation and management of bradycardia.

Therapeutic Interventions

Bradycardia can be a medical emergency if associated with hemodynamic compromise. We recommend that all patients be assessed for airway, breathing, and circulation. The airway should be secured, and the patient intubated if necessary, especially if signs of respiratory arrest are present. The patient should be immediately placed on a cardiac monitor, and pacer pads should be attached for possible transcutaneous pacing. Pacemaker capture should always be confirmed by matching the pulse with the pulse oximetry. Artificial pacing remains the management of choice for symptomatic second-degree type-II heart block and complete heart block. In patients with hemodynamic instability, atropine or epinephrine can be used depending on institutional guidelines. Inotropes such as epinephrine or dopamine should be started as vasopressor support; however, if unavailable, norepinephrine can be used for immediate support. Antidotes can be considered if the patient has a known history of using a specific medication, such as glucagon for beta-blockers, calcium chloride for calcium channel blockers, FAB fragments for digoxin (refer to Chapter 11), and naloxone for clonidine toxicity. All unstable patients should be transferred to ICU for further care. An urgent cardiology consultation should be obtained for temporary transvenous pacing.

SUMMARY OF A STEPWISE APPROACH TO A PATIENT WITH BRADYCARDIA

Step 1: Assess for airway and hemodynamic status. Attach cardiac monitor and place pacer pads. Secure airway if indicated.

Step 2: Obtain stat EKG to evaluate underlying rhythm. Compare to the native rhythm on prior EKGs, if hemodynamics allow.

Step 3: Obtain baseline lab work. Obtaining lab work should not delay other resuscitative measures.

Step 4: Administer atropine/epinephrine per advanced cardiac life support (ACLS) protocol and institutional guidelines.

Step 5: Initiate artificial pacing per ACLS protocol and institutional guidelines.

Step 6: Use IV fluids, pressors, and reversal agents for AV nodal blocking drugs (if the appropriate history of use of such medications is available) as indicated.

CODING A PATIENT WITH BRADYCARDIA

If a patient with bradycardia has a cardiac arrest, we suggest following the ACLS protocol to ensure that the airway is secured and effective cardiopulmonary resuscitation is initiated per the guidelines. In patients with a pulse, atropine 0.5 mg IV should be given every 3-5 min. If the patient has no IV access, then transcutaneous pacing should be initiated until adequate IV access has been established. If atropine is unsuccessful, either transcutaneous pacing, epinephrine, or dopamine infusion can be started. Specific reversal agents can be considered if history points toward the use of specific AV nodal blocking agents.

Suggested Reading

Bradycardia S. Part 7.3: Management of symptomatic bradycardia and tachycardia. *Circulation*. 2005;112(24 Suppl). https://doi.org/10.1161/CIRCULATIONAHA.105.166558.

Burri H, Dayal N. Bradycardia acute management. 2018;21(4):98-104. Cardiovascular Medicine. https://doi.org/10.4414/cvm.2018.00554.

Haghjoo M. In: Maleki M, Alizadehasl A, Haghjoo MBT-PC, eds. *Bradyarrhythmias*. Elsevier; 2018:261–268. https://doi.org/10.1016/B978-0-323-51149-0.00015-8.

Zaidi SAA, Shaikh D, Saad M, Vittorio TJ. Ranolazine induced bradycardia, renal failure, and hyperkalemia: a BRASH syndrome variant. *Case Rep Med*. 2019;2019. https://doi.org/10.1155/2019/2740617.

CHAPTER 10

Bradycardia in a Patient With Myocardial Infarction

Abdelrhman M. Abo-zed ▓ Kainat Saleem ▓ Firas Abdulmajeed
▓ Mohammad Adrish

Case Study

A rapid response event was initiated by the bedside nurse for a patient with new-onset fatigue, lightheadedness, and substernal pain at rest. On prompt arrival of the rapid response team, the patient's telemetry showed that he was gradually getting bradycardic to 50-60 beats per min (bpm). He was a 70-year-old male with a known history of coronary artery disease, hyperlipidemia, type 2 diabetes, and hypertension. He was admitted earlier for a syncopal event that was currently being evaluated.

VITAL SIGNS

Temperature: 98.2 °F, axillary
Blood Pressure: 100/52 mmHg
Heart Rate: 51 bpm - regular rhythm (Fig. 10.1)
Respiratory Rate: 22 breaths per min
Pulse Oximetry: 94% oxygen saturation on room air

FOCUSED PHYSICAL EXAMINATION

The patient was an elderly male in moderate distress, altered, pale, and diaphoretic grabbing the center of his chest. Appropriate personal protective equipment was established, and the patient was examined. A cardiac exam showed normal heart sounds with no murmurs. He had an elevated jugular vein distention. His lung exam showed minimal bibasilar crackles. His abdomen was soft, non-tender, and non-distended. His extremities were warm to the touch, and no peripheral edema was noted. Capillary refill was <2 s.

INTERVENTIONS

A cardiac monitor and pacing pads were attached immediately to the patient. Then, a 1000 mL of normal saline fluid bolus was started. One dose of 2 mg IV morphine was administered because of severe pain. A stat electrocardiogram (EKG) was obtained, which showed sinus bradycardia with elevated ST segments in leads II, III, and aVF concerning for an inferior wall myocardial infarction. A stat page was sent to interventional cardiology for review of the EKG. Troponin levels, complete blood count, comprehensive metabolic panel, and lactate level were obtained. The patient's hemodynamics deteriorated during the rapid response event, and his heart rate dropped to the mid-30s, with blood pressure dropping to 82/50 mmHg. Atropine 0.5 mg was administered per advanced cardiac life support (ACLS) protocol, and transcutaneous pacing was initiated, which improved the BP to 102/59 mmHg. Cardiology was consulted, and the patient was

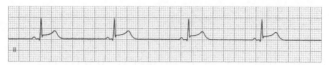

Fig. 10.1   Telemetry strip showing lead II–sinus bradycardia with ST changes.

immediately sent to the cardiac catheterization lab for possible percutaneous coronary intervention and from there to the intensive care unit for further care.

FINAL DIAGNOSIS

Second-degree atrioventricular (AV) block in the setting of inferior myocardial infarction.

Bradycardia – Heart Block After Myocardial Infarction

The cardiac conduction system is discussed in detail in Chapter 9. The sinoatrial (SA) node is the cardiac pacemaker, and following atrial activation, the electrical impulse reaches the AV node. The AV nodal depolarization is mediated by a slow calcium-mediated action potential which slows down the conduction speed. The impulse passes to the Bundle of His and then to the ventricles through the right and left bundle branches from the AV node. In the setting of myocardial infarction, certain parts of electrical conduction systems get ischemic (Table 10.1). The right coronary artery is the source of the blood supply to both the SA and AV nodes. Occlusion of this artery would cause ischemia and dysfunction of both these critical checkpoints in the cardiac impulse pathway. This AV nodal dysfunction is exacerbated by the enhanced release of acetylcholine from the inferoposterior myocardium in the setting of ischemia, which can result in the progression of bradycardia to heart block.

DEFINITION AND DIAGNOSIS

Bradycardia is defined as a resting heart rate <60bpm. This heart rate can be asymptomatic if adequate compensatory mechanisms are present. However, in the absence of adequate compensatory mechanisms, it can produce lightheadedness, syncope, exertional intolerance, dyspnea, and fatigue. Bradycardia may be pathologic or physiologic (details available in Chapter 9). Bradycardia is one of the most common arrhythmic complications of inferior wall myocardial infarction (Table 10.2). It is crucial to differentiate the transient events from those likely to progress to irreversible or high-degree AV block.

Suggested Approach to a Patient With Sinus Bradycardia in the Setting of Myocardial Infarction

For inpatient scenarios where sinus bradycardia as a complication of myocardial infarction is suspected, the following approach can be used to evaluate and manage the patient acutely. The ultimate management decisions are based on the treating clinician's discretion, expertise, and institutional guidelines. The usual sequence of history taking, physical exam, investigations, and resuscitative interventions are often not followed during a rapid response; these measures often run parallel to each other in a code situation. The following components of the rapid response are discussed in the traditional sequence only to ease understanding. See Fig. 10.2 for a basic flowchart to assess and manage a patient with acute onset bradycardia because of myocardial infarction.

TABLE 10.1 ■ **Blood supply of the cardiac conduction system**

Segment of the conduction pathway	Blood supply
SA Node	60% by the right coronary artery; 40% by left circumflex artery
AV Node	90% by the right coronary artery; 10% by the left circumflex artery
His Bundle	Right coronary artery (AV nodal branch)
Main Left Bundle Branch	Left anterior descending artery with some collateral flow from the right coronary artery or left circumflex artery
Left Posterior Fascicle	AV nodal branch and septal branches of the left anterior descending artery
Left Anterior Fascicle	Left anterior descending artery with some contribution from right coronary artery and left circumflex artery
Right Bundle Branch	Septal perforators from the left anterior descending artery with some contribution from right coronary artery and left circumflex artery

TABLE 10.2 ■ **Conduction abnormalities seen in inferior wall MI**

Conduction abnormality	Features
Sinus Bradycardia	• Most common arrhythmia • Normal PR interval • 40% occurs in the first 4 h. The frequency decreases to 20% in 24 h • Usually because of an increase in vagal tone
First Degree AV Block	• Prolongation of the PR interval >200 ms • Usually transient and resolves within five to seven days without intervention
Second Degree AV Block	• Intermittent atrial conduction to the ventricle, often in a regular pattern (2:1, 3:1, or higher degrees of block) ***Mobitz Type I ~ Wenckebach*** • PR interval that progressively prolongs until a beat is dropped ~ group beats. ***Mobitz Type II*** • Intermittent non-conducting P waves with unchanged PR interval. • The patient should be monitored with pacer pads attached given the propensity of progression to complete heart block • If the patient is symptomatic, transvenous pacing is indicated • Usually transient and resolves after percutaneous coronary intervention
Complete Heart Block	• Complete ventricular dissociation from atria • May require temporary pacing, however in the setting of myocardial infarction, this can be transient and usually resolves after percutaneous coronary intervention

FOCUSED HISTORY AND PHYSICAL EXAMINATION

- Evaluate for hypothermia
- The acuity of signs and symptoms (see Chapters 1 and 2 for a detailed discussion of the evaluation of chest pain and acute coronary syndromes, respectively)
- Native cardiac rhythm (review prior EKGs if available)
- History of recent use of AV nodal blocking agents
- Physical exam should begin with an assessment of airway, breathing, and circulation. Assess for signs of shock and decreased end-organ perfusion

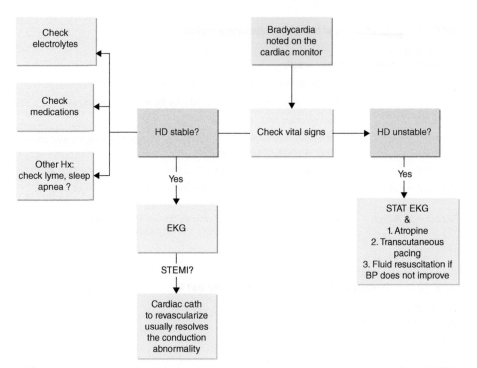

Fig. 10.2   Basic flowchart for the assessment and management of patients with bradycardia and STEMI.

LABORATORY TESTS

- Troponin level to evaluate for cardiac ischemia
- Electrolyte panel including glucose level to evaluate for severe electrolyte derangements
- Arterial blood gas with lactate to evaluate for acidemia
- A coagulation profile can be obtained in anticipation of any further interventions
- Thyroid-stimulating hormone level and free T4 level to evaluate for severe hypothyroidism
- Digoxin level can be considered if there is a history of use of this medication

ELECTROCARDIOGRAM

- EKG should be obtained in all cases for the following reasons:
  - To identify the site of pacemaker based on the QRS morphology (sinus bradycardia vs. high-grade AV block vs. junctional escape vs. ventricular escape)
  - To evaluate for inferior wall myocardial infarction (ST changes in leads II, III, aVF)

IMAGING STUDIES

- There is no specific role of imaging in acute evaluation and management of bradycardia

THERAPEUTIC INTERVENTIONS

Bradycardia can be a medical emergency if associated with hemodynamic compromise. We recommend that all patients be assessed for airway, breathing, and circulation. The airway should be

TABLE 10.3 ▪ Indications for transcutaneous/transvenous pacing

Indication	Description
High-grade AV nodal block	Mobitz type II or third-degree heart block can cause symptomatic bradycardia Those with frequent ventricular escapes are at risk of progression to complete heart block
RV infarction	Can cause decreased pre-load and symptomatic bradycardia
New bundle branch block	Can cause symptomatic bradycardia if associated with high-grade AV nodal block

secured and the patient intubated if necessary, especially if signs of respiratory arrest are present. The patient should be immediately placed on a cardiac monitor, and transcutaneous pacer pads should be attached. In patients with hemodynamic instability, atropine should be used per institutional guidelines. Transcutaneous pacing should be initiated, and pacemaker capture should always be confirmed by matching pulse with the pulse oximetry (Table 10.3 lists some indications of artificial pacing). IV fluids boluses should be considered carefully for treatment of hypotension as right ventricular failure is volume dependent. Nitroglycerin should be avoided as it can decrease the cardiac pre-load and worsen hypotension. Norepinephrine in combination with dopamine can be used for the treatment of cardiogenic shock. Reversal agents can be considered if the patient has a known history of using a specific medication, such as glucagon for beta-blockers, calcium chloride for calcium channel blockers, and Fab fragments for digoxin (refer to Chapter 11). An emergent cardiology consultation should be obtained for bradycardia associated with myocardial infarction.

SUMMARY OF A STEPWISE APPROACH TO A PATIENT WITH BRADYCARDIA

Step 1: Assess for airway and hemodynamic status. Attach cardiac monitor and place pacer pads. Secure airway if indicated.

Step 2: Obtain stat EKG to evaluate underlying rhythm. Compare to the native rhythm on prior EKGs, if hemodynamics allow.

Step 3: Obtain baseline lab work. Obtaining lab work should not delay other resuscitative measures.

Step 4: Administer atropine per ACLS protocol and institutional guidelines.

Step 5: Initiate transcutaneous pacing per ACLS protocol and institutional guidelines.

Step 6: Use IV fluids, pressors, and reversal agents for AV nodal blocking drugs (if an appropriate history of use of such medications is available) as indicated.

Step 7: Obtain immediate cardiology evaluation for revascularization if cardiac ischemia is suspected as the underlying cause.

CODING A PATIENT WITH BRADYCARDIA

If a patient with bradycardia has a cardiac arrest, we suggest following the ACLS protocol to ensure that the airway is secured and effective cardiopulmonary resuscitation is initiated per the guidelines. In patients with a pulse, atropine 0.5 mg IV should be given every 3-5 min. If the patient has no IV access, then transcutaneous pacing should be initiated until adequate IV access has been established. If atropine is unsuccessful, either transcutaneous pacing, epinephrine, or dopamine infusion can be started. Specific reversal agents can be considered if history points toward the use of specific AV nodal blocking agents. An emergent cardiology consultation should be obtained for revascularization if there is suspicion of underlying myocardial infarction.

Suggested Reading

Gang UJO, Hvelplund A, Pedersen S, et al. High-degree atrioventricular block complicating ST-segment elevation myocardial infarction in the era of primary percutaneous coronary intervention. *EP Eur.* 2012;14(11):1639–1645. https://doi.org/10.1093/europace/eus161.

Zimetbaum PJ, Marine JE. Conduction abnormalities after myocardial infarction. http://www.uptodate.com/contents/conduction-abnormalities-after-myocardial-infarction.

CHAPTER 11

Bradycardia in a Patient With Heart Failure

Syed Arsalan Akhter Zaidi   ▓   Mohammad Adrish   ▓   Firas Abdulmajeed

Case Study

A rapid response event was initiated by the bedside nurse for a patient with a heart rate of 44 beats per min (bpm) on the telemonitor. On prompt arrival of the rapid response team, it was noted that the patient was a 64-year-old male with comorbidities of chronic systolic heart failure, atrial fibrillation, and osteoarthritis, who was admitted three days ago for severe gastroenteritis and dehydration. The patient was receiving IV fluids since admission but was unable to get any fluids this day since he refused to be hooked up to continuous infusion. He had also refused any blood draws this morning. The patient was receiving metoprolol, apixaban, aspirin, lisinopril, and digoxin. Pacer pads were attached to the patient in preparation for any need for cardiac pacing.

VITAL SIGNS

Temperature: 98.6 °F
Blood Pressure: 90/60 mmHg
Heart Rate: 45 beats per min – with junctional bradycardia and narrow QRS complexes on telemonitor (Fig. 11.1)
Respiratory Rate: 14 breaths per min
Pulse Oximetry: 94% oxygen saturation on room air

FOCUSED PHYSICAL EXAMINATION

The patient was a middle-aged man sitting up in bed, leaning forward in obvious distress. The room was filled with an unmistakable smell of fecal matter. Before examining the patient, it was ensured that everyone had proper protective gowns, surgical gloves, and surgical masks on. The patient's heart auscultation revealed bradycardia, no prominent murmurs. Chest auscultation was clear. His abdominal exam showed diffuse tenderness. When asked, the patient reported that this started a few hours ago, and he did not report this to the nurse as he thought this might be from his continued diarrhea. He denied pain anywhere else in the body.

INTERVENTIONS

A stat electrocardiogram (EKG) was ordered, along with a troponin level and electrolytes. The patient was given 1000 cc Plasma-Lyte bolus. EKG obtained showed sinus bradycardia, with occasional breaks of junctional rhythm, depressed T waves, and ST depression in the lateral leads. His last laboratory tests showed that he was hypokalemic with a potassium of 2.8. Patient's potassium was being corrected intravenously till one day ago; however, he had refused medications and fluids today. With this history in mind, it was decided that this patient might be suffering

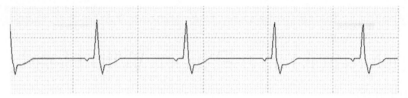

Fig. 11.1   Telemetry strip showing junctional bradycardia with inverted P and T waves with a narrow QRS complex.

from hypokalemia induced digitalis toxicity. He was given one dose of atropine (0.5 mg IV) and started on intravenous potassium supplementation. His heart rate and blood pressure improved to 55 bpm and 100/60 mmHg, respectively. Further labs were sent, including a lactate level, digoxin level, and magnesium level. It was decided to transfer him to the cardiac care unit for closer monitoring and possible need of digoxin-specific Fab fragments.

FINAL DIAGNOSIS:

Hypokalemia Induced Digoxin Toxicity Resulting in Sinus Dysfunction

Digoxin Toxicity

Digoxin is one of the oldest drugs for the treatment of heart failure. It was first described for heart failure treatment in 1785 as a component of the plant digitalis purpura. Although it has been in and out of favor by different cardiology guidelines, we have been seeing more and more physicians prescribing digoxin as a treatment for heart failure because of its inotropic effects on cardiac myocytes and rate-controlling agent in atrial fibrillation. The drug works by reversibly inhibiting Na-K-ATPase, leading to increased intracellular sodium and decreased intracellular potassium. Since digoxin binds to the potassium site of Na-K-ATPase, low potassium levels can lead to increased effects of digoxin, leading to toxicity. This mechanism and its interactions with multiple electrolytes have led to the establishment of a very narrow therapeutic index. When the patient is receiving digoxin, the optimal levels of potassium are supposed to be between 4 meq/dL and 5 meq/dL. Explanation of the complete pharmacokinetics for the development of toxicity from digoxin is out of the scope of this chapter, but we will explain what to look for in a patient on digoxin who has cardiac rhythm abnormalities or other signs of toxicity.

DEFINITION AND DIAGNOSIS

Digoxin toxicity, also known as digoxin poisoning, is when digoxin acts at an excess to its desired level of activity. This definition is broad, but it tells us that a person does not need to ingest more digoxin to get toxic levels in the system, such as in our case, the therapeutic dose of digoxin was continued, but because of hypokalemia, there was a disproportionate effect of digoxin on the heart.

Digoxin toxicity is a clinical diagnosis based on a history of exposure, suggestive clinical features, and electrocardiac manifestations (Table 11.1). Serum digoxin levels do not always correlate with toxicity, and toxicity can develop with normal serum levels of digoxin. See Table 11.2 for a list of common differential diagnoses of digoxin toxicity.

Suggested Approach to a Patient With Suspected Digoxin Toxicity

For inpatient scenarios where digoxin toxicity is being considered as the primary diagnosis of acute symptoms, the following approach can be used to evaluate and manage the patient. This

TABLE 11.1 ■ Signs and symptoms of digoxin toxicity

Cardiac	• Paroxysmal atrial tachycardia with AV nodal blockage • Pre-mature ventricular contractions • Bradycardia with a junctional escape rhythm • Bidirectional ventricular tachycardia • Sinus bradycardia with pre-mature ventricular contractions (PVC)
Neurologic	• Fatigue • Headache • Delirium • Confusion and disorientation
Visual	• Blurred or double vision • Altered color perception • Greenish-yellow halos around lights
Digestive	• Vomiting and nausea • Abdominal pain • Anorexia • Diarrhea

TABLE 11.2 ■ Differential diagnosis of digoxin toxicity

Diagnosis that mimicks digoxin toxicity	How to differentiate from digoxin toxicity?
• Poisoning with calcium channel blockers • Poisoning with beta-blockers • Poisoning with clonidine • Sick sinus syndrome • Hypothermia • Hypothyroidism • Myocardial infarction • Hyperkalemia	• Digoxin toxicity will have elevated serum levels of digoxin • Hypoglycemia seen in calcium channel blocker poisoning • Clonidine causes more central nervous system depression and miosis than is seen with digoxin • TSH, troponin usually normal in digoxin toxicity • Less respiratory depression in digoxin toxicity

approach is based on a thorough literature search and updated guidelines. This can be applied to emergency room scenarios as well, as the management is universal. See Fig. 11.2 for a basic flow-chart for the assessment and management of a patient with digoxin toxicity.

FOCUSED HISTORY AND PHYSICAL EXAMINATION

- Digoxin exposure/ingestion, and any other atrioventricular (AV) nodal blockers if ingested?
- Any new recent medication changes were made on admission to the hospital or just before that?
- Any other acute illnesses, e.g., gastroenteritis? which may cause dehydration, hypokalemia, and renal failure – leading to toxicity.
- Clinical manifestations from suspected digoxin toxicity (Table 11.1), especially neurologic, visual, and gastrointestinal? Ask about cardiac manifestations, but you are more likely to find those on EKG.
- Physical examination should begin with an assessment of airway, breathing, and circulation. Assess primarily for signs of hypotension like cool, clammy skin, and cyanosis. Also, acute mesenteric ischemia can cause severe abdominal pain in these patients.

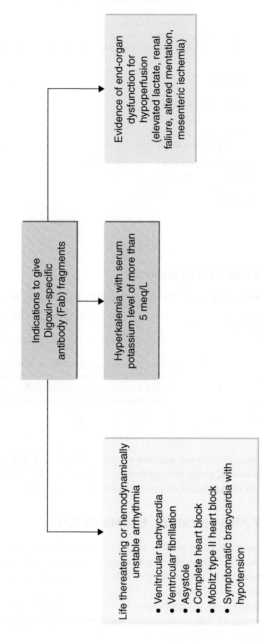

Fig. 11.2 Basic flowchart for the assessment and management of patients with digoxin toxicity.

LABORATORY TESTS

- Serum digoxin levels – although not necessary as the levels can be deceiving.
- Serum potassium and magnesium levels.
- Creatinine and blood urea levels for renal function assessment.
- Finger-stick glucose to rule out hypoglycemia.
- Urine and serum toxicology screen to assess for any other co-ingestions.

ELECTROCARDIOGRAM

- EKG should be obtained in all cases; digoxin toxicity can lead to any and all arrhythmias.
- PVCs are most common.
- Look for AV nodal blockage; this can be life-threatening.
- Look for ventricular fibrillation and ventricular tachycardia; this can also be life-threatening.
- Ventricular bigeminy.
- Junctional escape rhythms.
- Tachyarrhythmias.
- Digitalis effect – T-wave flattening or inversion, QT interval shortening, scooped ST segments and ST depression in lateral leads, increased amplitude of U waves. This is a common finding in patients on chronic digoxin therapy and does not correlate with clinical manifestations of this toxicity.

IMAGING STUDIES

- Imaging is usually not required in patients showing clinical manifestations of digoxin toxicity.

THERAPEUTIC INTERVENTIONS

Interventions for digoxin toxicity are based on the level of symptoms. In cases where rapid response teams are activated, this is mostly in the setting of cardiac rhythm abnormalities being seen on telemonitor. We suggest that all patients be assessed for airway, breathing, and circulation. Secure airway, intubate if necessary. Place patient on a cardiac monitor, and attach pacer pads if the patient is bradycardic. No matter the real cause, the first step in severely bradycardic patients with hypotension is to give atropine IV 0.5 mg, or if not available, give epinephrine IV infusion at 2 mcg/min (after consultation with intensivist). This should improve the heart rate and cardiac output, thus increasing blood flow. If these interventions fail to improve the patient's hemodynamics, the patient's heart should be paced artificially using transcutaneous pacer pads, which can be switched to a temporary transvenous pacer till the inciting cause can be determined and corrected. IV fluid boluses can also be given if needed to support blood pressure, although its use should be judicial in patients with heart failure. In academic centers where digoxin specific Fab fragments are available, they should be administered in hemodynamically unstable patients (Fig. 11.3). Once the patient is stabilized hemodynamically, correction of electrolytes, particularly potassium and magnesium, should be done. For patients with supraventricular tachycardia, ventricular tachycardia, or ventricular fibrillation, follow the advanced cardiac life support (ACLS) protocol in addition to Fab fragments.

SUMMARY OF STEPS TO APPROACH A PATIENT WITH DIGOXIN TOXICITY

Step 1: Patient with signs and symptoms of digoxin toxicity on focused history and physical?

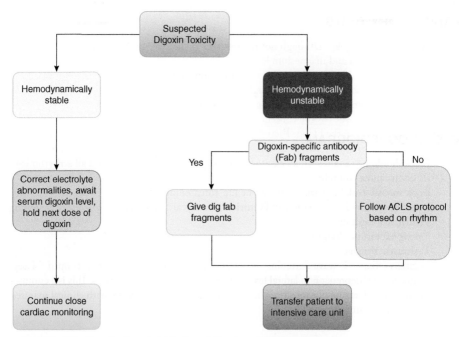

Fig. 11.3 Indications for the administration of digoxin specific Fab fragments.

Step 2: Assess for hemodynamic status.

Step 3: Obtain and evaluate the EKG for life-threatening abnormalities.

Step 4: If hemodynamically unstable, attach pacer pads, start artificial pacing, and give digoxin specific Fab fragments. If this is unavailable, give atropine, and/or epinephrine, and IV fluids, transfer this patient to the intensive care unit (ICU) immediately.

Step 5: If hemodynamically stable, evaluate electrolyte abnormalities and correct potassium and magnesium levels; patient can be monitored on the medical floor.

Step 6: A cardiology consult should be placed for all patients.

CODING A PATIENT WITH CARDIAC TOXICITY FROM DIGOXIN

If a patient with suspected cardiac toxicity has a cardiac arrest, we suggest following the ACLS protocol to make sure arrhythmias are dealt with as per guidelines, in addition to the digoxin specific Fab fragments. Patients with ventricular fibrillation will require defibrillation, while bradycardic patients will require atropine, epinephrine, and possibly transcutaneous pacing. The airway should be secured appropriately. We suggest immediate transfer to the ICU for closer monitoring and stat consult to cardiology. We also recommend stat consult to nephrology in case of life-threatening electrolyte abnormalities.

Suggested Reading

Ary L, Goldberger M. Cardiac arrhythmias due to digoxin toxicity. UpToDate.com. http://www.uptodate.com/contents/cardiac-arrhythmias-due-to-digoxin-toxicity.

Bradycardia S. Part 7.3: management of symptomatic bradycardia and tachycardia. *Circulation.* 2005;112(24 Suppl). https://doi.org/10.1161/CIRCULATIONAHA.105.166558.

Givens ML. Toxic bradycardias in the critically ill poisoned patient. *Emerg Med Int.* 2012;2012:1–6. https://doi.org/10.1155/2012/852051.

MacLeod-Glover N, Mink M, Yarema M, Chuang R. Digoxin toxicity: case for retiring its use in elderly patients? *Can Fam Physician.* 2016;62(3):223–228.

Pincus M. Management of digoxin toxicity. *Aust Prescr.* 2016;39(1):18–20. https://doi.org/10.18773/austprescr.2016.006.

CHAPTER 12

Hypotension in a Patient With Heart Failure

Abdelrhman M. Abo-zed ▪ Mohammad Adrish ▪ Firas Abdulmajeed

Case Study

A rapid response event was initiated by the bedside nurse after the patient had sudden acute shortness of breath and severe chest pain. On prompt arrival of the rapid response team, the patient's telemetry showed tachycardia with a regular rhythm. Chart review showed a 70-year-old male with a known history of coronary artery disease with coronary artery bypass grafting in the past, peripheral vascular disease, hyperlipidemia, type 2 diabetes, and hypertension. He was admitted earlier for chest pain and a syncopal event, which was being evaluated.

VITAL SIGNS

Temperature: 96.2 °F, axillary
Blood Pressure: 70/42 mmHg
Heart Rate: 120 beats per min (bpm) – regular rhythm
Respiratory Rate: 30 breaths per min
Pulse Oximetry: 86% oxygen saturation on room air, with saturation improving to 93% on 15 L/min via non-rebreather

FOCUSED PHYSICAL EXAMINATION

The patient was an elderly man in severe distress. He was alert but not oriented, responding to questions with yes and no intermittently. His cardiac exam showed tachycardia with normal heart sounds. He had distended neck veins, cold skin, and decreased intensity of the distal pulses. No peripheral edema was noted. Hepatojugular reflex was not checked because of patient distress. A lung exam showed tachypnea and fine bibasilar crackles. His abdomen was soft, non-tender, and non-distended.

INTERVENTIONS

A cardiac monitor and pacer pads were attached immediately. A stat electrocardiogram (EKG) showed tachycardia, irregular rhythm with a narrow QRS complex. He was also noted to have ST elevations in leads V5, V6, and leads I and aVL. The patient was given 2 mg intravenous (IV) morphine for dyspnea and pain. Norepinephrine and dopamine infusions were started for vasopressor support in the setting of suspected cardiogenic shock. Laboratory tests included complete blood count, chemistry panel, electrolytes, troponins, lactate, prothrombin time, international normalized ratio, and type and screen were ordered. A stat chest X-ray was obtained, which showed diffuse pulmonary infiltrates (Fig. 12.1). The patient was given 40 mg of IV furosemide. A stat consult was called to cardiology, and a working diagnosis of acute ST-elevation myocardial

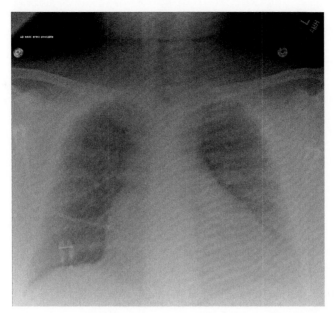

Fig. 12.1　Chest X-ray in an anteroposterior view showing pulmonary vascular congestion and globular heart.

infarction with cardiogenic shock was established. The patient was transferred to the cardiac catheterization lab immediately for revascularization.

FINAL DIAGNOSIS

Cardiogenic shock in the setting of STEMI.

Acute Cardiogenic Shock

Shock is a state of circulatory failure defined as a state of hypoxia at a tissue and cellular level because of either reduced delivery of oxygen, increased consumption of oxygen leading to mismatch, or inability to utilize the delivered oxygen adequately. Shock is classified into four etiologies based on the underlying pathophysiology: distributive, cardiogenic, hypovolemic, and obstructive (Table 12.1). Undifferentiated shock is the presence of shock without a clearly defined underlying mechanism.

Acute decompensated heart failure or cardiogenic shock is the sub-type of shock caused by an inability of the heart to pump an adequate amount of blood. The reduction in tissue perfusion results in decreased oxygen and nutrient delivery to the tissues and can lead to end-organ damage and multi-system failure if present for a long time.

PATHOPHYSIOLOGY

Failure of the left ventricle (LV) or right ventricle (RV) to pump an adequate amount of blood is the primary cause of cardiogenic shock. The fall in cardiac output leads to a compensatory rise in systemic vascular resistance (SVR) in an effort to maintain the mean arterial pressure. This response is mediated by endogenous vasoconstrictors such as epinephrine, norepinephrine, and angiotensin II.

TABLE 12.1 ■ Etiologies and hemodynamics of shock

Type of shock	Cardiac output	Systemic vascular resistance	Mean arterial pressure	Pulmonary capillary wedge pressure	Central venous O₂ saturation	Examples
Distributive	High/Normal	Low	Low	Low/Normal	Normal/High	Sepsis, anaphylaxis
Cardiogenic	Low	High	Low	High	Low	Acute MI
Hypovolemic	Low	High	Low	Low	Low	Hemorrhage
Obstructive	Low	High	Low	High/Normal	Low	Pulmonary embolism, tamponade

TABLE 12.2 ■ Etiologies of cardiogenic shock

Mechanism	Examples
Cardiomyopathic	• Acute myocardial infarction • Involving ≥40% of the left ventricule (LV) • Myocardial infarction of any size accompanied by severe coronary artery disease • Massive right ventricular (RV) infarct • Stunned myocardium following cardiac arrest • Myocardial suppression from severe sepsis or acidosis • Myocarditis • Drug toxicity
Arrhythmic	• Tachyarrhythmias • Bradyarrhythmias
Mechanical	• Acute valvulopathies • Acute mitral regurgitation from ruptured chordae tendineae or papillary muscle rupture • Acute aortic regurgitation from retrograde aortic dissection • Chronic valvulopathies • Severe aortic stenosis • Severe mitral regurgitation • Ruptured ventricular aneurysm • Ruptured ventricular free wall • LV outflow obstruction • Myocardial contusion

An increase in SVR exerts a strain on the already strained heart even further, leading to a vicious cycle and further fall in cardiac output, producing the classical "cold and wet" appearance.

Acute myocardial infarction (MI) is the most common cause of cardiogenic shock (see Table 12.2 for different etiologies of cardiogenic shock). Older age, co-morbidities such as hypertension, diabetes, multi-vessel coronary artery disease, prior MI, prior history of heart failure, and infarction of the anterior wall of the LV are risk factors for the development of heart failure in acute MI. The diagnosis of cardiogenic shock in the setting of acute MI can be made clinically with reasonable surety based on history, presentation, lab work, EKG, and chest X-ray. Specific diagnostic studies can be obtained in equivocal cases (Table 12.3).

TABLE 12.3 ■ Advanced diagnostic studies for the evaluation of cardiogenic shock

Study	Features and findings
Echocardiogram	• Most used diagnostic investigation • Can show severely depressed global left or right ventricular systolic function (or both), valvulopathies, and other mechanical etiologies • Point-of-care ultrasound can be used as a quick guide in a pinch
Invasive hemodynamic monitoring	• Balloon-tipped pulmonary artery catheter (Swann-Ganz) can be used to measure right-sided cardiac pressures, cardiac output, cardiac index, and pulmonary capillary wedge pressure • Especially useful in determining etiology in cases of undifferentiated shock
Coronary angiography +/–ventriculography	• Coronary angiography should be performed in all patients where acute myocardial infarction is suspected and who are candidates for revascularization • Left ventricular ventriculogram can give an estimate of the left ventricular function

Suggested Approach to a Patient With Cardiogenic Shock

Based on the literature review, the following approach can be used to evaluate and manage a patient suspected of having cardiogenic shock. This approach can be applied to emergency departments, and the management is universal. The usual sequence of history taking, physical exam, investigations, and resuscitative interventions is often not followed during a rapid response event; these measures often run parallel to each other in a code situation. The following components of the rapid response are discussed in the traditional sequence only to ease understanding.

FOCUSED HISTORY AND PHYSICAL EXAM

- The acuity of signs and symptoms.
- Association with chest pain.
- History of coronary artery disease, heart failure, prior MI, valvulopathies, arrhythmias.
- Physical exam should begin with the assessment of airway, breathing, and circulation.
- Detailed cardiovascular and pulmonary exam to evaluate the overall volume status and development of new murmurs.

LABORATORY TESTING

The diagnosis of acute decompensated heart failure and cardiogenic shock can be made clinically. The following testing should be obtained to support the diagnosis and guide further management.

- CBC – to evaluate for anemia (precipitant) and thrombocytopenia (to guide anti-platelet therapy).
- Chemistry including liver enzymes – to evaluate for electrolyte derangements and end-organ damage.
- Cardiac enzymes – to evaluate for underlying cardiac ischemia.
- Brain natriuretic peptide (BNP)/pro-BNP – to assess for myocardial strain.
- Lactate level – to assess for the degree of ischemia. However, normal values do not rule out shock.
- Arterial blood gases – to assess for acidosis and degree of hypoxia.

EKG

- Emergent EKG should be obtained in all patients to assess for cardiac ischemia and new arrhythmias.

IMAGING STUDIES

- A chest X-ray should be obtained in all patients to assess for pulmonary edema once the patient has been stabilized. The pattern of pulmonary edema (asymmetric) can sometimes point to etiologies like acute mitral regurgitation.

THERAPEUTIC INTERVENTIONS

Cardiogenic shock is a medical emergency. Prompt recognition is necessary to avoid end-organ damage. Cardiac monitor and pacer pads should be attached immediately. All patients should be assessed for airway, breathing, and circulation. The airway should be secured, and advanced airways should be used if necessary. Maintain O_2 saturation above 90%. Hypotension should be addressed; volume status should be determined as soon as possible as excessive IV fluid administration can worsen myocardial demand ischemia. Vasopressor support should be initiated with norepinephrine in combination with dopamine, dobutamine, or milrinone per institutional guidelines. Diuretics should be used to decrease cardiac afterload as appropriate, ideally after inotropic support is established. Diuretic therapy should be avoided if inferior wall infarction is suspected. Emergent investigations should be ordered to evaluate for acute coronary syndrome as MI is the most common cause of acute decompensated heart failure. Cardiogenic shock secondary to acute MI requires an emergent attempt at revascularization, and stat cardiology consult should be sought. Depending on the institutional protocol, the patient should be transferred to a cardiac stepdown unit or critical care unit.

STEPWISE APPROACH TO A PATIENT WITH SUSPECTED CARDIOGENIC SHOCK

Step 1: Assess airway, breathing, and circulation. Secure airway by invasive vs. non-invasive means as indicated. Correct hypoxia.

Step 2: Assess volume status to determine whether the patient will require IV fluids vs. diuretics. Preload-reducing therapy should be avoided if RV failure is suspected.

Step 3: Hypotension should be addressed; ionotropic support should be initiated with dopamine or dobutamine. Non-selective vasopressors such as norepinephrine can be considered as an alternative in ambiguous cases or where immediate ionotropic support is not available.

Step 4: Stat labs and EKG should be ordered to evaluate for acute coronary syndrome.

Step 5: Imaging studies including chest X-ray and point-of-care ultrasound can be done depending on the clinical picture and patient stability.

Step 6: Stat cardiac consultation should be obtained for coronary revascularization if the workup is indicative of acute MI.

Suggested Reading

Gaieski DF, Mikkelsen ME. Definition, classification, etiology, and pathophysiology of shock in adults. UpToDate.com. https://www.uptodate.com/contents/definition-classification-etiology-and-pathophysiology-of-shock-in-adults.

Jones TL, Nakamura K, McCabe JM. Cardiogenic shock: evolving definitions and future directions in management. *Open Hear.* 2019;6(1):e000960. https://doi.org/10.1136/openhrt-2018-000960.

Vahdatpour C, Collins D, Goldberg S. Cardiogenic Shock. *J Am Heart Assoc.* 2019;8(8):1–12. https://doi.org/10.1161/JAHA.119.011991.

Van Diepen S, Katz JN, Albert NM, et al. Contemporary Management of Cardiogenic Shock: A Scientific Statement from the American Heart Association. *Circulation.* 2017;136. https://doi.org/10.1161/CIR.0000000000000525.

CHAPTER 13

Hypotension in a Patient With Myocardial Infarction

Abdelrhman M. Abo-zed ▪ Syed Arsalan Akhter Zaidi ▪ Kainat Saleem

Case Study

A rapid response event was initiated by the bedside nurse for a patient who had a syncopal event, hypotension, and new tachyarrhythmia on the monitor. On prompt arrival of the rapid response team, chart review suggested that the patient was a 70-year-old female admitted for the management of myocardial infarction (MI) in the left anterior descending artery territory, requiring a percutaneous coronary intervention with a drug-eluting stent. She was four days post-procedure. She had a history of stage III chronic kidney disease, hypertension, type 2 diabetes, valvular heart disease, and coronary artery disease.

VITAL SIGNS

Temperature: 98.2 °F, axillary
Blood Pressure: 60/44 mmHg
Heart Rate: weak low volume pulse, at a rate of 140 beats per min (bpm)
Respiratory Rate: 26 breaths per min
Pulse Oximetry: 85% oxygen saturation on room air, up to 92% on 6 L NC.

FOCUSED PHYSICAL EXAMINATION

The patient was an elderly female holding her chest in apparent distress. On auscultation of her chest, diffuse bilateral crackles were evident, along with prominent jugular venous distension. Central cyanosis was seen. Her abdomen was soft and non-distended. No peripheral edema was noted, and her extremities were cool to the touch.

INTERVENTIONS

A cardiac monitor and pads were attached immediately, with telemetry showing narrow, complex, regular tachycardia. The patient was given a fluid bolus. EKG was obtained, which showed sinus tachycardia with persistent ST elevations in anterior leads. A complete blood count (CBC), electrolytes, lactate, and troponin levels were ordered. Chest X-ray revealed a globular cardiac shadow which was not present before. Stat consult page was sent to intensivist and cardiology for evaluation, as the patient was status post-cardiac intervention. In-house intensivist performed a bedside ultrasound which revealed a large pericardial effusion with evidence of chamber compression. Emergency pericardiocentesis was performed by the cardiothoracic surgery team at the bedside, with frank hemorrhagic output. The patient was provided with fluids and inotropic support and transferred urgently to the operating room for direct closure of suspected ventricular wall defect and a prosthetic pericardial patch.

FINAL DIAGNOSIS

Ventricular free wall rupture post-MI.

Mechanical Complications After MI

Mechanical complications of ST-segment elevation MI carry high morbidity and mortality. Fortunately, the rate of these complications is low, owing to the recent advances in early coronary revascularization. Common mechanical complications include left ventricular free wall rupture, right ventricular infarction, ventricular septal defect, and acute mitral regurgitation. Acute MI results in the loss of functioning ventricular myocardium. As the amount of healthy myocardium decreases, there is a progressive fall in the ventricular ejection fraction. Left ventricular free wall rupture, right ventricular infarction, ventricular septal defect, and acute mitral regurgitation are often grouped together, as they have rupture or tearing of necrotic myocardium as part of their underlying pathophysiology. See Table 13.1 for more information on the risk factors and clinical findings.

PATHOPHYSIOLOGY

Infarction of the myocardium leads to the formation of necrotic tissue. This necrotic area is vulnerable to rupture or tear because of the increased intracardiac pressures and volume, resulting in ventricular wall rupture, interventricular septal rupture, or mitral regurgitation from papillary muscle necrosis.

The diagnosis of mechanical complications of MI mainly depends on clinical suspicion and is confirmed by imaging (Fig. 13.1). An echocardiogram is the gold standard for diagnosing mechanical complications, but this can be difficult to obtain in emergency circumstances. A bedside point-of-care ultrasound (POCUS) might be done by credentialed individuals as allowed by institutional guidelines (intensivists, cardiologists, cardiothoracic surgeons, or interventional radiologists).

Suggested Approach to a Patient With a Suspected Mechanical Complication of MI

The following approach can be used for inpatient scenarios where a mechanical complication is suspected in a patient with a recent MI. The ultimate management decisions are based on the treating clinician's discretion and institutional guidelines. See Fig. 13.2 for a flowchart of management of such patients. The usual sequence of history taking, physical exam, investigations, and resuscitative interventions is often not followed during a rapid response; these measures often run parallel to each other in a code situation. The following components of the rapid response are discussed in the traditional sequence only to ease understanding.

HISTORY AND PHYSICAL EXAMINATION

- Assess for the timing of onset and duration of signs and symptoms.
- Details of chest pain – location and severity, as compared to how the pain was on initial presentation.
- Relevant medical history, especially recent cardiac history and other risk factors described in Table 13.1.
- Location of MI and the vessel of intervention. Usually, free wall ruptures are more commonly seen in those with anterior transmural infarctions.

TABLE 13.1 ■ **Associations and clinical findings of various mechanical complications of myocardial infarction (MI)**

Ventricular wall rupture	Interventricular septal rupture	Papillary muscle rupture
Risk factors: • First large transmural infarction • Anterior wall MI • Age >70 years • Female sex • Extensive myocardial damage	Risk factors: • Single-vessel disease (especially left anterior descending artery) • Extensive myocardial damage • Poor collateral septal circulation	Risk factors: • Single-vessel disease (especially left anterior descending artery) • Extensive myocardial damage • Poor collateral septal circulation
Clinical manifestations: This often occurs within the first five days after MI. Complete rupture of the left ventricular free wall can present as sudden profound right heart failure and shock, often progressing rapidly to pulseless electrical activity Incomplete/sub-acute rupture of the left ventricular free wall may be manifested clinically by persistent or recurrent chest pain, particularly pericardial pain, nausea, restlessness and agitation, abrupt, transient hypotension, and/or electrocardiographic features of localized or regional pericarditis.	Clinical manifestations: The ruptured septum may present with a wide range of symptoms and signs, from mild compromise with dyspnea at exertion to severe cardiogenic shock. A new cardiac murmur is nearly always present. The new murmur is typically harsh, loud, and holosystolic and is heard best at the lower left and usually at the right sternal border.	Clinical manifestations: Significant papillary muscle rupture includes the acute onset of hypotension and severe pulmonary edema The precordium may be hyperactive on physical examination, and a systolic murmur may be present. Typically, a mid-, late-, or holosystolic murmur is present that may have widespread radiation. Although the murmur may be loud, a thrill is generally not present.

Clinical features/risk factors

Early rupture <48h	Persistent pain (>4-6h)
	Acute arterial hypertension
	Persistent ST-segment elevation (except lateral leads)
	Delayed hospital admission
Late rupture >48h	Recurrent chest pain
	Persistent ST elevations
	"Undue" physical exercise

- All patients should be evaluated for airway, breathing, and circulation.
- Elevated jugular vein distention with cool extremities and crackles in the lungs are clinical signs that point to cardiogenic shock in patients with the above presentation.
- A new holo-systolic murmur suggests interventricular septal rupture.

LABORATORY TESTING

Laboratory investigations are not required for the diagnosis of mechanical complications of MI. Ancillary testing can be pursued to rule out other differentials.

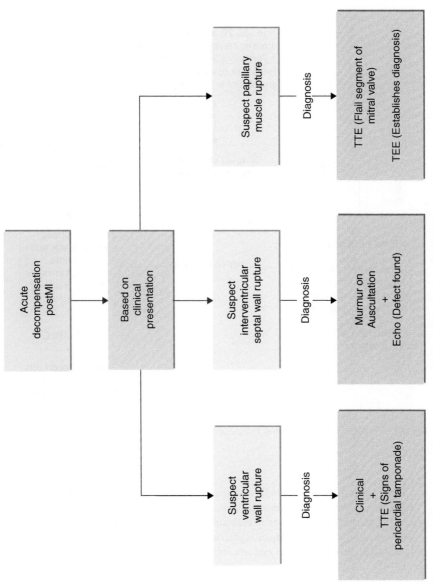

Fig. 13.1 Diagnosis and management of mechanical complications of myocardial infarction.

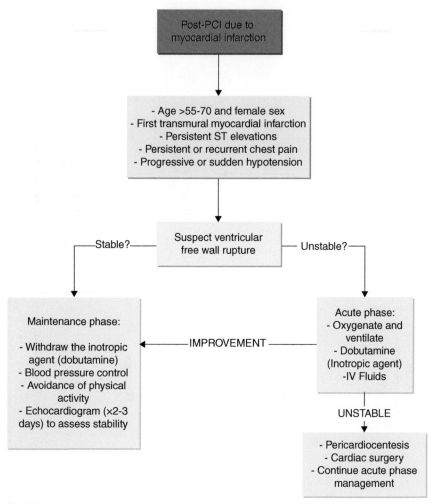

Fig. 13.2 Flowchart for the management of suspected ventricular free wall rupture.

- CBC – can be done to evaluate for severe anemia as the cause of hypotension, possibly from acute bleeding from the catheter insertion site.
- Electrolyte panel – can be done to evaluate for volume depletion.
- Troponin – can be done if suspicion of new myocardial ischemia or in-stent thrombosis.
- Lactate level – can be done to evaluate for shock.

EKG

- EKG should be obtained to assess for new ischemic changes, but this might be delayed when clinical suspicion is high for wall rupture and the patient is unstable.
- If obtained, EKG might show worsening ST elevations in anterior and/or inferior leads.

IMAGING

- An echocardiogram is the gold standard to diagnose mechanical complications following MI.
- Since patients with these complications are often clinically unstable, a bedside POCUS of the heart is often sufficient if done by an experienced provider such as a cardiologist or intensivist per institutional guidelines.
- An echocardiogram might show pericardial fluid collection with ventricular wall collapse during diastole, among other signs of tamponade.
- In case of new mitral regurgitation and after ensuring clinical stability, a transesophageal echocardiogram (TEE) could be obtained to assess for papillary muscle rupture. Chest X-ray at the bedside could show asymmetric pulmonary edema, which is indicative of acute heart failure from severe mitral regurgitation.

THERAPEUTIC INTERVENTIONS

Management of mechanical complications of MI depends on the severity of signs of symptoms and the patient's clinical stability. Unfortunately, most of these complications are surgical emergencies and require emergent surgical intervention.

Airway and breathing should be secured per advanced cardiac life support guidelines. Endotracheal intubation should be pursued if indicated. Circulation is often the most challenging aspect of management. Most patients with ventricular free wall rupture and interventricular septum rupture are hemodynamically unstable and require rapid infusions of fluid boluses and inotropic/vasopressor support to maintain blood pressure. In case of free wall rupture, emergency pericardiocentesis is indicated if the fluid is visualized. This procedure should be attempted only by an experienced and credentialed provider with ultrasound guidance (cardiothoracic surgery, cardiology, or critical care physician). If the patient stabilizes after pericardiocentesis and bleeding in the pericardial space stops, a conservative approach can be pursued with the patient being observed in an intensive care unit setting. If ventricular rupture persists and the patient remains unstable, immediate cardiac surgery should be considered for direct wall repair and pericardial patch. Most unstable patients are too critical at initial presentation, and death is often immediate.

In case of interventricular septum rupture, surgery is almost always required. Even with emergent surgery, this diagnosis carries a high mortality rate. Patients with overt cardiogenic shock will need to be stabilized by fluid resuscitation and inotropic/vasopressor support as a bridge to surgery.

For papillary muscle rupture, initial medical therapy may include afterload reduction using nitrates, sodium nitroprusside, and diuretics in case of adequate blood pressure. However, patients might present in various cardiogenic shock stages, which mandates inotropic and vasopressor support. Emergent surgical intervention remains the treatment of choice for papillary muscle rupture, and cardiothoracic surgery should be engaged emergently for evaluation.

SUMMARY OF A STEPWISE APPROACH TO A PATIENT WITH HYPOTENSION AND CHEST PAIN FOLLOWING MI AND SUSPICION OF A MECHANICAL COMPLICATION

Step 1: Assess for airway and hemodynamic status. Attach cardiac monitor and place pacer pads. Secure airway if indicated.

Step 2: For hypotensive patients, start fluid resuscitation and vasopressor support, +/− inotropic support.

Step 3: Stat consults to intensivist and cardiologist for bedside POCUS to evaluate for signs of tamponade and appropriate management.

Step 4: If wall rupture is suspected – pericardiocentesis, followed by surgery, is indicated if the patient remains unstable. Surgical repair should be performed if a septal or papillary muscle rupture is suspected. Cardiothoracic surgery should be engaged urgently for evaluation.

Suggested Reading

Damluji AA, van Diepen S, Katz JN, et al. Mechanical complications of acute myocardial infarction: a scientific statement from the American Heart Association. *Circulation*. 2021:CIR0000000000000985. https://doi.org/10.1161/CIR.0000000000000985.

Gong FF, Vaitenas I, Malaisrie SC, Maganti K. Mechanical complications of acute myocardial infarction: a review. *JAMA Cardiol*. 2021;6(3):341–349. https://doi.org/10.1001/jamacardio.2020.3690.

Kutty RS, Jones N, Moorjani N. Mechanical complications of acute myocardial infarction. *Cardiol Clin*. 2013;31(4):519–531. vii-viii. https://doi.org/10.1016/j.ccl.2013.07.004.

CHAPTER 14

Cardiac Arrest in a Patient With Pulseless Electrical Activity

Waliul Chowdhury ▓ Syed Arsalan Akhter Zaidi ▓ Firas Abdulmajeed ▓ Mohammad Adrish

Case Study

A rapid response event was initiated by the bedside nurse for a patient with sudden unresponsiveness. On prompt arrival of the rapid response team, it was noted that the patient was a 69-year-old male with a known history of type 2 diabetes, hypertension, COPD (on 4 L/min of oxygen at home), and tobacco abuse disorder, who was admitted with ST-elevation myocardial infarction and was two days post-coronary artery bypass grafting. Upon arrival, the bedside nurse was already performing cardiopulmonary resuscitation (CPR), and the attached cardiac monitor showed pulseless electrical activity (PEA).

VITAL SIGNS

Temperature: 95.7 °F, axillary
Blood Pressure: 80/40 mmHg while CPR being performed
Pulse: could not be palpated
Respiratory Rate: Ambu-bagged at ten breaths per min
Pulse Oximetry: 88% on 100% oxygen with Ambu-bag

FOCUSED PHYSICAL EXAM

A limited exam was done in the setting of cardiac arrest. It showed a pale, elderly appearing male undergoing chest compressions and bag-valve ventilation. No spontaneous activity was present, and the patient was pulseless. No other examination was performed during CPR.

INTERVENTIONS

The patient was intubated emergently to secure the airway. A total of two rounds of CPR were performed, and a total of two ampules of 1 mg (1:10,000) epinephrine were administered. A sine wave pattern was seen on the cardiac monitor during CPR (Fig. 14.1). Return of spontaneous circulation (ROSC) was achieved after 5 min, and normal sinus rhythm was restored. Examination after the achievement of ROSC showed that the patient was responding appropriately to painful stimuli. A stat electrocardiogram (EKG) was obtained and showed peaked T waves in the precordial leads (Fig. 14.2). Stat point-of-care (POC) electrolytes were obtained, which showed hyperkalemia with a potassium level of 7.2 mmol/L. Intravenous (IV) calcium gluconate, IV insulin and dextrose, albuterol nebulization, and 40 mg IV Lasix were administered. A stat basic metabolic panel was obtained and confirmed the POC electrolyte derangements. Serum magnesium and troponin levels were unremarkable. The glucose level was normal. He was transferred to the intensive care unit for further monitoring.

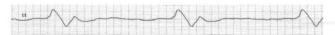

Fig. 14.1   Sine wave of hyperkalemia seen on the cardiac monitor during cardiopulmonary resuscitation.

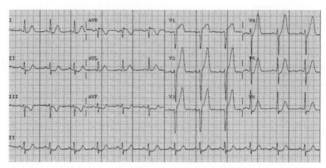

Fig. 14.2   Post-return of spontaneous circulation electrocardiogram showing peaked T waves in the precordial leads.

FINAL DIAGNOSIS

PEA secondary to hyperkalemia.

Pulseless Electrical Activity

DEFINITION AND DIAGNOSIS

PEA is the presence of an organized electrocardiographic rhythm without any myocardial contractility to produce a palpable pulse or measurable blood pressure. The complete absence of electrical or mechanical cardiac activity is called asystole. Both asystole and PEA are non-perfusing rhythms that do not respond to defibrillation. The management of PEA and asystole focuses on establishing effective CPR and identifying the underlying causes of PEA arrest. See Table 14.1 for some reversible causes of PEA and asystole.

PEA has often been divided into three main classes:

- *Primary PEA*: when the initial rhythm seen on the monitor in a cardiac arrest is typical of PEA, it is called a primary PEA arrest. If there is any residual left ventricular (LV) contraction at this time, organized QRS complexes might be seen on the monitor, but this LV contraction is not sufficient enough for organ perfusion. If there is no LV contraction at all, there might still be QRS complexes, usually wide, with no LV motion present.
- *Secondary PEA*: this is seen in post-shock situations, where a patient might receive shock for a shockable rhythm, leading to an organized rhythm without a pulse (PEA).
- *Agonal PEA*: this is seen on the monitor as a slow rhythm of wide QRS complexes. This is usually an irregular rhythm.

Suggested Approach to a Patient With PEA/Asystole

The following approach can be used for inpatient scenarios where PEA or asystole is being managed. This approach is based on a thorough literature search and updated guidelines. This can be applied to emergency room scenarios, as the management protocol for PEA/asystole

TABLE 14.1 ■ Reversible causes of PEA and asystole

Hs and Ts	Causes
Hypovolemia	Significant burns, diabetes, gastrointestinal losses, hemorrhage, malignancy, sepsis, trauma
Hypoxia	Upper airway obstruction, hypoventilation (central nervous system dysfunction, neuromuscular disease), pulmonary disease
Hydrogen ions (acidosis)	Diabetes, diarrhea, drug overdose, renal dysfunction, sepsis, shock
Hyper or hypokalemia	Hyperkalemia: drug overdose, renal dysfunction, hemolysis, excessive potassium intake, rhabdomyolysis, major soft tissue injury, tumor lysis syndrome
	Hypokalemia: alcohol abuse, diabetes mellitus, diuretics, drug overdose, profound gastrointestinal losses
Hypothermia	Alcohol intoxication, significant burns, drowning, drug overdose, elderly patient, endocrine disease, environmental exposure, spinal cord disease, trauma
Tension pneumothorax	Central venous catheter, mechanical ventilation, pulmonary disease (e.g., asthma, chronic obstructive pulmonary disease), thoracentesis, thoracic trauma
Cardiac tamponade	Post-cardiac surgery, malignancy, post-myocardial infarction, pericarditis, trauma
Pulmonary thromboembolism	Immobilized patients, recent surgical procedures (e.g., orthopedic), peripartum, risk factors for thromboembolic disease, recent trauma, presentation consistent with acute pulmonary embolism
Thrombosis, cardiac	Cardiac arrest
Toxins	History of alcohol or drug abuse, altered mental status, occupational exposure, psychiatric disease

is universal based on the advanced cardiac life support (ACLS) guidelines. See Fig. 14.3 for a flowchart of the ACLS algorithm for PEA arrest. The usual sequence of history taking, physical exam, investigations, and resuscitative interventions is often not followed during a rapid response, especially in a cardiac arrest situation; these measures often run parallel to each other. The following components of the rapid response are discussed in the traditional sequence only to ease understanding.

FOCUSED HISTORY AND PHYSICAL EXAMINATION

- Last known well state of the patient (time and condition).
- History of Hs and Ts preceding the arrest.
- Native cardiac rhythm and rhythm on the cardiac monitor during the arrest.
- The pre-test probability of PE (Well's score).

LABORATORY TESTING

- Troponin to evaluate for a significant preceding cardiac event.
- Electrolyte panel including glucose level to evaluate for serious electrolyte derangements.
- Arterial blood gas with lactate to evaluate for the degree of acidosis.
- A coagulation profile can be obtained in anticipation of any further interventions.

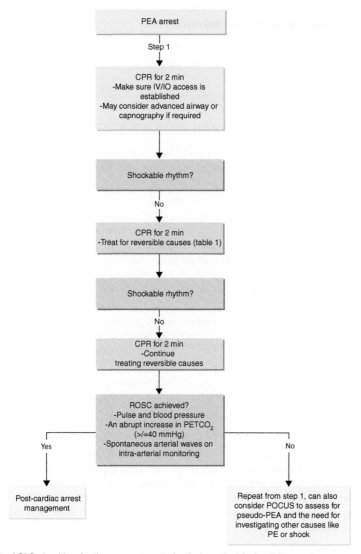

Fig. 14.3 ACLS algorithm for the management of pulseless electrical activity arrest.

ELECTROCARDIOGRAM

- EKG can be obtained after ROSC is achieved. CPR should not be interrupted to obtain EKG.

IMAGING STUDIES

- Doppler's can be used to assess pulses in obese patients where manual palpation might be difficult.
- Chest X-ray can be obtained after ROSC is achieved and the airway is secured.

THERAPEUTIC INTERVENTIONS

PEA arrest is a life-threatening medical emergency, and chest compressions should be started as soon as cardiac arrest is suspected. The airway should be secured with an advanced airway; a supraglottic airway can be used where endotracheal tube placement is not available emergently. Cardiac rhythm should be established, and the ACLS protocol should be followed regarding resuscitation. Atropine is no longer recommended for treating either PEA or asystole. Cardiac pacing is ineffective and is not recommended. Lab testing should be obtained, and electrolyte derangements should be treated as able. If tension pneumothorax or cardiac tamponade are suspected, immediate needle thoracostomy or pericardiocentesis can be considered, respectively, as these two underlying causes are easily reversible and will make CPR ineffective if not corrected. However, in most scenarios, the correction of these underlying causes requires an experienced provider and expert consultation with cardiology, cardiothoracic surgery, or critical care.

Suggested Readings

Kim Y-M, Park JE, Hwang SY, et al. Association between wide QRS pulseless electrical activity and hyperkalemia in cardiac arrest patients. *Am J Emerg Med*. 2021;45:86–91. https://doi.org/10.1016/j.ajem.2021.02.024.

Mark S, Link M. Approach to sudden cardiac arrest in the absence of apparent structural heart disease. UpToDate.com. https://www.uptodate.com/contents/approach-to-sudden-cardiac-arrest-in-the-absence-of-apparent-structural-heart-disease.

Myerburg RJ, Halperin H, Egan DA, et al. Pulseless electric activity: definition, causes, mechanisms, management, and research priorities for the next decade: report from a national heart, lung, and blood institute workshop. *Circulation*. 2013;128(23):2532–2541. https://doi.org/10.1161/CIRCULATIONAHA.113.004490.

Niemann JT, Cairns CB. Hyperkalemia and ionized hypocalcemia during cardiac arrest and resuscitation: possible culprits for postcountershock arrhythmias? *Ann Emerg Med*. 1999;34(1):1–7. https://doi.org/10.1016/s0196-0644(99)70265-9.

Parish DC, Goyal H, Dane FC. Mechanism of death: there's more to it than sudden cardiac arrest. *J Thorac Dis*. 2018;10(5):3081–3087. https://doi.org/10.21037/jtd.2018.04.113.

Van den Bempt S, Wauters L, Dewolf P. Pulseless electrical activity: detection of underlying causes in a prehospital setting. *Med Princ Pract*. 2020:212–222. https://doi.org/10.1159/000513431.

CHAPTER 15

Cardiac Arrest in a Patient With Ventricular Fibrillation

Waliul Chowdhury ▩ Syed Arsalan Akhter Zaidi ▩ Mohammad Adrish ▩
Firas Abdulmajeed

Case Study

A rapid response event was initiated by the bedside nurse for a patient with acute onset chest pain. Upon prompt arrival of the response team, the patient was noted to be a 59-year-old male with a history of coronary artery disease (CAD) status post-percutaneous coronary intervention with stent placement five years ago, newly diagnosed type 2 diabetes, and chronic liver cirrhosis. Moreover, 15 min before the rapid response was initiated, the patient started experiencing severe, crushing central chest pain, which had gotten worse in intensity and was now associated with shortness of breath, nausea, dizziness, and diaphoresis. The patient became unresponsive as a cardiac monitor was being attached to his chest, and cardiopulmonary resuscitation (CPR) was initiated.

VITAL SIGNS

Blood Pressure: not assessed as CPR was initiated
Pulse: could not be palpated
Respiratory Rate: Ambu-bagged at 10-12 breaths per min
Pulse Oximetry: 79% on 100% oxygen with Ambu-bag

Vital signs prior to the arrest:
Temperature: 95.8 °F, axillary
Blood Pressure: 178/97 mmHg
Pulse: 178 beats per min (bpm)
Respiratory Rate: 32 breaths per min
Pulse Oximetry: 88% oxygen saturation on room air

FOCUSED PHYSICAL EXAM

A limited exam showed an unresponsive, pale, middle-aged male undergoing chest compressions and Ambu-bagging. No other examination was performed during CPR.

INTERVENTIONS

CPR was continued. The cardiac monitor showed a jagged, wavy rhythm consistent with ventricular fibrillation (VF) (Fig. 15.1). The airway was secure with endotracheal intubation. Return of spontaneous circulation (ROSC) was achieved in 12 min after three defibrillation attempts at 360 J, four rounds of CPR, three doses of intravenous (IV) epinephrine, and one loading dose of 300 mg IV amiodarone. Normal sinus rhythm was restored. The exam after the achievement of

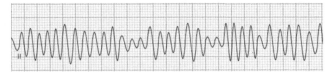

Fig. 15.1 Telemetry strip showing coarse ventricular fibrillation.

TABLE 15.1 ■ **Predisposing factors for ventricular fibrillation (VF)**

Predisposing factors and associations	
Ischemic	• Coronary artery disease (most commonly associated with VF)
Structural	• Dilated cardiomyopathy • Hypertrophic cardiomyopathy • Arrhythmogenic right ventricular dysplasia • Severe uncorrected valvular heart disease • Myocarditis
Abnormal excitation	• Ventricular ectopy (> ten premature ventricular complexes in 1 hour) • Hypoxia, hyperkalemia, hypercalcemia • Use of ionotropic medications (epinephrine, norepinephrine), especially in the setting of myocardial infarction or decompensated heart failure • Illicit drugs (cocaine, amphetamines) • Long QT syndrome • Catecholaminergic polymorphic ventricular tachycardia • Wolff–Parkinson–White syndrome • Brugada syndrome

ROSC showed that the patient was responding appropriately to painful stimuli. Stat point of care arterial blood gas analysis showed severe metabolic acidosis with pH 6.7, lactate 21 mmol/L, and bicarbonate level of 4 meq/L. The patient was immediately administered two ampules of 8.4% sodium bicarbonate and started on maintenance sodium bicarbonate drip. Epinephrine infusion was started for hemodynamic support. Post-ROSC electrocardiogram (EKG) was obtained, which showed ST-elevations in anterolateral leads concerning for acute myocardial infarction (MI) in the left anterior descending artery territory. Stat consultation with cardiology was obtained, and the patient was immediately transferred to the cardiac catheterization lab for revascularization.

FINAL DIAGNOSIS

Cardiac arrest in the setting of VF.

Ventricular Fibrillation

VF is a malignant non-perfusing cardiac arrhythmia that results from the replacement of coordinated ventricular myocardial depolarization by chaotic, disorganized excitation. This results in the loss of the ventricular myocytes' synchronous contractility, and the heart loses its ability to pump blood. CAD and myocardial ischemia are the most common precipitants of VF. In the hospital setting, VF is commonly seen in association with recent MI and can be the first sign of a new myocardial event. See Table 15.1 for common predisposing factors for VF.

Compared to cardiac arrest from other arrhythmias, the chances of resuscitation are higher when VF precipitates the arrest. Early defibrillation is the key to the restoration of sinus rhythm, and perfusion and diagnosis of VF are some of the few instances where CPR should be interrupted to deliver a shock. The chances of successful defibrillation go down by 5%-10% per min from the onset of VF. If allowed to progress naturally, VF deteriorates into pulseless electrical activity, which is a non-shockable rhythm and has poor outcomes.

Medications such as amiodarone or lidocaine can be used to restore sinus rhythm and are a part of the advanced cardiac life support (ACLS) algorithm for the treatment of VF. Amiodarone decreases the speed of conduction in all parts of the cardiac conduction system, prolongs the action potential, increases the refractory period of myocytes (both atrial and ventricular), and reduces the sensitivity of myocytes to adrenergic stimulation. Lidocaine increases the threshold of electrical stimulation of the ventricles and suppresses the automaticity of myocytes. It can be of particular use in VF with high suspicion of underlying acute myocardial ischemia.

Suggested Approach to a Patient With VF

The following approach can be used for in-hospital cases of VF arrest and is based on a thorough literature search and updated guidelines. This can also be applied to emergency room scenarios, as the management protocol is universal. See Fig. 15.2 for the ACLS algorithm for VF arrest. The usual sequence of history taking, physical exam, investigations, and resuscitative interventions is often not followed during a rapid response; these measures often run parallel to each other in a code situation. The following components of the rapid response are discussed in the traditional sequence only to ease understanding.

FOCUSED HISTORY AND PHYSICAL EXAMINATION

- Time of last known well state of the patient.
- History of recent myocardial event or signs and symptoms suggestive of ongoing myocardial event.
- History of any precipitating factors.

LABORATORY TESTING

- Troponin to evaluate for any significant preceding cardiac event.
- Electrolyte panel including glucose level to evaluate for serious electrolyte derangements.
- Arterial blood gas with lactate to evaluate for the degree of acidosis.
- A coagulation profile can be obtained in anticipation of any further interventions.

ELECTROCARDIOGRAM

- EKG should be obtained in all patients after ROSC is achieved. Acute coronary syndrome and myocardial ischemia is the most common trigger for VF and should be ruled out. CPR should not be interrupted to obtain EKG.

IMAGING STUDIES

- Imaging studies are not required for the management of VF.

THERAPEUTIC INTERVENTIONS

VF arrest is a life threatening medical emergency, and chest compressions should be started as soon as cardiac arrest is suspected. The airway should be secured with advanced airway placement. A supraglottic airway can be used if endotracheal tube placement is not available emergently.

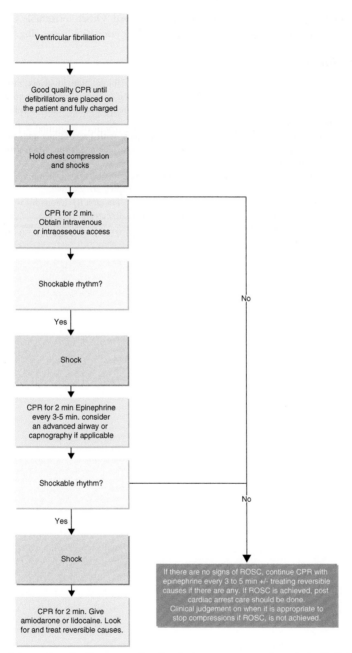

Fig. 15.2 Advanced cardiac life support algorithm for the management of ventricular fibrillation arrest.

Cardiac rhythm should be established, and the ACLS protocol should be followed regarding resuscitation. Early defibrillation is key to successful restoration of sinus rhythm, and CPR should be interrupted to deliver the shock as soon as VF is identified and the defibrillator is charged. Amiodarone or lidocaine should be administered per the ACLS protocol. All patients should be assessed for myocardial ischemia after ROSC is achieved. Other correctable causes such as hypoxia and electrolyte imbalance should be treated while resuscitation is ongoing.

Suggested Reading

Podrid PJ, Ganz LI. Ventricular arrhythmias during acute myocardial infarction: incidence, mechanisms, and clinical features. UpToDate.com. 2021. https://www.uptodate.com/contents/ventricular-arrhythmias-during-acute-myocardial-infarction-prevention-and-treatment?search=sustained-monomorphic-ventricular-tachycardia-diagnosis-and-evaluat.

Podrid PJ, Ganz LI. Ventricular arrhythmias: overview in patients with heart failure and cardiomyopathy. UpToDate.com. 2021. https://www.uptodate.com/contents/ventricular-arrhythmias-overview-in-patients-with-heart-failure-and-cardiomyopathy.

Szabó Z, Ujvárosy D, Ötvös T, Sebestyén V, Nánási PP. Handling of centricular fibrillation in the emergency setting. *Front Pharmacol*. 2020;10:1640. https://doi.org/10.3389/fphar.2019.01640.

Visser M, Van Der Heijden JF, Doevendans PA, Loh P, Wilde AA, Hassink RJ. Idiopathic ventricular fibrillation: the struggle for definition, diagnosis, and follow-up. *Circ Arrhythmia Electrophysiol*. 2016;9(5):1–11. https://doi.org/10.1161/CIRCEP.115.003817.

CHAPTER 16

Cardiac Arrest in a Patient With Torsades de Pointes

Waliul Chowdhury ▨ Syed Arsalan Akhter Zaidi ▨ Firas Abdulmajeed ▨ Mohammad Adrish

Case Study

A rapid response event was initiated by the bedside nurse for a patient with sustained ventricular tachycardia. On prompt arrival of the rapid response team (RRT), it was noted that the patient was a 66-year-old female who was admitted for acute exacerbation of congestive heart failure and was being treated with intravenous diuretics. Per the nurse, the patient had been drowsy, with recurrent episodes of palpitations and dizziness. A basal metabolic panel drawn 2 h prior to the event showed a serum magnesium level of 1.1 meq/L and potassium level of 1.9 mmol/L. The patient subsequently became pulseless while the RRT was making its initial assessment.

VITAL SIGNS

Noted before cardiopulmonary arrest:
Temperature: 98.6 °F, axillary
Blood Pressure: 80/40 mmHg
Pulse: 180 beats per min (bpm)
Respiratory Rate: 18 breaths per min
Pulse Oximetry: 85% oxygen saturation on 4 L nasal cannula

FOCUSED PHYSICAL EXAMINATION

The pre-arrest examination showed a middle-aged female in mild distress. The patient appeared drowsy with slowed responses. Appropriate personal protective equipment was established, and the patient was examined. Her cardiac exam showed tachycardia with normal heart sounds, and no new murmurs were appreciated. Her lung exam showed decreased breath sounds bilaterally with prominent crackles at lung bases. The patient became unresponsive and lost her pulse during the exam, and cardiopulmonary resuscitation (CPR) was started.

INTERVENTIONS

A cardiac monitor and defibrillator pads had already been attached when the RRT arrived at the patient's room. Telemetry findings were consistent with Torsades de Pointes (TdP) with cyclical alterations of the QRS complex around the isoelectric line (Fig. 16.1). Based on recent labs, 2 g of intravenous magnesium had already been ordered by patient's primary team and was in the process of being administered. After the patient's rhythm degenerated to pulseless ventricular fibrillation, CPR was initiated immediately. The airway was secured via endotracheal intubation. The patient was defibrillated at 200 J, and one ampule of 1 mg epinephrine was administered. Return

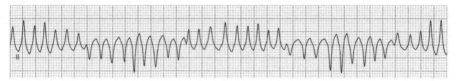

Fig. 16.1   Telemetry showing polymorphic tachycardia with alternating QRS complexes, or "twisting of the points."

of spontaneous circulation was achieved in under 2 min. Post-arrest telemetry strip showed sinus tachycardia. A 20 meq IV bolus of potassium was given, followed by an infusion rate of 20 meq/h via a central line. The patient was started on an infusion of norepinephrine for hemodynamic support and transferred to the intensive care unit for further care.

FINAL DIAGNOSIS

Torsades de Pointes (TdP) because of electrolyte abnormalities.

Torsades de Pointes (TdP)

DEFINITION AND DIAGNOSIS

Torsades or polymorphic ventricular tachycardia is defined as a ventricular rhythm that is greater than 100 bpm with alternating QRS complex morphology and/or axis. TdP usually runs between 160 and 250 bpm and can be either congenital or acquired, acquired being more common. Medications are the most common cause of acquired long QT syndrome and TdP. Other typical features include irregular RR intervals and an alternating QRS axis every 5 to 20 beats. TdP is usually self-terminating, but episodes can recur, which can degenerate into ventricular fibrillation and/or sudden cardiac death.

RISK FACTORS

- Medications: Drugs that prolong the QT interval directly or by slowing the metabolism of other QT-prolonging drugs by inhibiting cytochrome P450 enzymes are implicated (Table 16.1).
- Hypomagnesemia or hypokalemia.
- Bradycardia.
- Female sex.
- Underlying cardiac conduction system disease.
- Impaired renal or liver function.

Suggested Approach to a Patient With TdP

For inpatient scenarios where TdP is considered as a primary diagnosis, the following approach can be used to evaluate and manage these patients. This approach is based on a thorough literature search and updated guidelines. This can be expanded and used in emergency room situations as well, as the management is universal. See Fig. 16.2 for a flowchart of the assessment and management of patients with TdP. As mentioned in previous chapters, the usual sequence of history taking, physical exam, investigations, and resuscitative interventions is usually not

TABLE 16.1 ■ **Drugs commonly associated with QT prolongation and Torsades de Pointes**

Drug class	Examples
Antibiotics	Ciprofloxacin, levofloxacin, moxifloxacin, azithromycin, clarithromycin, erythromycin
Antifungals	Fluconazole, ketoconazole, pentamidine, voriconazole
Antiarrhythmics	Disopyramide, procainamide, quinidine, sotalol
Antipsychotics	Haloperidol, thioridazine, ziprasidone
Antidepressants	Citalopram, escitalopram
Antiemetics	Dolasetron, droperidol, granisetron, ondansetron
Opioids	Methadone
Diuretics	Lasix, hydrochlorothiazide

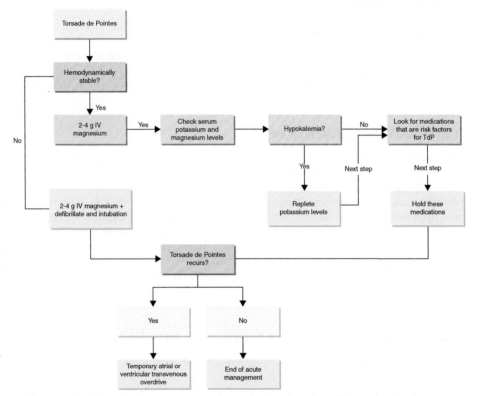

Fig. 16.2 Basic flowchart for assessment and management of a patient with torsades de pointes.

followed during a rapid response, especially in a cardiac arrest situation; these measures often run parallel to each other. If a palpable pulse is not found at any point of evaluation and management of these patients, CPR should be started per the advanced cardiac life support (ACLS) protocol.

FOCUSED HISTORY AND PHYSICAL EXAMINATION

- Vital signs, looking for signs of hemodynamic instability like low blood pressure and hypoxia. This will help decide whether defibrillation is required.
- Mental status and oxygen requirement, assessing the need for intubation.
- History of medications that are known to cause QT prolongation.
- Assess for underlying cardiac abnormalities which could potentiate TdP.

LABORATORY TESTS

- Electrolyte panel including magnesium and potassium levels since hypokalemia and hypo-magnesemia can precipitate TdP.
- Troponin level to assess for myocyte ischemia.
- TSH, free T3, and T4, since thyroid dysfunction can be a potential risk factor.

ELECTROCARDIOGRAM (EKG)

- EKG should be obtained in all cases (but should not delay life-saving measures including CPR). The following features are characteristic:
  - Polymorphic ventricular tachycardia with a ventricular rate typically between 160 and 250 bpm.
  - Irregular RR intervals and an alternating QRS axis every 5 to 20 beats or "twisting of the points."

THERAPEUTIC INTERVENTIONS

TdP can become a life threatening medical emergency. We recommend that all patients be assessed for airway, breathing, and circulation. In patients without a pulse, chest compressions, followed by defibrillation, are the most critical steps in resuscitation. Empiric magnesium supplementation should be considered – 2 mg magnesium push over 2 min is used. In patients with a pulse, magnesium should be infused over 15 min to prevent hypotension and asystole. Potassium supplementation should be done if indicated. Any culprit medications associated with TdP should be held. Sedation can be used to decrease sympathetic drive. As mentioned above, TdP is usually self-terminating and responds well to IV magnesium. Overdrive pacing can be used in refractory cases or cases associated with bradycardia. However, this is difficult to accomplish with transcutaneous pacers as the required pacing rate should exceed 100 bpm. Generally, expert cardiological consultation is required for the placement of an emergent transvenous pacer for this purpose.

SUMMARY OF A STEPWISE APPROACH TO A PATIENT WITH TDP

Step 1: Identify telemetry findings of polymorphic ventricular tachycardia with alternating QRS complex with a prolonged QTc interval.

Step 2: Assess airway and hemodynamic status.

Step 3: Bolus dose of intravenous magnesium 2-4 g.

Step 4: If hemodynamically unstable, administer prompt defibrillation. Follow the ACLS protocol.

Step 5: Check potassium levels along with magnesium.

Step 6: Hold medications that can potentially cause prolonged QTc intervals.

Step 7: If the patient does not respond to intravenous magnesium, temporary atrial or ventricular transvenous overdrive pacing can be used.

Note: For patients who become severely altered and/or hypoxic at any step mentioned above, establish an advanced airway for airway protection.

Suggested Reading

Berul CI. Acquired long QT syndrome: definitions, causes, and pathophysiology. UpToDate.com. https://www.uptodate.com/contents/acquired-long-qt-syndrome-definitions-causes-and-pathophysiology.

Danielsson B, Collin J, Nyman A, et al. Drug use and torsades de pointes cardiac arrhythmias in Sweden: a nationwide register-based cohort study. *BMJ Open*. 2020;10(3):e034560. https://doi.org/10.1136/bmjopen-2019-034560.

Drew BJ, Ackerman MJ, Funk M, et al. Prevention of torsade de pointes in hospital settings: a scientific statement from the American Heart Association and the American College of Cardiology Foundation. *Circulation*. 2010;121(8):1047–1060. https://doi.org/10.1161/CIRCULATIONAHA.109.192704.

Jankelson L, Karam G, Becker ML, Chinitz LA, Tsai M-C. QT prolongation, torsades de pointes, and sudden death with short courses of chloroquine or hydroxychloroquine as used in COVID-19: a systematic review. *Hear Rhythm*. 2020;17(9):1472–1479. https://doi.org/10.1016/j.hrthm.2020.05.008.

Kallergis EM, Goudis CA, Simantirakis EN, Kochiadakis GE, Vardas PE. Mechanisms, risk factors, and management of acquired long QT syndrome: a comprehensive review. *Sci World J*. 2012 https://doi.org/10.1100/2012/212178.

Li M, Ramos LG. Drug-induced QT prolongation and torsades de pointes. *P T*. 2017;42(7):473–477.

Semedo E, Kapel GF, van Opstal J, van Dessel PFHM. Drug-induced "torsade de pointes" in a COVID-19 patient despite discontinuation of chloroquine. Importance of its long half-life: a case report. *Eur Hear J Case Rep*. 2020;4(FI1):1–5. https://doi.org/10.1093/ehjcr/ytaa218.

PART 2

Cases With Respiratory Pathologies

CHAPTER 17

Tachypnea in a Patient With Severe Anemia

Rahul R. Bollam ▩ Syed Arsalan Akhter Zaidi ▩ Kainat Saleem

Case Study

A rapid response event was activated by the bedside nurse for a patient who developed acute respiratory distress. Upon the arrival of the rapid response team, it was found that the patient was a 55-year-old male with a history of alcohol abuse, chronic obstructive pulmonary disease (COPD), congestive heart failure (most recent left ventricular ejection fraction 20%) who initially presented for evaluation of chest pain. Emergent cardiac catheterization was performed through the femoral artery, and two coronary stents were placed. Overnight, the patient developed increasing difficulty breathing associated with tachycardia.

VITAL SIGNS

Temperature: 37.4 °F
Blood Pressure: 90/60 mmHg
Heart Rate: 120 beats per min – with sinus tachycardia on tele-monitor
Respiratory Rate: 35 breaths per min
Pulse Oximetry: 85% on room air, improved to 97% on 2 L oxygen

FOCUSED HISTORY AND PHYSICAL EXAMINATION

A middle-aged male who was visibly in distress was seen. Lungs and heart were clear on auscultation. However, the patient appeared dyspneic and was using accessory muscles of respiration. Abdominal examination was unremarkable, but inguinal examination showed bruising around the puncture site with associated swelling. The remaining examination was unremarkable.

INTERVENTIONS

Based on the history and physical examination, the patient appeared to be in acute hypoxic respiratory failure. He was placed on 2 L of supplemental oxygen through a nasal cannula, and 1 L of IV fluid bolus was initiated. A cardiac monitor was attached. Stat chest X-ray, arterial blood gas, EKG, brain natriuretic peptide (BNP), troponin, and basic labs were ordered. The chest X-ray was negative for any acute infiltrates. Arterial blood gas showed a pH of 7.59, pCO_2 of 22, and pO_2 of 52, which was significant for alkalosis and hypoxemia. Basic labs showed hemoglobin 4.1 mg/dL. His other labs were unremarkable. Computed tomography (CT) angiography of chest, abdomen, and pelvis was ordered stat to assess for an occult bleed. The patient was given an urgent blood transfusion and admitted to the intensive care unit for closer monitoring. Interventional radiology was consulted to evaluate for possible embolization.

FINAL DIAGNOSIS

Respiratory distress as an early feature of hemorrhagic shock and symptomatic anemia.

Tachypnea

The average breathing rate for an adult is 12-20 breaths per min. Tachypnea is defined as a breathing rate greater than 20 breaths per min. In contrast, dyspnea is the perception of an inability to breathe comfortably. Both these terms are often used interchangeably in the clinical setting. A wide variety of reasons can cause tachypnea. Clinicians must work through a comprehensive list of differentials to promptly identify the underlying cause and rule out life-threatening causes of tachypnea (Table 17.1).

Tachypnea is mediated through two different mechanisms. Pulmonary pathologies such as COPD, asthma, and congestive heart failure drive tachypnea by stimulating primary pulmonary mechanisms such as alveolar wall stretch and by activating lower airway receptors. Extrapulmonary factors drive tachypnea by stimulating medullary and carotid body chemoreceptors, the details of which can be found in Fig. 17.1. A systematic approach is required when evaluating a patient with tachypnea.

TABLE 17.1 ▪ Common and life-threatening causes of tachypnea

Life-threatening causes of tachypnea	Common causes of tachypnea
• Upper airway obstruction	• Obstructive airway disease
• Foreign body	• Chronic obstructive pulmonary disease
• Angioedema	• Asthma
• Hemorrhage	• Heart failure
• Tension pneumothorax	• Ischemic heart disease
• Acute coronary syndrome	• Pneumonia
• Pulmonary embolism	• Psychogenic
• Neuromuscular weakness	• Pain
• Myasthenia Gravis	
• Guillain-Barre's syndrome	
• Botulism	
• Fat embolism	

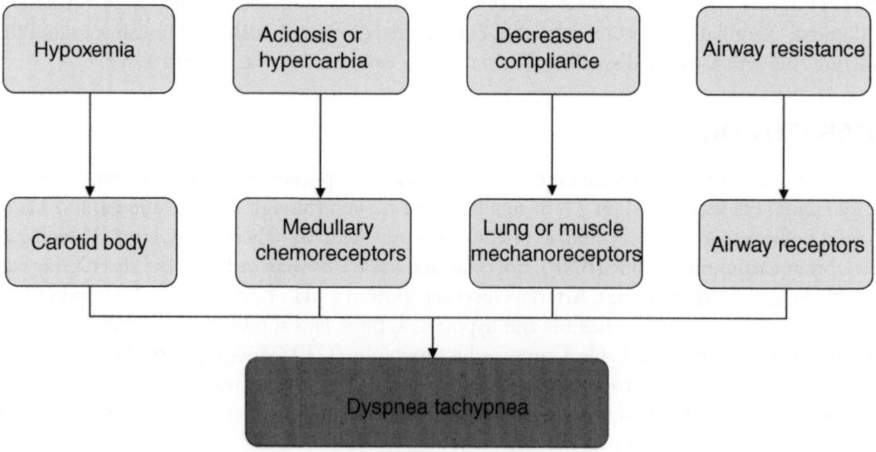

Fig. 17.1   Driving factors and receptors mediating tachypnea.

1. **Pulmonary causes:** The pulmonary system is the first organ system that should be evaluated in a tachypneic patient. Common causes include:
   - **Asthma/COPD:** These patients usually present with difficulty breathing. Classic exam findings include wheezing and prolonged expiratory phase on auscultation. Chest X-ray is usually without infiltrates with hyper-inflated lungs and a flattened diaphragm (Fig. 17.2).
   - **Pneumonia:** These patients usually present with fever/chills, difficulty breathing, cough with or without sputum production, and constitutional symptoms. The physical examination can show regional/diffuse rhonchi with bronchial breathing. Chest X-ray findings include interstitial infiltrates (Fig. 17.3).

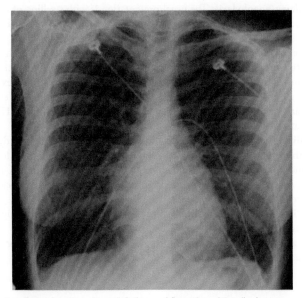

Fig. 17.2   Chest radiography shows hyperinflation and flattening of the diaphragm.

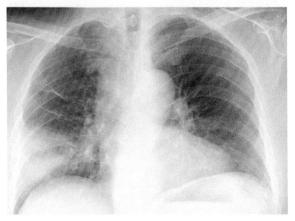

Fig. 17.3   Chest X-ray shows right lower lobe consolidation. Consolidation refers to the alveolar airspaces being filled with fluid, cells, tissue, or other material.

- **Pneumothorax:** Usual presentation is with difficulty breathing. Physical examination would show absent breath sounds on the affected side. Loss of pulmonary markings extending to the peripheral lung border would be seen on chest X-ray (Fig. 17.4). Lung ultrasound would show the loss of lung sliding.
- **Pulmonary embolism (PE):** These patients usually present with difficulty breathing. Chest pain is another typical finding. Isolated lower extremity swelling would point toward possible deep vein thrombosis. CT angiogram of the chest is the diagnostic test of choice.
- **Foreign body aspiration:** The usual presentation is with a choking sensation and difficulty breathing. The physical examination can show wheezing, which is the loudest in the throat. This cause of tachypnea is more common in children compared to adults.
- **Angioedema/anaphylaxis:** The usual presentation is with swelling of the lips, posterior pharynx, and larynx. The physical exam can show stridor and drooling. Low oxygen saturation is a late sign and signals impending airway compromise.
2. **Cardiovascular causes:** Common causes include:
   - **Congestive heart failure:** Common presenting symptoms include orthopnea, paroxysmal nocturnal dyspnea, and swelling of the lower extremities. Physical examination findings include basilar crackles, distended jugular vein, and pitting lower extremity edema. Pulmonary vascular congestion can be seen on a chest X-ray (Fig. 17.5). Pulmonary edema can also be seen.
   - **Pericardial effusion/tamponade:** The usual presentation is generally dyspnea on exertion, with hypotension and syncope in severe cases. EKG would show low voltage complexes and in moderate to large effusions, electrical alternans. Chest X-ray can show an enlarged cardiac silhouette in large pericardial effusions; however, it can be normal in smaller collections (Fig. 17.6).
   - **Cardiac ischemia:** Occasionally, dyspnea, also called the "angina equivalent," can be a presenting sign of cardiac ischemia. EKG is diagnostic.
   - **Cardiac arrhythmia:** Tachyarrhythmias such as atrial flutter, atrial fibrillation, tachyarrhythmias can lead to dyspnea. EKG can usually diagnose these.

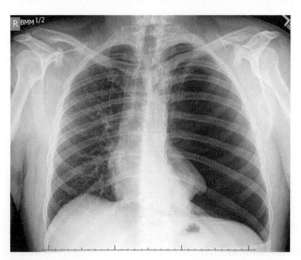

Fig. 17.4 Left-sided pneumothorax.

- **Valvular dysfunction:** Aortic stenosis, mitral regurgitation, or ruptured chordae tendinae can present with acute dyspnea. The physical examination will show a murmur; however, a lack of findings does not exclude the diagnosis.
3. **Hematological causes:** Hemoglobin is the primary transporter of oxygen in the blood, and any drop in hemoglobin can reduce the oxygen-carrying capacity of the blood, leading to

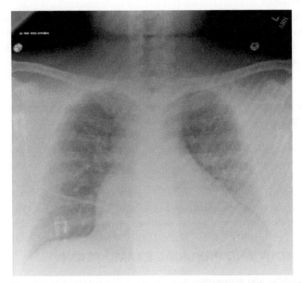

Fig. 17.5   Chest X-ray showing vascular congestion consistent with congestive heart failure.

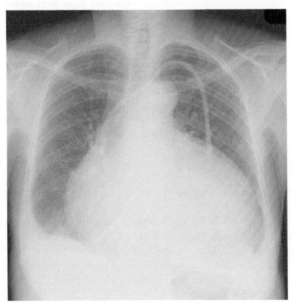

Fig. 17.6   Globular heart, which could be seen in pericardial effusion. This finding can also be seen in dilated cardiomyopathy.

compensatory tachypnea/dyspnea. Neurological and carotid chemoreceptors are stimulated to maintain oxygenation by increasing minute ventilation.

4. **Metabolic causes:**
   - **Metabolic acidosis:** Lungs are the initial compensatory organ for metabolic acidosis. The respiratory rate is increased to increase the elimination of acid in the form of CO_2.
   - **Poisoning:** Drugs such as salicylates, organophosphates, and petroleum are associated with tachypnea.
5. **Neuro-psychogenic causes**: Several neuromuscular diseases, including multiple sclerosis, Guillain-Barre's syndrome, and myasthenia gravis, can cause weakness of the respiratory muscles leading to respiratory distress. Anxiety and panic attacks can also lead to tachypnea.
6. **Miscellaneous causes:** Fever and pain can also lead to tachypnea.

Suggested Approach to Tachypnea of Unknown Cause in a Rapid Response Setting

For inpatient scenarios where tachypnea is being evaluated, we suggest the following for immediate risk assessment and management. This stepwise approach can be used to evaluate emergency room patients as well. The usual sequence of history taking, physical exam, investigations, and resuscitative interventions is often not followed during a rapid response; these measures often run parallel to each other in a code situation. The following components of the rapid response are discussed in the traditional sequence only to ease understanding.

FOCUSED HISTORY AND PHYSICAL EXAMINATION

- The acuity of signs and symptoms.
- A detailed description of tachypnea (timing, setting, alleviating/aggravating factors, positional variations, associated symptoms – pleuritic pain, fever or cough, prior similar symptoms).
- Prior cardiac history.
- Prior history of malignancy, PE, or deep vein thrombosis. A quick Wells score can be calculated for the likelihood of PE (refer to Chapter 19 for details).
- History of recent procedures (cardiac, thoracic, or esophageal procedures) – to evaluate for the possibility of a procedural complication, like pneumothorax.
- Physical exam should begin with an assessment of airway, breathing, and circulation. Assess for hypoxia (oxygen saturation <90%), breath sounds (absence of breath sounds might suggest pneumothorax), tachycardia, or a new cardiac murmur.

LABORATORY TESTS

- Complete blood count – to look for anemia or infection causing an increased respiratory rate.
- Basic metabolic panel/comprehensive metabolic panel, magnesium – looking for electrolyte abnormalities, specifically metabolic acidosis.
- Arterial blood gasses with lactate – to evaluate for acidosis.
- Troponin – looking for signs of necrosis of cardiac myocytes. Troponins can take up to 6 h from the onset of ischemia to become positive in a blood test.
- d-dimer – to rule out PE.
- Pro-BNP – to evaluate right ventricular dysfunction.

EKG

- EKG should be obtained based on the clinical suspicion of a cardiac cause of tachypnea and can evaluate for the following:
  - Acute coronary syndrome (ACS) – ST segment and T waves changes can be seen.
  - PE – Sinus tachycardia, S1Q3T3, RBBB can be seen.
  - Pericardial tamponade – Low voltage QRS complexes, electrical alternans can be seen.
  - Acute pericarditis – Widespread ST elevations, PR depressions can be seen.

IMAGING

- Chest X-ray should be done in most patients as it can be done at the bedside in a relatively small amount of time and can evaluate for a wide variety of differentials such as pneumonia, pneumothorax, pleural effusion, and heart failure.
- CT angiogram chest can be done per clinician judgment depending on clinical suspicion of PE.

INTERVENTIONS

We recommend that all patients be assessed for airway, breathing, circulation based on the advanced cardiac life support algorithm. The airway should be secured with advanced airway placement if indicated. A supraglottic airway can be used if endotracheal intubation is delayed. Hypoxia should be corrected with supplemental oxygen. Fever and pain should be addressed. Therapy should be directed toward addressing the underlying cause (please refer to the appropriate chapters for evaluating and managing individual causes). Morphine can be considered to improve air hunger in appropriate scenarios. Low doses of lorazepam can be considered per institutional guidelines in appropriate clinical scenarios, e.g., if the patient has a known history of anxiety, is hyperventilating, or showing other signs of anxiety. It is paramount to ensure the hemodynamic stability of the patient before attempting sedation of any kind.

Suggested Reading

Ahmed A, MD, Graber MA. Evaluation of the adult with dyspnea in the emergency department. UpToDate. com. https://www.uptodate.com/contents/evaluation-of-the-adult-with-dyspnea-in-the-emergency-department.
Sarkar M, Niranjan N, Banyal PK. Mechanisms of hypoxemia. *Lung India*. 2017;34(1):47–60. https://doi.org/10.4103/0970-2113.197116.

CHAPTER 18

Tachypnea in a Patient With Asthma

Rahul R. Bollam   Syed Arsalan Akhter Zaidi   Mohammad Adrish
Firas Abdulmajeed

Case Study

A rapid response code was activated for a patient who developed severe dyspnea at rest. On arrival of the condition team, it was found that the patient was a 30-year-old female with a history of asthma who was admitted two days ago for acute cholecystitis. She had undergone laparoscopic cholecystectomy a few hours prior and was successfully extubated without incident. She developed acute severe dyspnea 15 min before the condition was called.

VITAL SIGNS

Temperature: 99.8 °F, axillary
Blood Pressure: 130/90 mmHg
Heart Rate: 120 beats per min (bpm)
Respiratory Rate: 40 breaths per min
Oxygen Saturation: 85% on room air, 95% on 6 L/min O_2 via nasal cannula

FOCUSED PHYSICAL EXAMINATION

A quick exam showed a young female sitting up in bed in severe respiratory distress. She appeared visibly dyspneic, using accessory muscles of respiration. The patient was alert and oriented. However, she was unable to speak in complete sentences. On auscultation, significant wheezing was present in bilateral lung fields. No crackles were heard. Her cardiac exam showed tachycardia with normal heart sounds. The rest of her physical exam was unremarkable.

INTERVENTIONS

A cardiac monitor and defibrillator pads were attached. Due to the patient's new-onset hypoxia and significant work of breathing, emergent intubation was done at the bedside. Once the airway was secured, the patient was given a stat dose of 125 mg intravenous (IV) methylprednisolone and 2 g IV magnesium sulfate. She was also started on albuterol nebulization. A post-intubation chest X-ray (CXR) was obtained, which showed clear lungs, and no acute infiltrates (Fig. 18.1). Arterial blood gas was obtained and showed pH 7.23, pCO_2 35, pO_2 110, % sat 98% on 100% FiO_2. The patient was transferred to the intensive care unit (ICU) for further care.

FINAL DIAGNOSIS

Acute severe asthma exacerbation in the setting of recent intubation and surgical procedure.

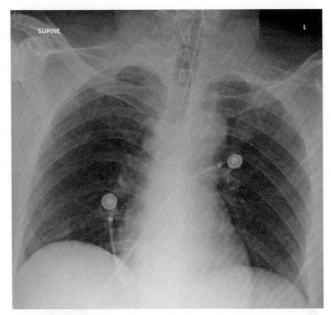

Fig. 18.1 Chest X-ray with clear lungs, no acute infiltrates – endotracheal tube in place.

Asthma Exacerbation

Asthma is a chronic disorder of the airways produced by recurring but reversible obstruction of airflow. The pathophysiology of this disorder is complex and involves various inflammatory mediators. The interactions between these mediators collectively result in bronchoconstriction, which is the primary underlying process of the disease. Allergen-mediated IgE-dependent degranulation of mast cells in airways leads to the release of histamine, tryptase, leukotrienes, and prostaglandins, which act directly on the bronchial smooth muscle to cause constriction. Other non-IgE-dependent mechanisms for the release of pro-inflammatory cytokines also exist, as seen in triggers like aspirin and non-steroidal anti-inflammatory drug-induced bronchoconstriction (see Table 18.1 for common triggers of acute asthma exacerbation). Some other important pathophysiological contributors include airway hyperresponsiveness, airway edema, mucous hypersecretion, hypertrophy and hyperplasia of bronchial smooth muscles, and eventual airway remodeling. Fig. 18.2 shows the vicious circle of interaction between mediators of asthma symptoms.

Exacerbation refers to an acute or sub-acute episode of increased asthma symptoms and poor pulmonary function. Symptoms include shortness of breath, tachycardia, cough, wheeze, and chest tightness. Signs such as a respiratory rate of >30 breaths per min, heart rate of >120 beats per min, use of accessory muscles of respiration, inability to speak in complete sentences, and impaired oxygenation are indicators of a severe exacerbation that requires prompt identification and intervention. Fig. 18.3 outlines the clinical signs to classify the severity of asthma exacerbation. About 50% of the patients can have a severe exacerbation even in the absence of these findings. An absence of wheezing or a "silent chest" is an ominous sign of status asthmaticus and impending respiratory failure.

The presence of signs and symptoms such as fever, chest pain, purulent sputum, or rash should alert the clinician of the presence of a co-morbid condition such as pneumonia, pneumothorax, or anaphylaxis (see Table 18.2 for common differentials of acute asthma exacerbation).

TABLE 18.1 ■ **Common triggers of asthma exacerbation**

Type	Examples
Allergic	• Inhaled – animal allergens, dust mites, cockroaches, mold, plant allergens • Food – usually as part of a more widespread allergic reaction • Occupational – toluene, enzymes, wood dust
Irritants	• Cigarette smoke, cannabis smoke • Air pollution and dust • Cleaning products
Miscellaneous	• Respiratory infections • Cold, dry air • Physical activity • Hormonal changes – pregnancy • Medications – beta-blockers, non-steroidal anti-inflammatory drugs, angiotensin-converting enzyme inhibitor • Anxiety, stress, gastroesophageal reflux disease • Medication non-compliance

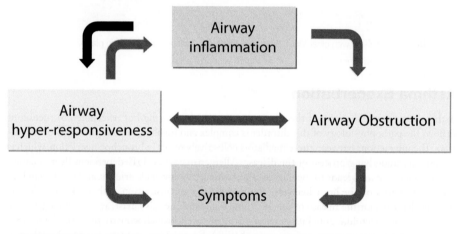

Fig. 18.2   Schematic diagram of the interaction between the mediators of asthma symptoms.

Suggested Approach to a Patient With Suspected Asthma Exacerbation

For inpatient scenarios where acute asthma exacerbation is suspected, we suggest the following approach to establish the diagnosis and initiate management. The final management decisions are ultimately up to the treating clinician's discretion based on their clinical judgment.

HISTORY AND PHYSICAL EXAMINATION

- The acuity of signs and symptoms.
- Signs and symptoms of comorbidities such as fever, purulent sputum, rash, angioedema.
- History of prior asthma attacks, including history of respiratory failure and intubation.
- History of allergies and medications used.

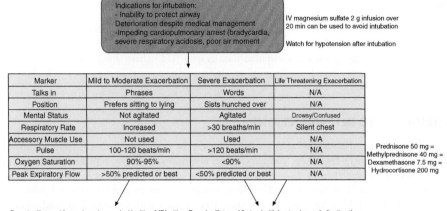

Fig. 18.3 Clinical signs to classify the severity of an acute asthma attack.

TABLE 18.2 ■ **Differentials of acute asthma exacerbation**

Disease	Features
COPD	Usually seen in the older age group with a history of smoking Difficult to differentiate from asthma clinically (overlap syndromes also present)
Allergic reaction/ anaphylaxis	History of allergy Presence of wheezing, facial swelling, rash, urticaria, hypotension Abrupt onset in case of anaphylaxis
Foreign body aspiration	History of aspiration Wheezing present in the upper airway rather than in the lungs
Congestive heart failure	History of heart disease Clinical and radiographic features of volume overload present
Vocal cord dysfunction	Mimics chronic asthma, very rare to see an "exacerbation" Does not respond to standard therapy

- Physical exam should start with an assessment of airway, breathing, and circulation.
  - Assess mental status and degree of hypoxia.
  - Assess for signs and symptoms of severe exacerbation – tachypnea, tachycardia, use of accessory muscles, ability to complete sentences.
  - Assess for presence of wheezing – silent chest is a sign of impending respiratory failure.

LABORATORY TESTING

- Lab work is not required to make the diagnosis of asthma exacerbation.
- Arterial blood gas can be obtained to assess for the degree of hypoxia, hypercarbia, and acidosis.

IMAGING

- A CXR is not required for the diagnosis of asthma exacerbation. However, it can be obtained to rule out comorbidities such as pneumothorax, pulmonary edema, and pneumonia.
- Advanced imaging such as computed tomography (CT) chest should be considered only if there is high clinical suspicion of an alternate diagnosis that requires a CT chest for identification.

THERAPEUTIC INTERVENTIONS

Severe asthma exacerbations and status asthmaticus are medical emergencies. All patients should be assessed for airway, breathing, and circulation. Hypoxia should be identified promptly and corrected with oxygen therapy. Non-invasive ventilation can be considered in patients who are not in emergent need of intubation. However, clinician judgment and institutional guidelines should be followed. If needed, the airway should be secured with endotracheal intubation. A large-sized endotracheal tube should be used to allow adequate ventilation. A growing body of evidence suggests that the use of propofol in intubated patients with status asthmaticus might be associated with bronchodilation. However, no large, randomized control trials exist to support this. Inhaled beta-2 agonists such as albuterol and muscarinic antagonists such as ipratropium bromide are the standard of care and should be administered early. IV steroid therapy should be initiated, although the effects would not be seen up until 6 hours from administration. The choice and dosing of steroids depends on institutional guidelines. IV magnesium sulfate can be administered in refractory cases. If comorbidities such as pulmonary edema, pleural effusion, pneumonia, or anaphylaxis are identified, directed management for these pathologies should also be initiated.

STEPWISE APPROACH TO THE MANAGEMENT OF A PATIENT WITH SUSPECTED ASTHMA EXACERBATION

Step 1: Assess airway, breathing, and circulation, with particular attention to signs of impending respiratory failure.

Step 2: Correct hypoxia with supplemental oxygen +/− non-invasive ventilation. Secure airway with endotracheal intubation if indicated.

Step 3: Obtain CXR to rule out co-morbid conditions such as pneumonia.

Step 4: Institute inhaled bronchodilators and IV steroids. IV magnesium can be used in refractory cases.

CODING A PATIENT WITH ASTHMA EXACERBATION AND RESPIRATORY ARREST

On presentation, these patients will require bag-mask ventilation. Aggressive bag-mask ventilation should be avoided since it can rapidly precipitate gas trapping which could cause simple or tension pneumothorax and hemodynamic compromise. Patients should be intubated emergently with a large endotracheal tube. Once the airway is secured, nebulized bronchodilators and IV steroids should be initiated. Further management should be done in an ICU.

Suggested Reading

Al-Shamrani A, Al-Harbi AS, Bagais K, Alenazi A, Alqwaiee M. Management of asthma exacerbation in the emergency departments. *Int J Pediatr Adolesc Med.* 2019;6(2):61–67. https://doi.org/10.1016/j.ijpam.2019.02.001.

Christopher H, Fanta M. Acute exacerbations of asthma in adults: emergency department and inpatient management. UpToDate.com. https://www.uptodate.com/contents/acute-exacerbations-of-asthma-in-adults-emergency-department-and-inpatient-management

Fergeson JE, Patel SS, Lockey RF. Acute asthma, prognosis, and treatment. *J Allergy Clin Immunol.* 2017;139(2):438–447. https://doi.org/10.1016/j.jaci.2016.06.054.

Israel E, Reddel HK. Severe and difficult-to-treat asthma in adults. *N Engl J Med.* 2017;377(10):965–976. https://doi.org/10.1056/nejmra1608969.

CHAPTER 19

Tachypnea in a Patient After Hip Repair Surgery

Syed Arsalan Akhter Zaidi ▥ Firas Abdulmajeed ▥ Mohammad Adrish

Case Study

Rapid response event was activated by bedside nurse for a patient with tachypnea and tachycardia (heart rate of 180 beats per min). On arrival of the rapid response team, the patient was quickly assessed along with a brief history from the bedside nurse. The patient was a 69-year-old male with no known comorbidities who was admitted to the hospital for the past five days after suffering a ground-level fall one week ago and a left femoral neck fracture. He underwent hip repair surgery four days ago and was doing fine with rehabilitation until the morning of this event when the nurse saw his elevated heart rate on routine vital monitoring.

VITAL SIGNS

Temperature: 98.4 °F, axillary
Blood Pressure: 110/78 mm of Hg
Heart Rate: 160 beats per min, sinus tachycardia on telemetry monitor (Fig. 19.1)
Respiratory Rate: 44 breaths per min
Oxygen Saturation: 82% on room air

FOCUSED PHYSICAL EXAMINATION

A quick exam showed a middle-aged man with moderate respiratory distress, who was tachypneic and sitting up in bed. His chest auscultation was not significant for wheezing or crackles, and his breath sounds were equal bilaterally. His heart sounds were difficult to comprehend because of severe tachycardia. He denied any chest pain or pain anywhere else in the body.

INTERVENTIONS

The patient was supplied with supplementary oxygen through a nasal cannula. A stat troponin, lactate level, complete blood count (CBC), arterial blood gas, and portable chest X-ray were ordered. Cardiac monitor pads were attached to the patient's chest. A 12-lead electrocardiogram (EKG) showed sinus tachycardia. Chest X-ray did not show any acute cardiopulmonary disease. Arterial blood gas showed a pH of 7.52, paO_2 of 50, pCO_2 of 30, and SPO_2 of 84%. At this time it was determined that the most likely (EKG) differential diagnosis for this event was an acute pulmonary embolism (PE). The patient was prophylactically started on a therapeutic heparin drip and sent down to the radiology department for computed tomography (CT) of the chest for the evaluation of PE. CT scan showed a large saddle embolus with signs of right ventricular (RV) strain. The patient was transferred to the intensive care unit (ICU) directly from the radiology department to monitor his hemodynamic status closely.

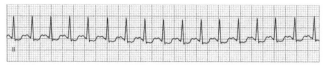

Fig. 19.1 Cardiac rhythm strip showing sinus tachycardia at a rate of ~180 beats per min, with ST-segment depression.

FINAL DIAGNOSIS

Acute submassive PE.

Alternative Diagnosis: Pulmonary fat embolism (can be primary diagnosis in a similar patient who did not get the fracture repaired); it can be differentiated from a PE on CT.

Pulmonary Embolism

PE is one of those clandestine conditions that occur in patients with decreased mobility and those with other risk factors that might provoke thrombosis. Our patient is one such prime example where he was immobile after suffering a fall and having a hip fracture. Although his fracture was repaired, his pain and post-operative status impaired his mobility level. Historical data suggests that PE and deep vein thrombosis (DVT) are most common in patients five to seven days after hip repair surgery, and to prevent this, almost all these patients are given high-dose prophylactic anticoagulation from post-operative day one. Enoxaparin is the preferred drug for this indication and although it reduces the incidence of PE, some patients still develop thrombosis post-operatively.

DEFINITION

Pulmonary embolism is defined as a sudden blockage in one of the pulmonary arteries. It is usually the result of DVT in one of the veins in extremities which gets dislodged and travels up toward the heart, crosses the right heart, and gets stuck in the pulmonary vasculature.

PE can be classified as massive, submassive, and low-risk PE (Table 19.1). Identifying different clinical signs and symptoms associated with PE is crucial for the prompt start of appropriate management and helping rule out other causes of hypoxia (Table 19.2).

Suggested Approach to a Patient With Suspected PE in a Rapid Response Event

For inpatient scenarios where acute PE is being considered as one of the top differentials, we suggest the following strategy for immediate risk assessment and management. See Fig. 19.2 for a basic flow-chart of the risk stratification and management of PE. This process might differ between institutions, and clinicians should always follow their institutional protocols and guidelines.

FOCUSED HISTORY AND PHYSICAL EXAMINATION

- The acuity of signs and symptoms?
- Medical vs. surgical admission, history of reduced mobility?
- On anticoagulation and antiplatelet therapy?

TABLE 19.1 ■ **Classification of pulmonary embolism per American Heart Association**

Massive PE	Submassive PE	Low Risk PE
Acute PE with sustained hypotension (SBP <90 mmHg) for more than 15 min or requiring inotropic support	Acute PE with SBP >90 mmHg and either: a) RV dysfunction (computed tomography, BNP/pro-BNP, electrocardiogram changes) or b) myocardial necrosis (elevated troponins)	Acute PE with an absence of systolic hypotension, right ventricular dysfunction, and myocardial necrosis
High mortality – 25%-65%	Low mortality – 3%	Lowest mortality –<1%
Also known as – PE with hypotension – High risk PE	Also known as – PE without hypotension – Intermediate risk PE	Known as low risk PE for all classifications
Therapy: systemic anticoagulation +/– thrombolysis	Therapy: systemic anticoagulation	Therapy: systemic anticoagulation. Some clinicians will decide not to anticoagulate patients with sub-segmental PE, as per the latest evidence
Setting: intensive care unit	Setting: better to monitor in an intensive care unit	Setting: can be monitored on a medical ward

Abbreviations: PE – pulmonary embolism, BNP – brain natriuretic peptide, SBP – systolic blood pressure

TABLE 19.2 ■ **Associated signs/symptoms/clinical tests for PE**

Sign/Symptom/Test	Value
Cool extremities and mottling	Signs of hypoperfusion – bad prognostic factor
Tachycardia	Common feature in PE, sinus tachycardia alone without hypotension, is not indicative of bad prognosis
Bradycardia	Bad prognosis: often indicates impending Brady-arrest
Hypotension	Shock index: heart rate/systolic blood pressure > one = low hemodynamic reserve = worse prognosis
Hypertension	Generally good prognosis, unless with other signs of submassive PE
Tachypnea	Higher the respiratory rate > worse the prognosis
Troponin	Indicates cardiac necrosis > bad prognosis
Lactate	Hemodynamic instability > bad prognosis
New S1Q3T3 on electrocardiogram	Right ventricular dysfunction – indicates possible PE
Point-of-care ultrasound visualized clot in transit	Mortality increased by five times
Large clot burden of deep vein thrombosis in extremity	Independent risk factor for mortality

Abbreviations: PE – pulmonary embolism

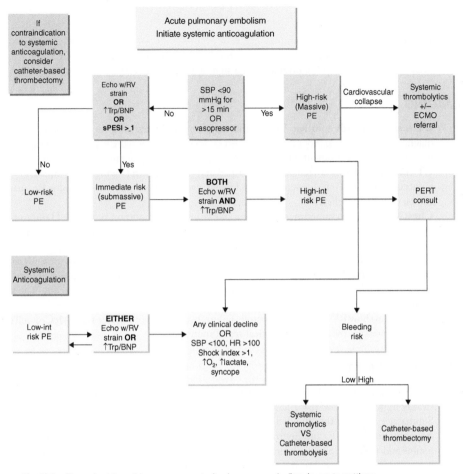

Fig. 19.2   Flow-chart to guide management of pulmonary embolism in acute settings.

- Prior history of PE or DVT.
- Family history of prothrombotic disorders.
- Vital signs: especially focus on blood pressure for risk stratification, and heart rate, respiratory rate, and pulse oximetry for supporting vitals.
- Duration of symptoms? Rapid onset and worsening symptoms are signs of evolving thrombus.
- Quick Wells' score for the likelihood of PE as the diagnosis.

LABORATORY TESTS

- Focus for risk stratification is on troponin (for signs of cardiac necrosis) and brain natriuretic peptide (BNP) (for RV dysfunction).
- Lactate – as an early sign of occult shock.
- CBC, basic metabolic panel, and coagulation panel should be drawn simultaneously.

EKG

- Sinus tachycardia – most common.
- S1Q3T3 sign – a sign of cardiac ischemia and RV dysfunction – predictor of PE.
- Generalized diffuse T wave inversions as a sign of cardiac ischemia.

IMAGING

- **CT scan chest with contrast**: This is the most important test and the *gold standard* for diagnosis of PE. CT angiogram of the chest is done with a special PE protocol to capture images right at the moment when contrast is passing through the pulmonary arteries.
- CT chest may also show signs of RV overload and dilation, with bowing of RV into LV.
- Contrast reflux into inferior vena cava and hepatic veins is also one of the signs for PE that can be seen on CT chest.
- **Chest X-ray** can also sometimes show signs of PE; one such important sign is the Hampton's hump. This refers to a pleural-based dome-shaped opacification in the lungs. This is most likely to be seen when a pulmonary infarct is present.
- If RV dysfunction is not apparent on CT, it can be seen by bedside **point-of-care ultrasound (POCUS)**. However, this may be challenging while in a rapid response event scenario, as it needs to be done by an experienced and credentialed provider only (cardiologist or intensivist).
- POCUS can show RV dilation, RV systolic failure, hypokinesis of RV free wall (McConnell's sign), RV pressure overload (paradoxical septal motion).

RISK STRATIFICATION SCORES

- PE severity score (PESI) – assesses demographics, comorbidities, lab tests, and vitals to stratify high risk vs. low-risk PE.
- Submassive PE is further divided into intermediate-low risk (RV abnormality or elevated troponins and/or BNP) and intermediate-high risk PE (RV abnormality plus elevated troponins and/or BNP). Some centers routinely assess patients with intermediate-high risk PE for systemic or catheter-directed thrombolytic therapy.

THERAPEUTIC INTERVENTIONS

Interventions should start with an assessment of airway, breathing, and circulation. Secure airway as appropriate. If, through relevant history, physical examination, EKG, and POCUS (if available through an experienced operator), PE is the top differential, we suggest starting systemic anticoagulation in patients who are hemodynamically stable while awaiting confirmation of PE via CT scan. For a hemodynamically unstable patient with a high suspicion of massive PE for which the patient will need thrombolysis or catheter-guided thrombectomy, the patient should be rushed to CT and a stat consult should be called to the ICU and PE response team (PERT). An increasing number of institutions are now encouraging the formation of a PERT team which deals with high-risk PEs. This team generally comprises of interventional radiology specialists, interventional cardiologists, cardiothoracic surgeons, and PE specialists. The main aim of this team is to assess a high-risk PE for indications of thrombectomy.

SUMMARY OF APPROACH TO A PATIENT WITH SUSPECTED PE IN A RAPID RESPONSE EVENT

Step 1: Assess airway, breathing, and circulation. Secure the airway as appropriate.

Step 2: Patient with signs and symptoms of PE (hypoxia, tachycardia, EKG changes, respiratory distress)?

Step 3: Assess hemodynamic status.

Step 4: Look for risk factors of PE and exclude other common causes of similar complaints, like cardiac ischemia (mainly rule out ST-elevation myocardial infarction on EKG, cardiac causes will have many more distinctive symptoms).

Step 5: Draw stat lactate, troponin, and pro-BNP.

Step 6: If hemodynamically stable –> start systemic anticoagulation and send for stat CT chest PE protocol.

Step 7: If hemodynamically unstable (hypotensive) –> start inotropic support to maintain blood pressure, send for stat CT chest w/contrast –> if positive send stat consults to ICU and PERT for thrombolysis. If the patient is very hypoxic, intubate and ventilate prior to performing other interventions.

WORST CASE SCENARIO

If, while evaluating this patient, they go bradycardic and then have a pulseless electrical activity arrest, it would be logical to give systemic thrombolysis (of course, while doing cardiopulmonary resuscitation per the advanced cardiac life support protocol!)

Suggested Reading

Bernal AG, Fanola C, Bartos JA. Management of PE. American College of Cardiology. https://www.acc.org/latest-in-cardiology/articles/2020/01/27/07/42/management-of-pe.

Duffett L, Castellucci LA, Forgie MA. Pulmonary embolism: update on management and controversies. *BMJ.* 2020;370. https://doi.org/10.1136/bmj.m2177.

Tapson VF, Weinberg AS. Treatment, prognosis, and follow-up of acute pulmonary embolism in adults. UpToDate.com. https://www.uptodate.com/contents/treatment-prognosis-and-follow-up-of-acute-pulmonary-embolism-in-adults.

CHAPTER 20

Hypoxia in a Patient After Repair of Femoral Fracture

Syed Arsalan Akhter Zaidi ■ Kainat Saleem

Case Study

A rapid response event was initiated for a patient in the post-op recovery unit by the charge nurse for acute onset of hypoxia and altered mentation. On arrival of the rapid response team, it was reported that the patient was a 62-year-old male who was 4 h post-op after intra-medullary nailing procedure of his left femoral shaft fracture. His comorbidities included chronic hypertension and type 2 diabetes. On a quick review of the chart, it was noted that the patient experienced a brief period of hypo-tension during surgery which responded appropriately to an intravenous fluid bolus. The nurse reported that the patient was doing fine in the recovery area and conversing with nursing staff when suddenly he became confused, and his oxygen saturation dropped to 80% on room air. He was then placed on supplemental oxygen via nasal cannula, and a rapid response code was activated.

VITAL SIGNS

Temperature: 98.4 °F, axillary
Blood Pressure: 100/58 mmHg
Heart Rate: 122 beats per min (bpm), sinus tachycardia on tele-monitor (Fig. 20.1)
Respiratory Rate: 36 breaths per min
Oxygen Saturation: 80% on room air, 90% on 6 L nasal cannula

FOCUSED PHYSICAL EXAMINATION

A quick exam showed a middle-aged man with moderate respiratory distress, who was tachypneic and lying on his back in bed. He was alert but not oriented to time and place. His chest auscultation was not significant for wheezing or crackles, and breath sounds were equal bilaterally. A cardiac exam revealed regular rhythm with tachycardia. He denied any chest pain or pain anywhere else in the body. His left leg was wrapped in a bandage marking the site of the recent procedure. There was evidence of a new petechial rash on his anterior chest going up to his neck and axillary areas bilaterally.

INTERVENTIONS

A cardiac monitor and pads were attached to the patient. Supplemental oxygen was continued, and an intravenous bolus of 1 L Plasma-Lyte was started. A stat complete blood count (CBC), basic metabolic panel (BMP), troponin, lactate level, arterial blood gas, and portable chest X-ray were ordered. A 12-lead electrocardiogram showed sinus tachycardia. His chest X-ray showed multiple bilateral patchy opacities, which were not present on admission imaging (Fig. 20.2).

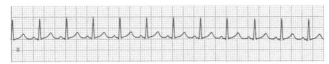

Fig. 20.1 Telemetry strip showing sinus tachycardia at almost 122 beats per min.

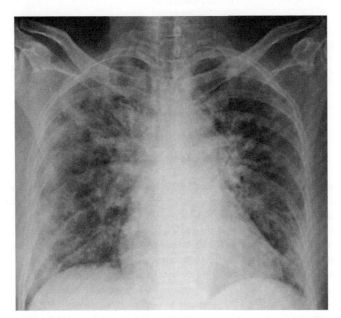

Fig. 20.2 Chest X-ray showing diffuse bilateral opacities.

Arterial blood gas (ABG) showed a pH of 7.52, paO_2 of 65, pCO_2 of 30, and SPO_2 of 92% on 8 L oxygen via nasal cannula. His CBC was remarkable for a hemoglobin level of 10.2 g/dL (dropped from 13 g/dL on admission) and a platelet level of 220,000/uL (dropped from 360,000/uL on admission). His white blood cell count, BMP, and troponin levels were unremarkable. The lactate level was slightly elevated at 2.2 mmol/L. At this time, it was determined that the most likely differential diagnosis for this event was fat embolism syndrome (FES), with acute pulmonary embolism (PE) as a differential diagnosis. The patient was sent for a stat computed tomography (CT) angiography of the chest with contrast, which was negative for acute PE, but revealed bilateral areas of consolidation and diffuse ground-glass opacities. The patient's hypoxia and confusion deteriorated abruptly in the scanner, and he was intubated for airway protection and respiratory support. A stat CT head at the same time revealed diffuse white matter petechial hemorrhages. The patient was transferred to the intensive care unit (ICU) for further monitoring and management of FES.

FINAL DIAGNOSIS

Fat embolism syndrome.

Fat Embolism Syndrome

Fat embolism is classically defined as the presence of fat globules in pulmonary microcirculation. Pulmonary fat embolism can be completely asymptomatic or present with pulmonary

TABLE 20.1 ▪ **Various traumatic and non-traumatic conditions associated with fat embolism syndrome**

Non-trauma related	Trauma related
Pancreatitis	Fractures:
Lipid infusion (e.g., total par-	• Long bone fractures
enteral nutrition)	• Pelvic fractures
Osteomyelitis	• Other fractures of marrow containing bones
Steroid therapy	Therapeutic procedures such as:
Bone tumor lysis	
Sickle cell hemoglobinopathies	• Bone marrow transplant/harvesting
leading to bone infarct	• Soft tissue injuries obtained during cardiopulmonary resuscitation/
Alcoholic liver disease	chest compressions
Diabetes mellitus	• Orthopedic procedures like hip arthroplasty
Intra-osseous infusions	• Liposuction
Mineral oil enemas	• Augmentation mammoplasty
Altitude illness	• Lymphangiography
Viral hepatitis	Burn injuries
	Liquefying hematoma

complications ranging from mild hypoxia to severe life-threatening hypoxic respiratory failure. FES is an ill-defined entity that comprises various systemic complications arising from the introduction of fat emboli in the circulation.

FES is most commonly seen after orthopedic trauma (especially after closed fractures of long bones of the lower extremities and pelvic fractures). Some other causes of FES are presented in Table 20.1. There are no universal diagnostic criteria for FES, but various authors have suggested different criteria for diagnosing FES. The most notable of these criteria were by Gurd et al., Lindeque et al., and Schonfeld et al.; these criteria are described in Table 20.2.

After the initial insult (Table 20.1), there is usually an asymptomatic interval of about 12 to 72 h, but symptoms can present earlier in some cases. The classical presenting features of FES are the triad of respiratory failure, neurological manifestations, and petechial rash. Various signs and symptoms of complications from FES are listed in Table 20.3. The mainstay of therapy for FES is supportive measures.

In most cases, the systemic complications of FES resolve within 7 to 14 days, with dermatologic findings resolving earliest, followed by pulmonary and neurological recovery (although neurological status might not return to baseline). Excellent supportive care and intensive monitoring have been shown to reduce the mortality associated with FES to under 10%.

Suggested Approach to a Patient With FES

For inpatient scenarios where FES is considered one of the top differentials, we suggest the following steps for immediate risk assessment and management. This process might vary between institutions, and clinicians should always follow their institutional protocols and guidelines. As mentioned before, the usual sequence of history taking, physical exam, investigations, and resuscitative interventions is often not followed during a rapid response; these measures often run parallel to each other in a code situation. The following components of the rapid response are discussed in the traditional sequence only to ease understanding.

FOCUSED HISTORY AND PHYSICAL EXAMINATION

- The severity and duration of signs and symptoms?
- Medical vs. surgical admission, history of reduced mobility? History of recent procedure or fracture?

TABLE 20.2 ■ **Different diagnostic criteria used for FES**

Gurd's Criteria[1]	Schonfeld's Criteria[2]		Lindeque's Criteria[3]
Major criteria • Petechial rash • Respiratory symptoms with a radiographic change • Central nervous system signs unrelated to trauma or other conditions Minor criteria • Tachycardia (heart rate 120 bpm) • Pyrexia (temperature >39 °C) • Retinal change (fat or petechiae) • Acute thrombocytopenia • Acute decrease in hemoglobin • High erythrocyte sedimentation rate • Fat globules in sputum	**Criteria**	**Points**	• Sustained $PaO_2 \leq 60$ mmHg • Sustained $PaCO_2$ of more than 55 mmHg or pH ≤ 7.3 • Sustained respiratory rate >35/min despite sedation • Increase work of breathing, dyspnea, accessory muscle use, tachycardia, and anxiety
	Petechiae	5	
	Chest X-ray change (diffuse alveolar change)	4	
	Hypoxemia ($PaO_2 <69$ mmHg)	3	
	Fever (temperature >100.4 °F)	1	
	Tachycardia (heart rate >120 bpm)	1	
	Tachypnea (>30 bpm)	1	
	Confusion	1	
Two major criteria or one major criterion plus two minor criteria are required for the diagnosis of FES	A total score of more than five is required for the diagnosis of FES		A patient with any one of these respiratory criteria, in the setting of long bone fracture, was judged to have FES

[1]Gurd AR, Wilson RI. The fat embolism syndrome. *J Bone Joint Surg Br*. 1974 Aug;56B(3):408–416. PMID: 4547466.
[2]Schonfeld SA, Ploysongsang Y, DiLisio R, et al. Fat embolism prophylaxis with corticosteroids. A prospective study in high-risk patients. *Ann Intern Med*. 1983 Oct;99(4):438–443. https://doi.org/10.7326/0003-4819-99-4-438. PMID: 6354030.
[3]Lindeque BG, Schoeman HS, Dommisse GF, Boeyens MC, Vlok AL. Fat embolism and the fat embolism syndrome. A double-blind therapeutic study. *J Bone Joint Surg Br*. 1987 Jan;69(1):128–131. https://doi.org/10.1302/0301-620X.69B1.3818718. PMID: 3818718.

FES, Fat embolism syndrome

TABLE 20.3 ■ **Systemic manifestations of FES, along with imaging and therapeutic interventions**

System involved	Respiratory	Neurologic	Dermatologic
Clinical manifestations	• Mild dyspnea • Tachypnea • Hypoxemia • Acute respiratory distress syndrome	• Headache • Acute confusion • Seizures • Coma	• Petechial rash that is more common in non-dependent areas, such as chest, axilla, neck, and scalp • Sub-conjunctival hemorrhages
Imaging Studies	• Chest X-ray • Chest CT angiogram	• CT of the head without contrast • Magnetic resonance imaging of the head	No specific imaging study
Therapeutic measures	Supplemental oxygen via non-invasive or invasive ventilation based on the appropriate clinical scenario	Supportive measures	Supportive measures

• Other systemic findings may include fever, thrombocytopenia, jaundice, lipuria, hematuria, and retinopathy.
• Severe cases of FES can be complicated by disseminated intravascular coagulation, right heart failure, circulatory shock, and even death.

FES, Fat embolism syndrome; *CT*, computed tomography

- Look for the presence of other associated conditions as mentioned in Table 20.1.
- Prior history of PE or deep vein thrombosis.
- Vital signs: especially focus on blood pressure for risk stratification, and heart rate, respiratory rate, and pulse oximetry for supporting vitals.
- Physical examination should begin with an evaluation of the airway, breathing, and circulation.
- Respiratory examination to look for clinical findings which might point to other differentials (e.g., aspiration pneumonia after surgery).
- Neurological examination to assess for the extent of neurological manifestations.
- Dermatologic examination to look for petechial rash (most common in non-dependent parts of the body).
- Eye examination to look for sub-conjunctival hemorrhages.

LABORATORY TESTS

- CBC can reveal acute anemia and thrombocytopenia.
- Coagulation profile to evaluate for baseline levels in case anticoagulation is needed, and to rule out disseminated intravascular coagulation (DIC), which can be a component of this syndrome.
- Fibrinogen level to rule out DIC.

EKG

- EKG is not needed for the diagnosis of FES but can be used to rule out cardiac ischemia.
- Sinus tachycardia can be seen.

IMAGING STUDIES

- Chest X-ray can be completely normal or show diffuse bilateral patchy infiltrates, consistent with acute respiratory distress syndrome (ARDS).
- CT angiogram chest to rule out PE and to better visualize any infiltrates seen on chest X-ray and differentiate them from pulmonary edema and pulmonary hemorrhage.
- CT scan of the head without contrast can sometimes reveal diffuse white matter petechial hemorrhages; this should be done in patients with worsening confusion.
- Magnetic resonance imaging of the brain can show hyperintense lesions in both white and gray matter that are diffuse but non-confluent. This pattern is also called the "star-field" pattern.

THERAPEUTIC INTERVENTIONS

Although rare, a fat embolism can lead to life-threatening complications. The management begins with the assessment of the airway, breathing, and circulation. The capability of the patient to maintain airway should be assessed. Patients with FES and neurological manifestations might often be at risk for aspiration; thus, if suspicion is present for inability to protect the airway, the patients should be intubated and transferred to ICU for further care. Respiratory manifestations can range from mild hypoxia to severe ARDS and should be managed with supplemental oxygen via non-invasive or invasive ventilation as appropriate. In cases of ARDS, a lung-protective ventilation strategy should be followed. Patients who are hemodynamically stable and do not require ICU care should still be monitored closely as they can deteriorate rapidly. Close monitoring of hemodynamic status and maintenance of blood volume is of paramount importance since a state of shock can exacerbate the lung injury caused by FES. The mainstay of therapy for FES is symptomatic and supportive. With excellent supportive care, the mortality rate can be reduced to below 10%.

STEPWISE APPROACH TO A PATIENT WITH FES

Step 1: Evaluation should begin with an assessment of the airway, breathing, and circulation; advanced airway should be placed in patients who cannot protect the airway or are severely hypoxic on non-invasive supplemental oxygen support.

Step 2: Appropriate history of inciting factors (Table 20.1) should be taken. A full physical examination should include a detailed respiratory, neurological and dermatological exam to look for signs and symptoms that point to FES.

Step 3: Lab work including CBC, BMP, coagulation panel, lactate level, and ABG should be obtained to assess for anemia, thrombocytopenia, DIC, acidosis, hypoxia, CO_2 retention, and electrolyte derangements.

Step 4: Chest X-ray should be obtained to evaluate for concomitant illnesses such as pneumonia and pulmonary edema and assess for typical features of FES on chest X-ray (bilateral diffuse opacities). However, a normal chest X-ray does not rule out the diagnosis. CT of the chest to rule out PE and CT of the head to evaluate for an acute bleed should be done in appropriate cases.

Step 5: Patients on non-invasive ventilation should be monitored closely for the first few hours. Endotracheal intubation should be pursued if the patient does not show signs of improvement or clinically deteriorates.

Step 6: Neurological monitoring should include frequent re-orientation and monitoring of intracranial pressure (this is not a part of rapid response management but can be done in ICU).

Step 7: In intubated patients, adequate anesthesia should be provided to limit sympathetic response to injury (this is part of ICU management).

Suggested Reading

Gerald L, Weinhouse M. Fat embolism syndrome. UpToDate.com. https://www.uptodate.com/contents/fat-embolism-syndrome.

Kosova E, Bergmark B, Piazza G. Fat embolism syndrome. *Circulation*. 2015;131(3):317–320. https://doi.org/10.1161/CIRCULATIONAHA.114.010835.

Rothberg DL, Makarewich CA. Fat embolism and fat embolism syndrome. *J Am Acad Orthop Surg*. 2019;27(8):e346–e355. https://doi.org/10.5435/JAAOS-D-17-00571.

Shaikh N. Emergency management of fat embolism syndrome. *J Emerg Trauma Shock*. 2009;2(1):29–33. https://doi.org/10.4103/0974-2700.44680.

CHAPTER 21

Hypoxia in a Patient With No Cardiac or Pulmonary History

Rahul R. Bollam ▦ Kainat Saleem ▦ Syed Arsalan Akhter Zaidi

Case Study

A rapid response event was activated by the bedside nurse for a patient who developed respiratory distress and required increasing oxygen supplementation. On arrival of the condition team, the patient was visibly dyspneic and using accessory muscles of respiration. Per the bedside nurse, the patient was a 40-year-old male with a history of hypertension and diabetes mellitus who was admitted to the hospital for treatment of community-acquired pneumonia. The patient was admitted with oxygen supplementation of 4 L via nasal cannula and treated with ceftriaxone and azithromycin.

VITAL SIGNS

Temperature: 98.3 °F, axillary
Blood Pressure: 130/90 mmHg
Pulse: 120 beats per min – sinus tachycardia on telemetry
Respiratory Rate: 32 breaths per min
Pulse Oximetry: 85% on 4 L, 95% on 15 L non-rebreather

FOCUSED PHYSICAL EXAMINATION

A quick exam showed a middle-aged male who appeared visibly dyspneic, using accessory muscles of respiration. The patient was unable to speak in complete sentences. On auscultation, significant crackles and rhonchi were present in bilateral lung fields. His cardiac exam revealed regular rhythm and tachycardia. No murmurs or added heart sounds were identified. The remaining physical examination was unremarkable.

INTERVENTIONS

A cardiac monitor and pads were attached to the patient. Due to hypoxemia and increased work of breathing, the patient was started on a high flow nasal cannula, which improved his work of breathing. Stat chest X-ray and arterial blood gas (ABG) were obtained. ABG showed a pH of 7.40, pCO_2 of 40, pO_2 of 70, on a 15 L non-rebreather mask, which was significant for hypoxemia. Chest X-ray revealed multi-focal pneumonia, worse than that was seen on admission imaging (Fig. 21.1). The case was discussed with the intensive care specialist, and the patient was transferred to the intensive care unit for closer monitoring of respiratory status with a low threshold for intubation.

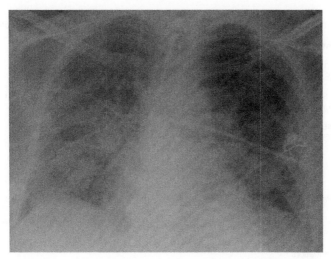

Fig. 21.1   Chest X-ray in an anteroposterior view showing bilateral infiltrates consistent with multi-focal pneumonia.

FINAL DIAGNOSIS

Acute hypoxic respiratory failure from community-acquired pneumonia.

Hypoxia/Hypoxemia

Hypoxia and hypoxemia are two interchangeably used terms in the clinical setting. Hypoxemia is defined as a low partial pressure of oxygen in arterial blood, while hypoxia is defined as insufficient global or local tissue oxygen content. See Table 21.1 for various parameters for assessing the degree of oxygenation of the blood. There is a wide range of causes of hypoxia in an acute setting, which should be narrowed down with a focused history, physical examination, and appropriate workup.

Various mechanisms underlie the development of hypoxia (Fig. 21.2):

1. **Hypoventilation** is a state in which a reduced amount of air enters the alveoli, leading to a decreasing amount of oxygen and increasing amount of carbon dioxide in alveoli as the gas exchange continues between alveoli and blood.
   - Hypoxemia because of pure hypoventilation can be corrected by supplemental oxygen.
   - Causes: central nervous system (CNS) depression (because of drug overdoses, CNS lesions that affect the respiratory center), obesity hypoventilation syndrome (i.e., Pickwickian's syndrome), impaired neural conduction (seen in amyotrophic lateral sclerosis, Guillain-Barre's syndrome, high cervical spine injury, phrenic nerve paralysis, and aminoglycoside blockade), muscular weakness (seen in myasthenia gravis, idiopathic diaphragmatic paralysis, polymyositis, muscular dystrophy, and severe hypothyroidism), poor chest wall elasticity (seen in flail chest and kyphoscoliosis), and airway obstruction (laryngeal edema or foreign body inhalation).

2. **Ventilation/perfusion mismatch (V/Q mismatch)** refers to an imbalance between blood flow and ventilation.
   - Ventilation and perfusion are dependent on gravity and intrathoracic pressure, and even under physiological conditions, there is a V/Q mismatch at both the apices and the bases of the lungs. The ideal V/Q ratio is found toward the middle of the lungs, where both

TABLE 21.1 ■ **Various parameters for assessing the degree of oxygenation of the blood**

Measurement	Features
Arterial oxygen saturation (SaO_2)	• Direct measurement of the percentage of oxyhemoglobin • Measured using arterial blood gas
Pulse oxygen saturation (SpO_2)	• Measurement of percent of saturated hemoglobin in the capillary bed • Measured with pulse oximetry
Partial pressure of oxygen (PaO_2)	• Represents the amount of oxygen dissolved in the plasma • Measured using an arterial blood gas
A-a gradient	• This is the difference between the amount of oxygen in the alveoli (PaO_2) and the amount of oxygen dissolved in the plasma (PaO_2) • PaO_2 can be calculated using the alveolar gas equation*
"PF ratio" or PaO_2/ FiO_2	• This is the ratio between the amount of oxygen dissolved in the plasma (PaO_2) and the fraction of oxygen in inhaled air • Mostly in mechanically ventilated patients where FiO_2 can be calculated accurately

*Alveolar gas equation:
$PaO_2 = (PB - PH_2O) FiO_2 - (PaCO_2 \div R)$
where PB = barometric pressure, PH_2O = water vapor pressure (usually 47 mmHg), FiO_2 = fractional concentration of inspired oxygen, and R = gas exchange ratio

ventilation and perfusion are in proportion to each other. Lung spaces with a low V/Q ratio (lung bases) will have low alveolar oxygen but a high CO_2 content. Similarly, lung spaces with a high V/Q ratio (lung apices) will have lower CO_2 content and higher oxygen content.

- Hypoxia because of V/Q mismatch can be initially corrected with supplemental oxygen. However, it needs to be followed by specific therapy for the cause of the mismatch.
- Causes: obstructive lung disease, pulmonary vascular disease (including pulmonary embolism), and interstitial lung diseases.

3. **Diffusion limitation** occurs when the movement of oxygen from the alveoli to the pulmonary capillaries is impaired. This disease process usually coincides with a V/Q mismatch.
   - Causes: alveolar and/or interstitial inflammation or fibrosis, where there is loss of functioning capillaries, or the capillary membrane has thickened, leading to stiffer vessels and faster blood flow. The faster blood flow across the diffusion bed does not give enough time for the oxygen to bind to enough sites on the hemoglobin in red blood cells.

4. **Right-to-left shunt** exists when blood passes from the right side of the heart to the left side without oxygenation. These shunts lead to V/Q mismatch, causing hypoxemia that does not improve with supplemental oxygen.
   - Causes: anatomic shunting (intra-cardiac shunts like septal defects, arterio-venous malformations, or hepato-pulmonary syndrome) or physiologic shunting (atelectasis, pneumonia, acute respiratory distress syndrome).

5. **Reduced inspired oxygen tension** is seen at high altitudes. Reduced atmospheric pressure directly reduces the oxygen tension in alveoli. This does not impair the A-a gradient.
   - Supplemental oxygen can treat hypoxemia in high-altitude settings.

Compensatory mechanisms for hypoxia include increased minute ventilation, pulmonary arterial vasoconstriction, and increased sympathetic tone. There are many systemic changes in response to hypoxia. The peripheral vessels dilate in response to low oxygen while the vessels in the pulmonary vasculature constrict to shunt the blood away from poorly ventilated regions to help

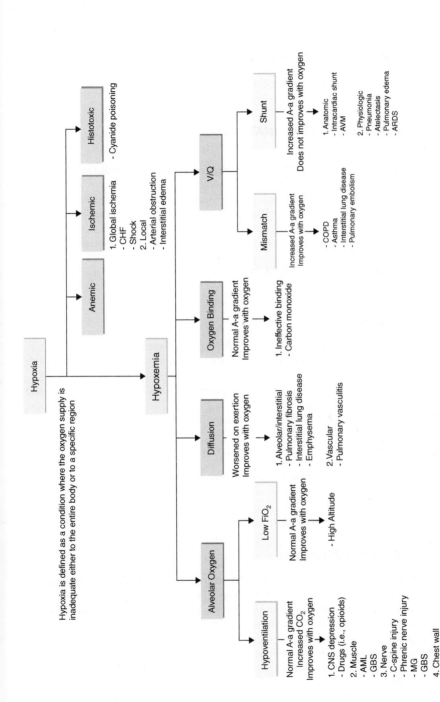

Fig. 21.2 Various mechanisms underlying hypoxia.

with the V/Q ratio. Hypoxia has hazardous effects on organ systems, especially in cases of stroke (cerebral ischemia) or myocardial ischemia.

Suggested Approach to a Patient With Hypoxia

For inpatient scenarios with acute onset hypoxia, we recommend the following approach based on a thorough literature review.

HISTORY AND PHYSICAL EXAMINATION

- The acuity of signs and symptoms.
- History of cardiac, pulmonary, CNS disease associated with reduced ventilation.
- History of any medication use that is associated with reduced ventilation.
- Physical exam should start with an assessment of airway, breathing, and circulation.
- Response to oxygen supplementation should be assessed. No response to supplemental oxygen would point toward shunting.
- A focused cardiac and pulmonary exam should be done to identify a primary cardiac or pulmonary cause of hypoxia.
- A focused neurological exam can be done to assess the ability to protect the airway and determine the need for intubation.

LABORATORY TESTING

- Complete blood count – should be done to evaluate for leukocytosis or severe anemia.
- Electrolyte panel – should be done to evaluate for acidosis, which is seen commonly with hypoxia.
- ABG – should be done for various O_2 measurements mentioned in Table 21.1. It will also give measurements of CO_2 and pH.
- Other testing – BNP, procalcitonin can be done in appropriate clinical scenarios.

IMAGING

- Chest X-ray – should be done in all patients. This quick bedside study can provide much helpful information, e.g., pulmonary edema, pleural effusion, consolidation, pneumothorax.
- Chest computed tomography (CT) – non-contrasted study vs. CT angiogram can be considered in appropriate clinical settings.

THERAPEUTIC INTERVENTIONS

In hypoxic patients, treatment should begin with the management of the airway, breathing, and circulation. This chapter will focus on the general management of hypoxia. For the management of specific causes of hypoxia, please refer to the relevant chapters. Hypoventilation should be addressed by ensuring the patency of the airway. An advanced airway should be placed if concern about airway patency is present. Diffusion capacity should be increased by therapy directed at the underlying cause, e.g., diuretics for pulmonary edema, steroids for obstructive lung disease. Supplemental oxygen should be used to increase the FiO_2 via low flow or high flow devices based on the patient's degree of hypoxia.

Mechanical ventilation devices are used to ensure improved oxygenation in cases of severe hypoxia not responsive to conservative therapy. These include:

Non-invasive positive pressure ventilation devices:

- Continuous positive airway pressure mask – delivers oxygen under preset pressure via a tightly fitted mask. Positive pressure is continuous to ensure the airway remains open. It can be used in obstructive sleep apnea and acute pulmonary edema
- Bi-level positive airways pressure – higher positive pressure on inspiration and lower positive pressure on expiration. This is mainly used in patients with acute hypercapnia with chronic obstructive pulmonary disease exacerbation and acute cardiogenic pulmonary edema.

Invasive ventilation devices:

- Ventilator/respirator – positive pressure is administered using an endotracheal tube or tracheostomy tube.

Suggested Reading

Ahmed A, Graber MA. Evaluation of the adult with dyspnea in the emergency department. UpToDate.com. https://www.uptodate.com/contents/evaluation-of-the-adult-with-dyspnea-in-the-emergency-department.

Sarkar M, Niranjan N, Banyal PK. Mechanisms of hypoxemia. *Lung India*. 2017;34(1):47–60. https://doi.org/10.4103/0970-2113.197116.

CHAPTER 22

Acute Hypoxia in a Patient With Stroke

Abdelrhman M. Abo-zed ▨ Mohammad Adrish ▨ Firas Abdulmajeed

Case Study

The bedside nurse initiated a rapid response event after the patient had an aspiration event where he had desaturated to the 70 s. Upon prompt arrival of the rapid response team, the patient was found to be a 77-year-old male with a known history of chronic obstructive pulmonary disease, coronary artery disease, type 2 diabetes mellitus, hypertension, and poor oral dentition. He was admitted a few hours earlier for right-sided weakness in the upper and lower extremities with a left-sided facial droop and was being evaluated for a stroke. The patient was still to be seen by speech therapy. His daughter had brought in some chicken noodle soup which he was eating, and started choking on it.

VITAL SIGNS

Temperature: 98.2 °F, axillary
Blood Pressure: 155/97 mmHg
Pulse: 110 beats per min (bpm) – regular rhythm.
Respiratory Rate: 28 breaths per min
Pulse Oximetry: 72% on room air, improved to 85% when placed on a 15 L/min (LPM)
    non-rebreather (NRB)

FOCUSED PHYSICAL EXAMINATION

A quick exam showed an elderly male sitting up in bed in significant respiratory distress. He was alert and oriented and followed all commands appropriately. A pulmonary exam showed tachypnea with coarse breath sounds in the right lung. Diffuse wheezing was also present in all lung fields. His cardiac exam was significant for tachycardia with normal heart sounds, no murmur. The patient had weakness of the right upper and right lower extremity, with a left-sided facial droop which was similar to prior documentation. A detailed neurological exam was not done given tenuous respiratory status.

INTERVENTIONS

A cardiac monitor and pads were attached immediately. Emergent endotracheal intubation was done at the bedside to secure the airway. Arterial blood gas was obtained, which later showed a pH of 7.19, pCO_2 of 118, pO_2 of 50, oxygen saturation of 85% on 15 LPM NRB. Stat chest X-ray (CXR) was obtained, which showed an endotracheal tube in the correct place. It also showed diffuse bilateral opacities/consolidation, most prominent in the left mid and lower lung zones, consistent with aspiration pattern (Fig. 22.1). Stat dose of ampicillin-sulbactam was ordered, and the patient was immediately transferred to the intensive care unit for therapeutic bronchoscopy and pulmonary toilet.

TABLE 22.1 ■ **Comparison between aspiration pneumonia and aspiration pneumonitis**

Features	Aspiration pneumonia	Aspiration pneumonitis
Inoculum	Oropharyngeal material colonized with flora	Sterile gastric contents
Mechanism of injury	Infection and inflammation of pulmonary parenchyma from bacteria	Inflammation of pulmonary parenchyma from gastric acid
Microbiological profile	Mixed gram-positive and gram-negative organisms, particularly anaerobes	Sterile initially, however, can develop superinfection later on
Pre-disposing factors	Dysphagia	Altered mental status, peri-procedural
Clinical features	Fever, cough, purulent sputum, hypoxia Pulmonary infiltrates on imaging take time to develop	Cough, wheezing, hypoxia Pulmonary infiltrates on imaging develop in about 2 h
Treatment	Broad-spectrum antibiotics that cover anaerobes, e.g., ampicillin-sulbactam in stable patients, carbapenems in sick patients	Observation and supportive care Antibiotics should be initiated if difficult to ascertain the absence of pneumonia or in the presence of clinical deterioration
Clinical course	Cure rate 76%-88% with broad-spectrum antibiotics	Rapid clinical recovery in 24-48 h Outcomes unchanged with antibiotics

FINAL DIAGNOSIS

Hypoxic respiratory failure secondary to aspiration of food contents.

Aspiration Pneumonia

Aspiration pneumonia is the inflammation and infection of the pulmonary parenchyma caused by the penetration of the respiratory tract by oropharyngeal or gastric secretions. In contrast, aspiration pneumonitis is the inflammation of lung parenchyma from sterile oro-gastric contents, especially gastric acid (Table 22.1). Risk factors associated with aspiration pneumonia include pathologies that lead to an inability to clear oral secretions. It can present in a variety of manners depending on different inoculums (Table 22.2).

Risk factors for aspiration pneumonia include:
- Reduced level of alertness – encephalopathy of any cause, seizures, head trauma, use of sedatives and opioids, anesthesia, alcohol intoxication, or illicit drug use.
- Dysphagia
  - Oropharyngeal causes – tracheoesophageal fistula, head and neck cancers, oropharyngeal surgery, or xerostomia.
  - Esophageal causes – esophageal strictures, achalasia, esophagitis, esophageal malignancies, or dysfunctional lower esophageal sphincter.
- Neurological disorders – stroke, Parkinson, myasthenia, or multiple sclerosis.
- Miscellaneous – pharyngeal anesthesia, vocal cord paralysis, intractable vomiting, e.g., vomiting associated with gastric outlet obstruction or small bowel obstruction, ascites, gastroparesis, poor positioning while eating, poor dental hygiene, advanced age, placement in long-term care facilities, or cardiac arrest.

TABLE 22.2 ■ Different presentations of aspiration pneumonia based on the type of inoculum

Inoculum	Pulmonary Sequelae	Clinical Features	Therapy
Acid	Chemical pneumonitis	Abrupt dyspnea, tachypnea with mild fever, hypoxemia	Tracheal suctioning Positive pressure breathing Intravenous fluids
Oropharyngeal Bacteria	Bacterial infection	Cough, fever, purulent sputum	Antibiotics
Inert Fluids	Mechanical obstruction, reflex airway closure	Acute dyspnea, cyanosis, apnea	Positive airway pressure Tracheal suctioning
Particulate Matter	Mechanical obstruction	Causes irritative cough to acute apnea/rapid death	Extract particulate via bronchoscopy Antibiotics for superimposed infection

Suggested Approach to a Patient With Suspected Aspiration

We suggest the following approach to a patient when an aspiration event is suspected. This approach is based on a thorough literature review, but eventual decision-making should be based on the clinician's judgment and expertise. This approach can also be utilized in the emergency department, as management is universal.

FOCUSED HISTORY AND PHYSICAL EXAM

- History should focus on risk factors for aspiration.
- History should be obtained regarding the contents of the aspirate: gastric contents vs. food.
- Physical exam should begin with an assessment of airway, breathing, and circulation.
- A pulmonary exam can show tachypnea, coarse breath sounds, and wheeze.
- The presence of new-onset dysphagia should raise concern for a new cerebrovascular accident, and a thorough neurological exam should be done once airway, breathing, and circulation are stabilized.

LABORATORY TESTING

- Complete blood count (CBC) – can be done to evaluate for leukocytosis; however, white is unlikely to rise immediately after an acute event.
- Arterial blood gas (ABG) – new-onset hypoxia should prompt ABG testing to assess the degree of hypoxia and concomitant acidosis.

IMAGING STUDIES

- CXR is usually done in all patients immediately. However, it should be kept in mind that imaging findings can take time to develop.

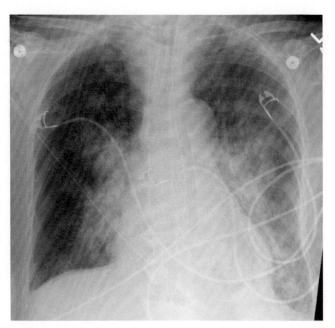

Fig. 22.1 Chest X-ray with bibasilar pneumonia, consistent with aspiration pattern. Also visible are an endotracheal tube in place, nasogastric tube in place, and multiple cardiac monitor chest leads.

THERAPEUTIC INTERVENTIONS

The broad aim of therapeutic interventions in suspected aspiration should be to prevent a recurrence. All patients should be evaluated for airway, breathing, and circulation. The airway should be secured with endotracheal intubation if necessary. Non-invasive ventilation can be considered in select cases. However, aspiration/inability to protect the airway is a relative contraindication to the use of bilevel positive airway pressure. Hypoxia should be addressed, and hemodynamics should be secured. Gastric decompression with a nasogastric tube should be considered in the appropriate setting. Patients can be clinically monitored without antibiotics in select cases. However, general practice is to initiate broad-spectrum antibiotics and de-escalate at a later point. Patients would require emergent pulmonology consult for pulmonary toilet in instances of food aspiration. Appropriate consultants should be engaged based on the underlying cause of aspiration.

STEPWISE APPROACH TO A PATIENT WITH SUSPECTED ASPIRATION

Step 1: Assess the patient for airway, breathing, and circulation.
Step 2: Secure the airway to prevent further aspiration.
Step 3: Determine the contents of aspirate: oral secretions vs. gastric contents vs. food.
Step 4: Determine the cause of aspiration. Consider gastric decompression in appropriate scenarios.
Step 5: Initiate broad-spectrum antibiotics as appropriate.
Step 6: The pulmonology team should be engaged for pulmonary toilet in case of aspiration of food contents.

Suggested Reading

Cruz-Jentoft AJ. Aspiration pneumonia. *Eur Geriatr Med.* 2011;2(3):179. https://doi.org/10.1016/j. eurger.2011.04.008.

DiBardino DM, Wunderink RG. Aspiration pneumonia: a review of modern trends. *J Crit Care.* 2015;30(1): 40–48. https://doi.org/10.1016/j.jcrc.2014.07.011.

Klompas M. Aspiration pneumonia in adults. UpToDate.com. https://www.uptodate.com/contents/ aspiration-pneumonia-in-adults.

CHAPTER 23

Hypoxia in a Patient With Chronic Obstructive Pulmonary Disease (COPD)

Abdelrhman M. Abo-zed ▪ Syed Zaidi ▪ Firas Abdulmajeed ▪ Mohammad Adrish

Case Study

The bedside nurse initiated a rapid response event after the patient was found to be in significant respiratory distress and with oxygen saturation in the 80s. On prompt arrival of the rapid response team, the patient was found to be a 65-year-old male with an extensive history of smoking, oxygen-dependent chronic obstructive pulmonary disease (COPD), hypertension, and heart failure with a preserved ejection fraction. The patient used 2 L/min (LPM) oxygen (O_2) at baseline. He reported progressive shortness of breath and increasing sputum production in the few days before admission and had been using 4 LPM O_2 through a nasal cannula at home. He was admitted earlier in the day after a friend found him confused at home. He was briefly trialed on bilevel positive airway pressure (BiPAP) in the emergency department (ED), which led to improved mental status, and the patient was admitted.

VITAL SIGNS

Temperature: 100.4 °F, axillary
Blood Pressure: 155/97 mmHg
Pulse: 101 beats per min (bpm) – regular rhythm.
Respiratory Rate: 30 breaths per min
Pulse Oximetry: 83% on 6 LPM O_2 through nasal canula

FOCUSED PHYSICAL EXAMINATION

A quick exam showed a frail, middle-aged male in respiratory distress. The patient was using accessory muscles of respiration and could not complete a sentence. The lung exam was significant for minimal breath sounds and absence of wheezing. His heart sounds were distant but unremarkable. The patient became increasingly somnolent and difficult to arouse during the evaluation. The rest of his exam was unremarkable.

INTERVENTIONS

A cardiac monitor and pads were attached to the patient. Then, 15 LPM of O_2 was administered through a non-rebreather mask which improved oxygen saturation to 96%. Stat arterial blood gas was ordered, which showed a pH of 7.28, pO_2 of 50 mmHg on 15 LPM non-rebreather, pCO_2 of 135 mmHg, lactate of 4.9 mmol/L, and oxygen saturation of 85%. A basic metabolic panel (BMP)

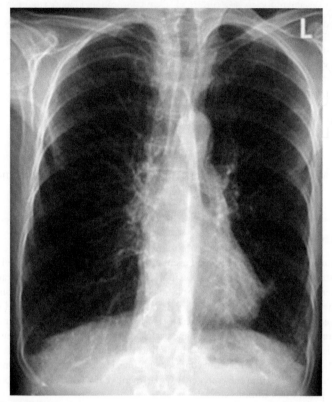

Fig. 23.1   Chest X-Ray in the anteroposterior view showing hyperinflated lungs.

drawn simultaneously showed a bicarbonate level of 26 meq/L. The patient was started on BiPAP at inspiratory pressure of 12 cm H_2O, expiratory pressure of 6 cm H_2O, and 100% FiO_2. A stat chest X-ray was obtained, which was negative for any acute pulmonary infiltrates (Fig. 23.1). The patient was ordered nebulizer treatment with ipratropium and albuterol. No glucocorticoids were administered as the patient had already received intravenous (IV) 125 mg methylprednisolone in the ED a few hours earlier. One dose of IV azithromycin was administered, and the patient was transferred to the intensive care unit (ICU) for further care.

FINAL DIAGNOSIS

Acute on chronic hypoxic and hypercapnic respiratory failure secondary to COPD exacerbation.

COPD Exacerbation and CO_2 Narcosis

COPD is a combination of two pulmonary pathologies: emphysema caused by the destruction of pulmonary parenchyma resulting in reduced surface area for gas exchange, and chronic bronchitis caused by chronic inflammation of the airways causing airflow obstruction. An exacerbation is an event characterized by an acute worsening of a patient's symptoms beyond the variation seen on a day-to-day basis. This change should be sufficient to warrant a change in management. Among patients with COPD, the frequency of exacerbation varies with the severity of the disease. Some patients have more frequent exacerbations than others, independent of other measures of disease severity. Table 23.1 outlines some symptoms, risk factors, and diagnostic criteria for COPD exacerbation.

An increase in airway inflammation is considered an important mechanism in the pathophysiology of exacerbation. Increased inflammation leads to increased bronchial tone, increased edema of the bronchial wall, and increased mucous production. These mechanisms lead to a ventilation-perfusion mismatch and reduced expiratory flow.

Hypercapnia is a classic feature of respiratory failure in COPD exacerbation and is produced by decreased minute ventilation and increased dead space ventilation in the setting of the poor pulmonary reserve. Classically called type-II respiratory failure, hypercapnic respiratory failure is associated with $paCO_2$ greater than 50 mmHg. Mild to moderate cases present with daytime sluggishness, headaches, or increased somnolence (Table 23.2). Severe cases are associated with confusion and decreased arousal, which can eventually progress to coma. Other comorbid illnesses and differentials of a simple COPD exacerbation should be ruled out appropriately (Table 23.3).

Acute respiratory failure secondary to acute exacerbation of COPD is one of the two conditions which are known to respond well to non-invasive ventilation, the other being acute cardiogenic pulmonary edema. A short trial of non-invasive ventilation is appropriate in respiratory failure from acute COPD exacerbations if no absolute contraindication to non-invasive

TABLE 23.1 ■ Symptoms, diagnosis, and risk factors for chronic obstructive pulmonary disease (COPD) exacerbation

Symptoms of exacerbation	Risk factors for exacerbation
The presence of two out of three of the following is required for diagnosis: • Increased cough • Increased sputum production • Increased sputum purulence Other symptoms: • Increased shortness of breath	Advanced age Productive cough Longer duration of COPD History of antibiotic therapy COPD related hospitalization within the previous year Chronic mucous hypersecretion Peripheral blood eosinophil count >0.3 × 10⁹ Presence of comorbidities

TABLE 23.2 ■ Various physiological changes seen with increased carbon dioxide tension in the blood

Physiological effects of hypercapnia	
Cerebral effects	• An initial increase in respiratory drive followed by decreased level of arousal and then decreased respiratory drive • Increased cerebral blood flow and increased intracranial pressure which can lead to seizures
Cardiorespiratory effects	• An initial feeling of dyspnea as a compensatory mechanism • Myocardial and diaphragmatic suppression leading to arrhythmia and arrest
Hematological effects	• Increased release of oxygen from hemoglobin in acute cases • Polycythemia in chronic cases
Metabolic effects	• Acute cases associated with acidosis, hyperkalemia, and increased ionized serum calcium. Bicarbonate does not change significantly • Chronic cases associated with increased renal retention of bicarbonate

TABLE 23.3 ■ **Differentials and comorbid illnesses of acute respiratory failure and chronic obstructive pulmonary disease (COPD) exacerbation**

Differentials	Features
Decompensated heart failure	• Acute vs. acute on chronic dyspnea • Fine inspiratory crackles on lung exam • Brain natriuretic peptide and chest X-rays consistent with volume load
Atrial fibrillation	• Common comorbidity in COPD patients • Irregular pulse on exam • Telemetry and electrocardiogram consistent with supraventricular tachycardia
Pneumonia	• Difficult to distinguish clinically from COPD exacerbation • Chest X-ray might show infiltrates consistent with a bacterial infection
Pneumothorax	• Presence of pleuritic chest pain • Decreased breath sounds on lung exam • Chest X-ray consistent with air in the pleural cavity
Pulmonary embolism	• Often has vague symptoms and is difficult to distinguish clinically from COPD exacerbation. Requires a high clinical suspicion • Computed tomography angiogram should be considered if clinical suspicion is high

TABLE 23.4 ■ **Contraindications to use of non-invasive ventilation**

Absolute contraindications	Relative contraindications
• Presence of a life-threatening cardiopulmonary condition • Cardiac or respiratory arrest • Severe respiratory distress • Malignant cardiac arrhythmia • Acute myocardial infarction	• Inability to protect the airway • Presence of a comorbid life-threatening non-cardiopulmonary condition • Active gastrointestinal bleed • Intracranial hemorrhage • Shock • Contraindication to use of high-pressure face mask • Facial trauma or fractures • Neurological surgery • Upper airway obstruction • Anticipated prolonged need for ventilatory support

ventilation (NIV) exists (Table 23.4). Patients should be monitored closely, preferably in an ICU setting, for deterioration and need for intubation.

Suggested Approach to a Patient With Respiratory Failure Secondary to COPD Exacerbation

For patients suspected of having acute respiratory failure secondary to COPD exacerbation, we suggest the following approach based on a thorough literature review. This approach can also be utilized in the ED, as management is universal.

FOCUSED HISTORY AND PHYSICAL EXAM

- The timing of onset and acuity of signs and symptoms.
- History of triggers for exacerbations.

- History findings such as chest pain, fever, lower extremity edema, or palpitations could point toward a concurrent illness or complication.
- Physical exam should begin with an assessment of airway, breathing, and circulation.
- A lung exam would show end-expiratory wheezing in an isolated COPD exacerbation. A "silent chest" should raise concern for severe exacerbation, minimal air movement, and impending respiratory failure.

LABORATORY TESTING

- Complete blood count (CBC) – to evaluate for worsening leukocytosis, which can point toward an infection.
- Electrolyte panel – to evaluate for acidosis or potassium derangements.
- Arterial blood gas – to assess the degree of hypoxia and hypercapnia. This would also help evaluate for compensated vs. uncompensated acidosis.
- Brain natriuretic peptide – can be obtained if suspicion of concomitant volume overload/ heart failure.
- d-dimer – can be obtained to rule out pulmonary embolism (PE) in appropriate cases.

IMAGING

- Chest X-ray – should be obtained in all patients to evaluate for pneumonia, pulmonary edema, pleural effusion, pneumothorax which are all comorbid illnesses in COPD exacerbations
- CT angiogram chest – can be obtained if there is clinical suspicion of PE.

EKG

- Should be obtained in all patients with tachycardia as atrial arrhythmias are a common complication of COPD and lung disease.

THERAPEUTIC INTERVENTIONS

Management begins with the assessment of the airway, breathing, and circulation. The capability of the patient to maintain the airway should be assessed. Acute exacerbation of COPD is one of the few conditions with known benefits from NIV. The assessment for the need for invasive airway via endotracheal intubation should be made as soon as possible. If the patient does not require emergent intubation, a short trial of BiPAP should be initiated after ensuring that the patient has no contraindication to NIV. Hypoxia should be corrected; O_2 can be delivered via NIV. Nebulized breathing treatments should be initiated to reduce bronchospasm. IV glucocorticoids should be initiated if the patient is not on them already. Higher doses of glucocorticoids have not shown any benefit over standard doses. Empiric antibiotics should be considered if there is clinical suspicion or evidence of concomitant pneumonia. Azithromycin can be used for its anti-inflammatory properties in the absence of frank pneumonia. Patients on NIV should be monitored closely in the first few hours, ideally in an ICU setting or step-down unit.

STEPWISE APPROACH TO A PATIENT WITH ACUTE RESPIRATORY FAILURE FROM COPD EXACERBATION

Step 1: Assess the airway, breathing, and circulation.
Step 2: If no contraindication to NIV, BiPAP should be initiated for respiratory support.

Step 3: Lab work including CBC, BMP, and arterial blood gas should be obtained to assess for leukocytosis, acidosis, hypoxia, CO_2 retention, and electrolyte derangements.

Step 4: A chest X-ray should be obtained to evaluate for concomitant illnesses such as pneumonia, pulmonary edema, and pneumothorax.

Step 5: EKG should be obtained in tachycardic patients to evaluate for atrial arrhythmias.

Step 6: Patients on NIV should be monitored closely for the first few hours. Endotracheal intubation should be pursued if the patient does not show signs of improvement or deteriorates clinically.

Suggested Reading

Crisafulli E, Barbeta E, Ielpo A, Torres A. Management of severe acute exacerbations of COPD: an updated narrative review. *Multidiscip Respir Med.* 2018 Oct 2;13:36. doi: 10.1186/s40248-018-0149-0. PMID: 30302247; PMCID: PMC6167788.

Halpin DM, Miravitlles M, Metzdorf N, Celli B. Impact and prevention of severe exacerbations of COPD: a review of the evidence. *Int J Chron Obstruct Pulmon Dis.* 2017;12:2891–2908. doi:10.2147/COPD.S139470.

Stoller JK. COPD exacerbations: management. UpToDate.com. https://www.uptodate.com/contents/copd-exacerbations-management

Mathioudakis AG, Janssens W, Sivapalan P, et al. Acute exacerbations of chronic obstructive pulmonary disease: in search of diagnostic biomarkers and treatable traits. *Thorax.* 2020;75(6):520–527. https://doi.org/10.1136/thoraxjnl-2019-214484.

Viniol C, Vogelmeier CF. Exacerbations of COPD. *Eur Respir Rev.* 2018;27(147). doi:10.1183/16000617.0103-2017.

CHAPTER 24

Hypoxia in a Patient With COVID-19

Rahul R. Bollam ▦ Kainat Saleem ▦ Syed Arsalan Akhter Zaidi

Case Study

A rapid response code was activated for a patient who developed acute dyspnea. On arrival of the condition team, the patient was found to be a 75-year-old male with a known history of chronic obstructive pulmonary disease (COPD), who was admitted to the hospital one day earlier for cough and fever secondary to coronavirus disease 2019 (COVID-19) pneumonia. The patient's oxygenation had been stable on room air since admission. He had ambulated to the bathroom 30 min before the rapid response event and was having difficulty catching his breath since then.

VITAL SIGNS

Temperature: 101.3 °F, axillary
Blood Pressure: 160/90 mmHg
Heart Rate: 120 beats per min (bpm)
Respiratory Rate: 35 breaths per min
Oxygen Saturation: 85% 4 L nasal cannula, 100% on a non-rebreather face mask

FOCUSED PHYSICAL EXAMINATION

After donning proper personal protective equipment (PPE), a quick exam showed an elderly male in visible respiratory distress, using accessory muscles of respiration. The patient was unable to speak in complete sentences. The lung exam was significant for inspiratory crackles and expiratory wheezing in all lung fields. The cardiac exam was notable for tachycardia but was unremarkable otherwise.

INTERVENTIONS

A cardiac monitor and pads were attached to the patient. A stat chest X-ray was ordered, and labs including complete blood count (CBC), electrolytes, and arterial blood gas were obtained. Chest X-ray showed multi-focal infiltrates that were worse than seen on the X-ray obtained admission (Fig. 24.1). Labs were significant for a pH of 7.22, pO_2 of 259, pCO_2 of 95, and lactate of 3.4. The patient was given a dose of IV ceftriaxone, IV azithromycin, and IV dexamethasone per institutional protocol. The patient was transferred to the intensive care unit for a trial of non-invasive ventilation.

FINAL DIAGNOSIS

Acute hypoxic respiratory failure secondary to COVID-19 infection.

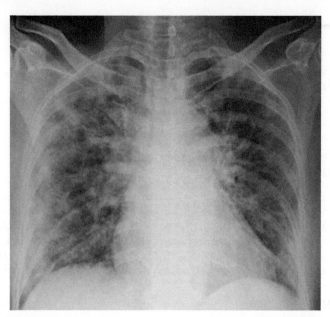

Fig. 24.1   Chest X-ray in the anteroposterior view showing bilateral infiltrates, consistent with multi-focal pneumonia. https://www.uptodate.com/contents/coronavirus-disease-2019-covid-19-critical-care-and-airway-management-issues.

COVID-19

Severe acute respiratory syndrome coronavirus 2 (SARS-CoV-2) is a part of the family of coronaviruses. The four coronaviruses, which are endemic, usually cause the common cold. However, SARS and Middle East respiratory syndrome have caused epidemics with high mortality rates. SARS-CoV-2 is closely related to SARS. The understanding of COVID-19, the disease caused by SARS-CoV-2, is evolving, and the information presented in this chapter is current as of February 2021. More up-to-date resources should be referred to for the latest information on the diagnosis and treatment of this illness.

The range of symptoms of COVID-19 varies from asymptomatic infection to severe respiratory failure requiring mechanical ventilation. Various risk factors have been identified which are associated with worse outcomes. These include older age, medical comorbidities such as cardiovascular disease, diabetes, hypertension, underlying lung disease, chronic kidney disease, obesity, history of smoking, and history of malignancies, particularly heme malignancies. Other factors such as viral mutations leading to the development of new variants have been associated with increased transmission and worse outcomes. However, this data is preliminary at this point and should be considered with caution.

As of the writing of this chapter, glucocorticoids such as dexamethasone are the only intervention that has been associated with a reduction in mortality associated with this illness. The antiviral agent remdesivir has been shown to reduce time to recovery in hospitalized adults. However, no reduction in mortality has been seen. Therapies such as interleukin-6 inhibitor tocilizumab, convalescent plasma, and antiviral antibodies are currently under investigation in clinical trials. The latest guidelines from the Centers for Disease Control and Prevention (CDC) should be sought for up-to-date SARS-CoV-2 directed therapy.

Hypoxia is the most common manifestation and acute complication of COVID-19. It is generally caused by ventilation-perfusion mismatch from consolidation. Other causes of V/Q mismatch, such as pulmonary embolism (PE; given the hypercoagulable state in active COVID infection) and intrapulmonary shunting, should also be considered in the differential for hypoxia. Based on current recommendations, a trial of non-invasive ventilation with a high-flow nasal cannula (HFNC) or bilevel positive airway pressure is preferred over direct intubation, depending on the patient's respiratory status. Non-invasive ventilation is associated with the risk of aerosolization of viral particles, and institutional guidelines should be followed regarding PPE use in such cases.

Suggested Approach to a Patient With Acute Hypoxia From COVID-19

Based on the current guidelines (as of February 2021), the following approach can be used for the evaluation and management of hypoxia and respiratory distress in patients with COVID-19. The writers want to emphasize that SAR-CoV-2 and COVID-19 are evolving topics, and the recommendations are current as of the writing of this chapter. The latest guidelines from the CDC and other societies should be referred to for the latest updates in the management of COVID-19.

FOCUSED HISTORY AND PHYSICAL EXAMINATION

- The acuity of signs and symptoms – acute worsening after initial recovery can be a sign of superimposed infection.
- History of underlying lung disease such as asthma and COPD.
- Physical exam should assess for airway, breathing, and circulation.
- A pulmonary exam should be done to identify concomitant causes of worsening respiratory status such as wheezing (COPD or asthma exacerbation), fine crackles (heart failure exacerbation), and decreased breath sounds (pleural effusion).

LABORATORY TESTS

- CBC – to evaluate for worsening white count, coagulopathy.
- Electrolyte panel – to evaluate for acidosis.
- Arterial blood gas, including lactate – to evaluate the degree of hypoxia and acidosis.
- Cultures including blood and sputum – if bacterial superinfection is suspected.
- Respiratory viral panel (NAAT) – can be considered if concurrent infection with other viral agents is suspected.
- d-dimer – can be obtained if suspicion of concomitant PE.
- Procalcitonin – can help rue out bacterial superinfections; however, it is rarely reported fast enough to be helpful in a rapid response setting.

IMAGING STUDIES

- Chest X-ray – should be obtained in patients with worsening respiratory status to evaluate for superinfection, concomitant pulmonary edema, and pleural effusions.
- CT angiogram – should be obtained if there is suspicion of PE, which is a known complication of COVID-19.

THERAPEUTIC INTERVENTIONS

The diagnosis and treatment options for COVID-19 are in constant flux. As the disease is relatively new, multiple aspects of this illness are still unknown. Very few COVID-19 directed therapies are established at this point, and numerous clinical trials are underway to determine what does and does not work. The latest CDC guidelines should be referred to for the up-to-date management essentials of COVID-19.

All patients should be assessed for airway, breathing, and circulation. Hypoxia should be treated to achieve blood oxygen saturation of 94% or above. Current guidelines recommend a trial of non-invasive ventilation to manage severe hypoxia, depending on clinical judgment and institutional policies. Empiric antibiotics for bacterial pneumonia can be considered if there is a high suspicion of bacterial superinfection or in immunocompromised patients. Again, clinical judgment should be used. Patients should be treated with low-dose dexamethasone (or equivalent) for new-onset hypoxia. Remdesivir has been approved by the Food and Drug Administration for COVID-19 and should be used per institutional policy. Other investigational therapies should be used per institutional guidelines. PE should be considered a contributor to hypoxia in the appropriate clinical setting.

STEPWISE APPROACH TO THE MANAGEMENT OF A PATIENT WITH COVID-19-RELATED RESPIRATORY FAILURE

Step 1: Appropriate PPE should be established per institutional guidelines.

Step 2: The patient should be assessed for airway, breathing, and circulation. Supplemental O_2 should be initiated with goal oxygen saturation $\geq$94%.

Step 3: A chest X-ray should be obtained to evaluate for concomitant causes of respiratory distress.

Step 4: CBC, basic metabolic panel, and arterial blood gas should be obtained.

Step 5: Non-invasive ventilation should be considered before intubation in appropriate scenarios.

Step 6: Low dose dexamethasone should be initiated. Remdesivir and investigational therapies should be used per institutional guidelines.

Coding a Patient With COVID-19 Pneumonia With Acute Hypoxic Respiratory Failure

In patients with confirmed COVID-19 infection, clinicians should establish appropriate PPE before entering the room. If the patient is awake and able to follow commands, a trial of HFNC or continuous positive airway pressure (CPAP) can be started to improve saturations. If the patient cannot maintain saturation while on HFNC/CPAP or is not awake, bag-mask ventilation should be done immediately, followed by advanced airway placement. Intubation should be attempted by the most experienced provider available to avoid multiple attempts and reduce the risk of aerosolization.

Suggested Reading

Kim AY, Gandhi RT. COVID-19: Management in hospitalized adults. UpToDate.com. https://www.upto-date.com/contents/covid-19-management-in-hospitalized-adults

CHAPTER 25

Hypoxia in a Patient With Hypertensive Emergency

Rahul R. Bollam ▓ Mohammad Adrish ▓ Firas Abdulmajeed

Case Study

A bedside nurse initiated a rapid response code for a patient who appeared to be in acute respiratory distress and was hypoxic. On arrival of the condition team, the patient was short of breath, sitting on the side of his bed. Per the bedside report, the patient was a 60-year-old male with a history of end-stage renal disease admitted earlier in the day for a two- to three-day history of dyspnea on exertion because of multiple missed dialysis sessions. Since calling the rapid response code, the patient's dyspnea had worsened acutely, and his shortness of breath was unrelieved by albuterol nebulizations.

VITAL SIGNS

Temperature: 98.6 °F, axillary
Blood Pressure: 240/140 mm of Hg
Respiratory Rate: 32 breaths per min
Heart Rate: 120 beats per min
Oxygen Saturation: 82% on room air; 97% on 8L/min (LPM) nasal cannula.

FOCUSED PHYSICAL EXAMINATION

A quick exam showed a middle-aged male in severe respiratory distress, tachypneic, and using accessory muscles of respiration. Significant crackles were present in all lung fields on auscultation, with trace edema present in the lower extremities. His cardiac exam showed tachycardia with no new murmurs. Trace bilateral lower extremity edema was present.

INTERVENTIONS

A cardiac monitor and associated pads were attached to the patient. Stat troponin, arterial blood gas (ABG), and chest X-ray were obtained. Possible causes of presentation were considered, including flash pulmonary edema in the setting of hypertensive crisis, acute exacerbation of congestive heart failure, acute coronary syndrome, or pulmonary embolism. ABG showed a pH of 7.55, paO_2 of 70, $paCO_2$ of 25, and oxygen saturation of 94% on 8 LPM. The chest X-ray was significant for bilateral pulmonary vascular congestion (Fig. 25.1), and telemetry showed sinus tachycardia. A point-of-care ultrasound (POCUS) exam done by an in-house intensivist showed Kirley B-Lines in bilateral lung fields. Based on the available information, the most likely differential diagnosis was flash pulmonary edema in the setting of uncontrolled hypertension. The patient was started on non-invasive positive pressure ventilation via continuous positive airway pressure and transferred to the intensive care unit for monitoring and emergent dialysis.

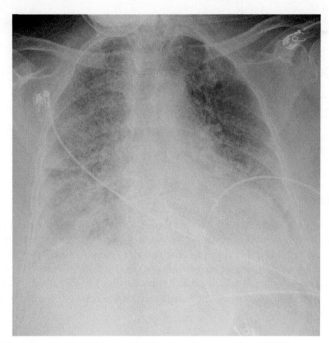

Fig. 25.1   Chest X-ray showing bilateral pulmonary vascular congestion.

FINAL DIAGNOSIS

Flash pulmonary edema.

Pulmonary Edema

Pulmonary edema is a condition caused by excessive fluid in the alveolar sacs causing interference with gas exchange. This interference can present as dyspnea and reduced blood oxygenation. Traditionally, pulmonary edema can be classified into cardiogenic and non-cardiogenic pulmonary edema (Table 25.1).

Definition and Diagnosis: Flash pulmonary edema (also called sympathetic crashing acute pulmonary edema) is caused by an acute increase in afterload, causing sudden onset pulmonary edema and poor peripheral perfusion. A sympathetic surge occurs because of decreased systemic perfusion, which further increases the cardiac afterload and leads to rapid respiratory and hemodynamic decompensation (Fig. 25.2). Well-established risk factors such as hypertension, coronary ischemia, and valvular diseases are associated with flash pulmonary edema. Other causes, such as severe neurological insult and naloxone administration, can also cause flash pulmonary edema.

Suggested Approach to a Patient With Flash Pulmonary Edema

For inpatient scenarios where acute pulmonary edema is being considered as the top differential, we suggest the following to determine the diagnosis and cause of pulmonary edema. See Fig. 25.3 for a flowchart of management of flash pulmonary edema. The usual sequence of history taking,

TABLE 25.1 ▣ **Pathophysiology and causes of pulmonary edema**

	Cardiogenic pulmonary edema	Non-cardiogenic pulmonary edema
Pathophysiology	Caused by increased pulmonary capillary hydrostatic pressure	Occurs because of increased pulmonary capillary endothelial permeability following direct or indirect lung injury
Causes	Heart failure, aortic/mitral disease, transfusion-associated circulatory overload, high dietary salt load, uncontrolled hypertension (sympathetic crashing edema), acute coronary syndrome, renal artery stenosis, pheochromocytoma	Acute respiratory distress syndrome, upper airway obstruction (also called negative pressure pulmonary edema), high altitude, central nervous system injury (neurogenic), ischemic/reperfusion injury (after lung transplant), re-expansion edema (after thoracentesis), or drug-induced pulmonary edema

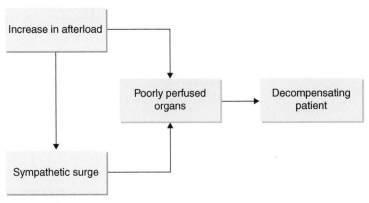

Fig. 25.2 Vicious cycle of sympathetic surge.

physical exam, investigations, and resuscitative interventions is often not followed during a rapid response; these measures often run parallel to each other in a code situation. The following components of the rapid response are discussed in the traditional sequence only to ease understanding.

FOCUSED HISTORY AND PHYSICAL

- History: Acuity of signs and symptoms. Past medical history of valvular disease, congestive heart failure, central nervous system injury, recent lung transplant, or recent thoracentesis.
- Physical examination: Physical exam should begin with an assessment of the airway, breathing, and circulation. Assess for signs of shock and decreased end-organ perfusion. A focused exam will include lung auscultation (presence of crackles?), cardiac auscultation (third heart sound, mitral regurgitation murmur?), signs of peripheral edema, and jugular venous distension.

LABORATORY TESTS

- ABG should be obtained to assess true oxygenation status.
- Troponin should be obtained to rule out cardiac ischemia.
- Brain natriuretic peptide should be done to evaluate for decompensated heart failure.

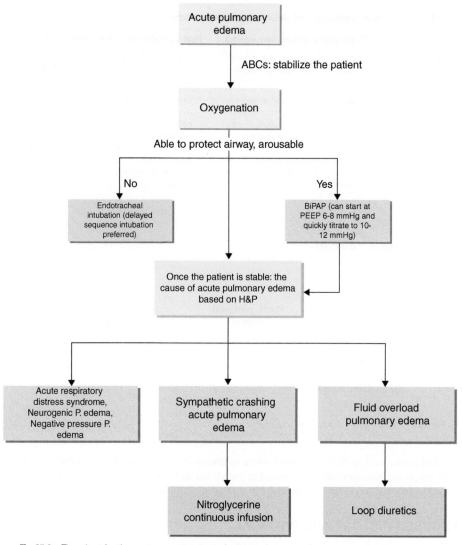

Fig. 25.3 Flowchart for the acute management of acute pulmonary edema.

IMAGING STUDIES

- Chest X-ray should be obtained in all cases as soon as airway and breathing are secured.
  - Look for findings such as cephalization, interstitial edema, pulmonary venous congestion.
  - Signs of pulmonary congestion may not be present for hours after acute flash pulmonary edema, so a normal chest X-ray is frequently seen. In a study of 45 patients with pulmonary edema in whom the cause was determined clinically, chest X-ray features were identified in 87% of patients with cardiogenic causes, while only in 60% of patients with non-cardiogenic causes.

- POCUS: An experienced and credentialed provider can perform this if present in the RRT.
  - A bedside lung ultrasound can be used to evaluate for pulmonary edema. B-lines are associated with pulmonary edema.
  - Bedside cardiac ultrasound can be used to evaluate for acute left ventricular dysfunction, new valvulopathy, or new wall motion abnormalities.

ELECTROCARDIOGRAM (EKG)

- EKG can be used to identify cardiac ischemia as an underlying cause of pulmonary edema.

THERAPEUTIC INTERVENTIONS

The primary goal in acute pulmonary edema is to reduce pulmonary fluid levels by shifting fluid from the lungs to the systemic circulation. We recommend that all patients be assessed for airway, breathing, circulation.

- Oxygenation/ventilatory support: Oxygen is provided to hypoxemic patients. Positive end-expiratory pressure (either non-invasive ventilation [NIV] or invasive ventilation) is used to improve gas exchange, reduce work of breathing and directly redistribute fluid from alveoli into pulmonary lymphatics for drainage. The positive pressure also reduces venous return and wedge pressure. Bilevel positive airway pressure can be started per institutional guidelines. NIV can be started with a PEEP of 6-8 mmHg and titrated quickly to 10-12 mmHg. If intubation is required, consider delayed sequence intubation.
- Medications: For patients with uncontrolled hypertension, vasodilators (such as nitrates or angiotensinogen converting enzyme inhibitors) should be used to reduce left ventricular filling pressure. Nitroglycerin can be started as 50-100 mcg/min, then titrated to 200-400 mcg/min. Doses >120 mcg/min are usually required to significantly decrease pulmonary capillary wedge pressure. Another method for administering nitroglycerin is starting with nitroglycerin bolus (400-800 mcg over 1-2 min), then starting continuous infusion at 100 mcg/min, titrate to effect. It has been found that 1-2 mg bolus doses are safe and effective. Sub-lingual nitroglycerin can be used if there is a delay in the initiation of nitroglycerin drip. Nitroprusside can be used as an alternative when there is an insufficient response to nitroglycerin; it can be started at 5 mcg/kg/min with titration based on blood pressure. Cyanide toxicity risk increases proportionately with infusion rate and the length of time.
- Loop diuretics (such as furosemide) are given to reduce circulating fluid volume, which are used in cases of volume overload.

SUMMARY OF A STEPWISE APPROACH TO FLASH PULMONARY EDEMA

Step 1: Patient with signs of flash pulmonary edema (respiratory distress, hypoxia, crackles on auscultation).

Step 2: Assess oxygenation and secure the airway. Start positive pressure ventilation with either invasive or non-invasive methods.

Step 3: Evaluate the cause of pulmonary edema based on the history, physical examination, and vital signs. Treat the underlying cause as appropriate.

Step 4: Use loop diuretics based on volume status.

Step 5: Transfer to the intensive care unit for closer monitoring.

CODING A PATIENT WITH PULMONARY EDEMA

Patients with pulmonary edema are more likely to undergo respiratory arrest than cardiac arrest. Early securement of the airway is of paramount importance. If a patient with pulmonary edema has a cardiac arrest, we suggest following the advanced cardiac life support protocol and initiation of effective cardiopulmonary resuscitation per guidelines. Post-cardiac arrest care should be initiated once the return of spontaneous circulation is achieved.

Suggested Reading

Agrawal N, Kumar A, Aggarwal P, Jamshed N. Sympathetic crashing acute pulmonary edema. *Indian J Crit Care Med*. 2016;20(12):719–723. https://doi.org/10.4103/0972-5229.195710.

Aronow WS. Treatment of hypertensive emergencies. *Ann Transl Med*. 2017;5(Suppl 1). https://doi. org/10.21037/atm.2017.03.34. S5-S5.

Brathwaite L, Reif M. Hypertensive emergencies: a review of common presentations and treatment options. *Cardiol Clin*. 2019;37(3):275–286. https://doi.org/10.1016/j.ccl.2019.04.003.

Meyer TE. Approach to diagnosis and evaluation of acute decompensated heart failure in adults. UpToDate. com. https://www.uptodate.com/contents/approach-to-diagnosis-and-evaluation-of-acute-decompensated-heart-failure-in-adults.

CHAPTER 26

Hypoxia in a Patient With Bullous Emphysema

Rahul R. Bollam ▦ Kainat Saleem ▦ Firas Abdulmajeed ▦ Mohammad Adrish

Case Study

The bedside nurse activated a rapid response code for a patient who appeared to be in acute respiratory distress and had new right-sided chest pain. On arrival of the rapid response team (RRT), the patient was found to be a 62-year-old male with a history of chronic obstructive pulmonary disease (COPD) who was admitted one day ago for COPD exacerbation. Overnight, the patient was placed on bilevel positive airway pressure (BiPAP) therapy for respiratory acidosis. In the 10 min before the RRT event, the patient became acutely dyspneic with increasing lethargy and right-sided chest pain.

VITAL SIGNS

Temperature: 37.4 °F, axillary
Blood Pressure: 90/50 mmHg
Heart Rate: 122 beats per min (bpm)
Respiratory Rate: 30 breaths per min
Oxygen Saturation: 70% on room air, 90% on 15 L/min (LPM) non-rebreather

FOCUSED PHYSICAL EXAMINATION

A quick exam revealed a middle-aged male lying in bed in obvious distress. The patient appeared drowsy and tachypneic, using accessory muscles of respiration. There was reduced air entry on the right lung field, and the left lung was clear to auscultation. His cardiac examination revealed tachycardia with normal heart sounds. His abdomen was non-tender and non-distended. The remaining examination was unremarkable.

WORKING DIAGNOSIS

Acute respiratory failure because of COPD exacerbation vs. acute respiratory distress syndrome vs. pneumothorax

INTERVENTIONS

A cardiac monitor and pads were attached to the patient. The patient was continued on 15 LPM via a non-rebreather mask, and a stat chest X-ray was ordered. Arterial blood gas (ABG), troponin, and electrocardiogram (EKG) were obtained. ABG showed reduced oxygen saturation with respiratory acidosis (pH 7.2/pCO_2 80 mmHg/pO_2 60 mmHg/SpO_2 91%). EKG was unremarkable for an acute ischemic event. Chest X-ray was significant for right-sided pneumothorax, which was not present on admission imaging (Fig. 26.1). Thoracic surgery was paged emergently for the need of a chest tube for pneumothorax. The chest tube was placed at the bedside by thoracic surgery with rapid improvement of symptoms. The patient was transferred to the intensive care unit for closer monitoring.

FINAL DIAGNOSIS

Secondary pneumothorax in the setting of COPD with possible bullae rupture because of BiPAP.

Pneumothorax

Pneumothorax is a collection of air in the pleural space separating the thoracic wall and lung. Air can enter the intra-pleural space through communication from the chest wall (e.g., after trauma) or through lung parenchyma across the visceral pleura (e.g., after rupture of an emphysematous bulla). Most pneumothoraces are simple, but tension pneumothorax is occasionally seen, which is a life-threatening emergency. Simple pneumothorax does not cause a mediastinal shift or hemodynamic instability. The different types of pneumothoraces are:

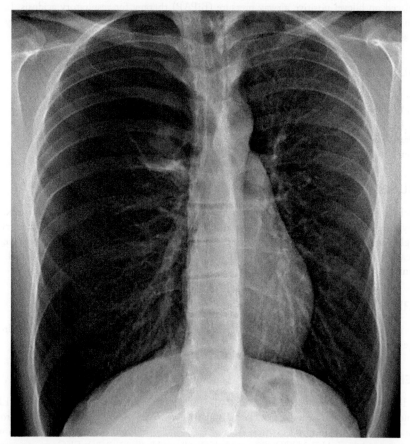

Fig. 26.1   Chest X-ray showing absence of lung markings in the right hemithorax, significant for right-sided pneumothorax.

1. Primary Spontaneous Pneumothorax
   a. These occur spontaneously without a known lung pathologic condition.
   b. These are most common in young, thin male adults.
2. Secondary Spontaneous Pneumothorax
   a. These occur in the setting of known pulmonary abnormality/pathologic condition.
   b. These are more common in older patients.
   c. Risk factors include COPD, cystic fibrosis, interstitial lung disease, and connective tissue disorders.
   d. Carry higher morbidity and mortality than primary pneumothoraces and have recurrence rates up to 43% in five years.
3. Traumatic Pneumothorax
   a. These occur secondary to traumatic injury or iatrogenic causes.
   b. The most common iatrogenic causes are transthoracic needle aspiration, subclavian needle stick, thoracentesis, transbronchial biopsy, and pleural biopsy.
   c. Pneumothoraces are the second most common complication after chest trauma; rib fractures are the most common complication.
4. Tension Pneumothorax
   a. A life-threatening complication of traumatic pneumothorax in which air accumulates and becomes trapped by a one-way valve that can compress the lung, displace mediastinal structures leading to hemodynamic instability (Fig. 26.2).
   b. In the combat setting, like warzones, tension pneumothorax is the second most common cause of death

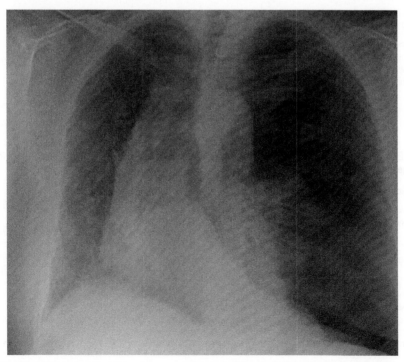

Fig. 26.2   Chest X-ray showing left tension pneumothorax pushing mediastinal structures to the right.

Pneumothorax can also be classified as closed pneumothorax or open pneumothorax; see Table 26.1 for the difference between closed and open pneumothoraces.

Patients with pneumothorax usually present with pleuritic chest pain and difficulty breathing. Characteristic physical findings include decreased chest wall motion, diminished breath sounds, and enlarged hemithorax on the affected side. Evidence of labored breathing and accessory muscle use suggests respiratory compromise from a sizable pneumothorax. Tracheal deviation away from the affected side is a late sign. Hemodynamic compromise (such as tachycardia and hypotension) suggests tension pneumothorax and/or impending cardiopulmonary collapse. The management of pneumothorax largely depends on the size of pneumothorax and the hemodynamic compromise caused by the pneumothorax (Table 26.2 and Fig. 26.3).

Suggested Approach to a Patient With Suspected Pneumothorax

For a patient presenting with signs and symptoms of respiratory distress and clinical suspicion of pneumothorax, we suggest the following approach to help guide management in rapid response

TABLE 26.1 ■ Features of closed and open pneumothorax

Closed Pneumothorax	Open Pneumothorax
The chest wall is intact	Chest wall has an opening after penetrating trauma
Commonly seen in rib fractures which puncture lungs	Commonly seen in gunshot wounds, stabbing
Not usually life-threatening unless advances to tension pneumothorax	It can be life-threatening as this often advances to tension pneumothorax
Signs and symptoms: • Dyspnea • Tachypnea • Chest pain	Signs and symptoms: • Dyspnea • Tachypnea • Chest pain • Sucking/gurgling sounds over the chest wall opening

TABLE 26.2 ■ Size of pneumothorax and management based on size and symptoms, per American College of Chest Physicians guidelines

Clinical Status	Size of Pneumothorax	Management
Stable[1] and/or Asymptomatic	Small[2]	No intervention
	Large[3]	Chest tube placement with negative pressure and water seal
Unstable and/or Tachypneic	Size does not determine therapy in unstable patients	Chest tube placement with negative pressure and water seal

[1]Respiratory rate <24 breaths per min, heart rate 60–120 bpm, oxygen saturation >90% on room air, blood pressure >90/60 mmHg, and can complete full sentences between breaths.
[2]Less than 3 cm apical inter-pleural distance, and presence of less than 2 cm rim between lung and chest wall in other areas of thorax.
[3]3 cm or more of apical inter-pleural distance, and presence of at least 2 cm rim between lung and chest wall in other areas of thorax.

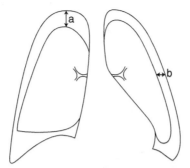

Fig. 26.3 Size of pneumothorax. a = apex to cupola disease, b = interpleural distance at the level of the hilum. Chest radiography is commonly used to quantify the size; Computed tomography is regarded as the best method for establishing size.

settings. This can be expanded and used in emergency room situations as well, as these suggestions are based on thorough literature research and updated guidelines for the management of pneumothorax. See Fig. 26.4 for a flowchart of management of a patient with pneumothorax. A credentialed specialist should do any imaging such as point-of-care ultrasound or intervention such as needle decompression and chest thoracostomy per institutional protocol.

HISTORY AND PHYSICAL EXAMINATION

- The timing and acuity of signs and symptoms?
- History of any underlying lung pathologic conditions? Recent non-invasive positive pressure ventilation? Recent gastric or thoracic procedures?
- Physical exam should begin with an assessment of airway, breathing, and circulation
- Air entry in both lung fields? Accessory muscles usage?
- Warning signs: hypoxia, hemodynamic instability, deviation of the trachea, distended neck veins.

LABORATORY TESTING

- Lab blood testing is not required for the diagnosis of pneumothorax.
- ABG can be obtained in patients with moderate to severe hypoxia to assess for the degree of hypoxia and acidosis.
- Ancillary testing can be done once the patient is hemodynamically stable to rule out other comorbid conditions such as a troponin level to rule out cardiac ischemia.

IMAGING

- The use of imaging will depend on clinical stability. Suppose the patient is unstable with high clinical suspicion of pneumothorax (e.g., with absent breath sounds on one side of the thorax); in that case, thoracic surgery should be called for evaluation and management. Occasionally surgical teams would perform a focused lung ultrasound to confirm pneumothorax location and size and to guide placement of chest drain. However, if the patient is more stable, chest radiography can be used for confirmation of pneumothorax. Pneumothoraces will present as hyperlucency in the lung fields. Tension pneumothorax features include depressed hemidiaphragm, increased volume of hemithorax, and tracheal deviation.

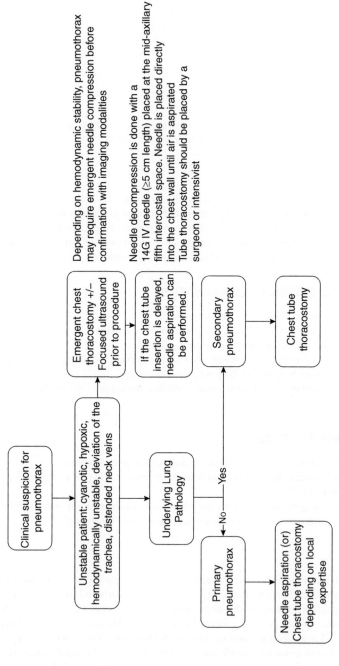

Fig. 26.4 Flowchart for management of pneumothorax.

- Chest X-ray: Most pneumothoraces will be detected on radiography; however, 20%-35% can be missed. Standing erect X-rays in inspiration are preferable; however, they are not practical in significantly symptomatic patients.
- Ultrasound: Mainly used as a guide to place drains by experienced providers. M-mode can be used to determine the movement of the lung within the rib interspace.
- Computed tomography (CT) chest without contrast can be done when there is a high clinical suspicion with negative ultrasound and X-ray.

THERAPEUTIC INTERVENTIONS

Management should begin with securing the airway, breathing, and circulation. Patients with pneumothorax are treated with supplemental oxygen and air removal from the pleural space, typically by chest tube thoracostomy. Thoracic surgery or critical care should be consulted immediately for intervention. Depending on the type and severity of pneumothorax, the treatment options may vary.

- Unstable patients require needle decompression immediately followed by chest tube placement.
- Stable patients with small pneumothoraces (<3 cm from the thoracic cupola to lung apex) who are significantly symptomatic can be treated with a catheter or tube thoracostomy. Otherwise, patients with small pneumothoraces can be given supplemental oxygen and observed. In patients with large pneumothoraces (≥3 cm), prompt drainage is indicated. Since secondary spontaneous pneumothorax is a complication of underlying lung disease, they may need to be treated together.

Re-expansion pulmonary edema is a known complication of fast, large volume pleural space evacuation. It presents as unilateral pulmonary edema after reinflation of the collapsed lung. This may occur if the drained volume is greater than 2 L, if suction is applied, or if the air is drained too rapidly. Many patients (especially primary spontaneous pneumothorax) present several days after onset of symptoms: the longer the elapsed period, the greater the risk of re-expansion pulmonary edema after evacuation.

STEPWISE APPROACH TO A PATIENT WITH ACUTE HYPOXIA FROM SUSPECTED PNEUMOTHORAX

Step 1: Assess airway, breathing, and circulation.

Step 2: Supplemental oxygen should be applied, and hypoxia should be corrected.

Step 3: In unstable patients with suspected tension pneumothorax, the surgical team or critical care team should be consulted for immediate bedside needle thoracostomy.

Step 4: In stable patients, a chest X-ray should be obtained to confirm the diagnosis and rule out other differentials such as pneumonia.

Step 5: ABG should be obtained in hypoxic patients. Acute coronary syndrome should be ruled out with troponin and EKG in appropriate cases.

Step 6: Surgical services or pulmonology should be consulted for possible chest tube placement and definitive management of pneumothorax.

CODING A PATIENT WITH ACUTE RESPIRATORY FAILURE FROM TENSION PNEUMOTHORAX

If the patient with suspected pneumothorax becomes acutely hypoxic, the first step would be to place the patient on 100% FiO_2 through a non-rebreather mask. Efforts should be made to avoid any forms of positive pressure ventilation since these can worsen the pneumothorax by increasing the inspiratory pressures. If non-invasive ventilation is unable to increase the oxygen saturation, and surgery service is not emergently available, the patient should be intubated for mechanical ventilation. The pneumothorax should be immediately treated using a needle decompression; this should be performed by a cardiothoracic surgeon or intensivist, depending on institutional credentialing and protocols. This can be done with a needle (14 or 16 G) directly inserted into the fifth intercostal space midaxillary line until the air is aspirated. Tube thoracostomy should be done by surgery or interventional radiology immediately afterward. If the patient's clinical status does not improve with decompression, the patient may require intubation followed by evaluating other causes of deterioration.

Suggested Reading

Imran JB, Eastman AL. Pneumothorax. *JAMA*. 2017;318(10):974. https://doi.org/10.1001/jama.2017.10476.

MacDuff A, Arnold A, Harvey J. Management of spontaneous pneumothorax: British Thoracic Society Pleural Disease Guideline 2010. *Thorax*. 2010;65(Suppl 2). https://doi.org/10.1136/thx.2010.136986.

Mendogni P, Vannucci J, Ghisalberti M, et al. Epidemiology and management of primary spontaneous pneumothorax: a systematic review. *Interact Cardiovasc Thorac Surg*. 2020;30(3):337–345. https://doi.org/10.1093/icvts/ivz290.

Zarogoulidis P, Kioumis I, Pitsiou G, et al. Pneumothorax: from definition to diagnosis and treatment. *J Thorac Dis*. 2014;6(Suppl 4):S372–S376. https://doi.org/10.3978/j.issn.2072-1439.2014.09.24.

CHAPTER 27

Hypoxia in a Patient With Myasthenia Gravis

Rahul R. Bollam ▪ Syed Arsalan Akhter Zaidi ▪ Firas Abdulmajeed ▪ Mohammad Adrish

Case Study

A rapid response code was activated for a patient who appeared to be in acute respiratory distress. On arrival of the condition team, the patient was found to be a 45-year-old male with a history of myasthenia gravis who was admitted to the hospital with possible pneumonia. The patient has been experiencing fever for one to two weeks associated with increased sputum production and purulence. On admission, the patient was empirically started on ceftriaxone and azithromycin. Overnight, the patient developed worsening blurry vision/double vision with worsening oxygen saturation requiring further assistance from the rapid response team.

VITAL SIGNS

Temperature: 96.5 °F, axillary
Blood Pressure: 110/75 mmHg
Heart Rate: 145 beats per min (bpm)
Respiratory Rate: 36 breaths per min
Oxygen Saturation: 80% on room air, 95% on 12 L/min (LPM) high flow nasal cannula.

FOCUSED PHYSICAL EXAMINATION

A quick examination showed a middle-aged gentleman in severe distress. He was alert and responsive to commands. Gurgling sounds could be heard coming from the patient's throat, and he was having difficulty swallowing or coughing up any secretions. His lung examination showed tachypnea, coarse breath sounds in all lung fields, and the use of accessory muscles of respiration. His cardiac exam showed tachycardia with normal heart sounds. No peripheral edema was appreciated. The patient had significant weakness of bilateral upper extremities and had considerable difficulty raising his arms against resistance. A detailed neurological exam was not done, given tenuous respiratory status.

THERAPEUTIC INTERVENTIONS

A cardiac monitor and pads were attached immediately. A 15 LPM non-rebreather facemask was applied, which improved the patient's oxygen saturation to 99%. An emergent chest X-ray was obtained at the bedside, which showed an opacity in the left lower lung. The clinical scenario was concerning for mucous plugging vs. aspiration, given the patient's poor respiratory effort and inability to clear secretions. Due to continued respiratory distress, the patient was intubated by an anesthesiologist at the bedside using rapid sequence intubation. Computed tomography (CT) chest was ordered to evaluate for pneumonia (Fig. 27.1), and the patient was taken to the intensive care unit after for therapeutic bronchoscopy and further management.

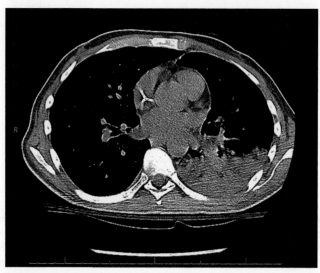

Fig. 27.1 Computed tomography scan showing the collapse of left lower lobe and questionable infiltrate because of suspected mucous plugging of left lower lobe bronchus.

FINAL DIAGNOSIS

Hypoxic respiratory failure secondary to mucous plugging in the setting of myasthenia crisis

Myasthenic Crisis

Myasthenia gravis is an autoimmune disorder affecting the neuromuscular (NM) junctions, which usually presents with painless, fluctuating weakness of the muscle groups and often begins with ocular signs (including ptosis and diplopia). Myasthenic crisis is a life-threatening condition defined as worsening myasthenic weakness requiring intubation or non-invasive ventilation. A myasthenic crisis will usually present with increasing generalized/bulbar weakness followed by respiratory failure. Myasthenic crisis can be precipitated by various factors, most common being infections, however, other conditions such as pregnancy/delivery, change in immunosuppressant medication, and certain medications can also trigger a crisis (Table 27.1).

The respiratory muscle strength should be monitored closely in patients with concern for a myasthenic crisis. If the clinical evaluation suggests impending respiratory failure, the patient can be electively intubated. The vital capacity (VC) and maximal inspiratory pressure are the main parameters used to monitor respiratory muscle strength. A fall in VC below 15-20 mL/kg, maximum insufflation capacity (MIC) between 0 and -10 cmH_2O, respiratory distress, worsening respiratory acidosis, inadequate clearance of secretions, and mucous plugging are indications for initiation of mechanical ventilation. It should be borne in mind that respiratory distress can "improve" as muscle weakness worsens, and clinicians should be aware that these patients are very near respiratory arrest. Non-invasive ventilation can be considered in patients with an adequate cough and in those who are expected to improve quickly. Close monitoring of respiratory status should be done if non-invasive ventilation is opted for.

NM blockade for rapid sequence intubation is somewhat challenging in patients with myasthenia. Depolarizing blockers like succinylcholine are safe for induction. However, patients with myasthenia are resistant to its effects given very few available acetylcholine receptors. These

TABLE 27.1 ■ **Some commonly used drugs that are associated with unmasking or worsening myasthenia gravis**

Drug class	Examples
Antibiotics	Aminoglycosides
	Fluoroquinolones
	Macrolides
Anesthetic agents	Non-depolarizing NM blockers
Cardiovascular drugs	Beta-blockers
	Procainamide
	Quinidine
Miscellaneous	Anti-PD-1 monoclonal antibodies
	Chloroquine
	Hydroxychloroquine
	Magnesium
	Penicillamine
	Glucocorticoids

patients require higher than normal doses of succinylcholine. In contrast, patients with myasthenia are overly susceptible to non-depolarizing NM blockers such as rocuronium or cisatracurium. For rapid sequence intubation, an experienced provider should use these drugs in incremental doses.

Mucous plugging because of inadequate cough and inability to clear secretions is a common cause of the respiratory collapse in myasthenia crisis. Occlusion of the airways leads to the collapse of alveoli and loss of lung volume. Aspiration of oral secretions can lead to pneumonia and should be kept in mind during management.

Suggested Approach to a Patient With Respiratory Failure From Myasthenic Crisis

We recommend the following approach to patients with myasthenia crisis who are suspected to be in respiratory failure. This approach can be employed in the emergency department, as management is universal.

FOCUSED HISTORY AND PHYSICAL

- The acuity of signs and symptoms
- History of use of precipitating medications including glucocorticoids for some other indication
- Physical exam should start with an assessment of airway, breathing, and circulation. Following signs should be looked for:
  - Inadequate clearance of oral secretions
  - Use of accessory muscles of respiration – the absence of this does not rule impending respiratory failure
- A focused neurological exam would show ptosis and weakness of extremities. Securing the airway should not be delayed for a neurological exam

LABORATORY TESTS

- Lab work is not necessary for the diagnosis of myasthenia crisis. Testing should be done to evaluate for consequences of the crisis
- Arterial blood gas – to evaluate for the degree of hypoxia and acidosis
- Complete blood count (CBC) – to assess for concomitant infection
- Electrolyte panel – to assess for the degree of acidosis and other concomitant electrolyte derangements

IMAGING STUDIES

- Chest X-ray is not required for the diagnosis of myasthenia crisis. It should be done to evaluate for complications such as pneumonia or collapsed lung lobe
- CT chest without contrast can be obtained; however, it should be done only after the airway has been secured and the patient has been stabilized. It can give a better idea about the presence and degree of any mucous plugging and can evaluate for aspiration and presence of concomitant pneumonia

THERAPEUTIC INTERVENTIONS

Myasthenia crisis is a medical emergency. We recommend that all patients should be assessed for airway, breathing, and circulation. Identification of impending respiratory arrest is critical as elective intubation is preferred over emergent intubation (Fig. 27.2). The airway should be secured with endotracheal intubation. Depolarizing NM blockers such as succinylcholine are safe but require high doses to overcome the limitation of very few acetylcholine receptors. Non-depolarizing NM blockers such as rocuronium and cisatracurium should be used in small incremental doses by an experienced provider, given the increased sensitivity of myasthenia patients toward these agents. Reversal of NM blockade should be considered afterward. Nebulized hypertonic saline can be given once the airway is secured and can help with pulmonary toilet. Antibiotics should be initiated if there is a suspicion of concomitant aspiration or pneumonia. Care should be taken in the choice of antibiotics (see Table 27.1). Any medications that can worsen the myasthenic crisis should be discontinued. Potassium, magnesium, and phosphate depletion can exacerbate the myasthenic crisis and should be repleted. Magnesium replacement should only be done enterally at a slow rate, as intravenous magnesium sulfate can further inhibit acetylcholine release. Patients should be transferred to the intensive care unit for pulmonary toilet and myasthenia-directed therapies. Non-invasive ventilation can be considered based on institutional guidelines in stable cases where rapid improvement is expected, and the patient has an adequate cough.

After establishing an airway, further management of the myasthenic crisis is done with intravenous immunoglobulins (IVIG) and/or plasma exchange (PE) therapy, with expert consultations. The details of these are not in the scope of this book, but briefly, a typical course of IVIG is 400 mg/kg for five days, and a typical course of PE is done over ten days, with a total of five exchanges done every other day. Patients who do not respond to one therapy can be tried on the other therapy. Some patients require corticosteroids in addition to the above. Cyclosporine can be used for patients who cannot tolerate corticosteroids. Thymectomy has shown promise as a therapy to reduce the frequency of myasthenic crisis, but large randomized controlled trials (RCTs) are still underway to investigate this.

SUMMARY OF A STEPWISE APPROACH TO PATIENTS WITH SUSPECTED MYASTHENIA CRISIS

Step 1: Assess airway, breathing, and circulation. Assess for signs of impending respiratory failure.

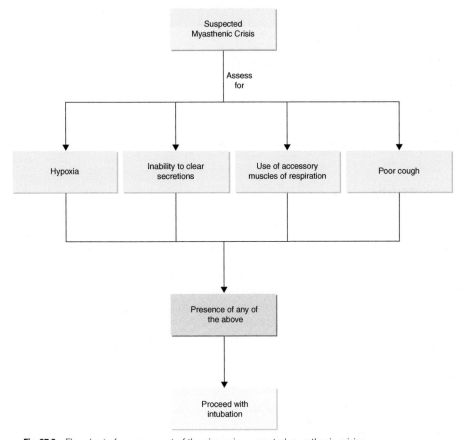

Fig. 27.2 Flowchart of management of the airway in suspected myasthenia crisis.

Step 2: Proceed with early endotracheal intubation if the deterioration of the condition is expected.

Step 3: Succinylcholine is safe for induction. However, it requires higher doses. Non-depolarizing NM blockers should be used with caution and in small incremental doses because of the higher sensitivity of these patients. Consider reversal of NM blockade with agents like sugammadex.

Step 4: Chest X-ray or CT chest should be obtained to evaluate for complications such as pulmonary collapse, aspiration, and pneumonia.

Step 5: Patient should be transferred to intensive care unit for bronchoscopy and pulmonary toilet.

Suggested Reading

Jayam Trouth A, Dabi A, Solieman N, Kurukumbi M, Kalyanam J. Myasthenia gravis: a review. *Autoimmune Dis.* 2012;2012:874680. https://doi.org/10.1155/2012/874680.

Nils E, Gilhus MD. Myasthenia gravis. *NEJM.* 2016. https://doi.org/10.1056/NEJMra1602678.

Shawn J, Bird MD, Joshua M, Levine M. Myasthenic crisis. UpToDate.com. https://www.uptodate.com/contents/myasthenic-crisis

Wendell LC, Levine JM. Myasthenic crisis. *Neurohospitalist.* 2011;1(1):16–22. https://doi.org/10.1177/1941875210382918.

CHAPTER 28

Hypoxia in a Patient With Sickle Cell Disease

Kainat Saleem ▪ Firas Abdulmajeed ▪ Mohammad Adrish

Case Study

A rapid response event was initiated by the bedside nurse for a patient with shortness of breath, hypoxia, and altered mental status. On prompt arrival of the rapid response team, it was noted that the patient was a 25-year-old female with a known history of sickle cell disease who was admitted to the hospital earlier in the evening for the evaluation of back pain, bilateral lower extremity pain, and chest pain. The patient's oxygen saturation was 95% on room air at the time of admission. A chest X-ray at the time was negative for any pulmonary infiltrates. The patient had been started on hypotonic fluids and had been receiving hydromorphone through a patient-controlled analgesia pump for the vaso-occlusive crisis. She had received roughly 700 cc of fluids by the time condition was called.

VITAL SIGNS

Temperature: 99.6 °F, axillary
Blood Pressure: 145/110 mmHg
Pulse: 136 beats per min (bpm) – sinus tachycardia on telemetry
Respiratory Rate: 38 breaths per min
Pulse Oximetry: 82% on 6 L/min (LPM) O_2 through a nasal canula

FOCUSED PHYSICAL EXAMINATION

A quick exam showed a young lady propped up in bed. She looked lethargic and in obvious respiratory distress. Appropriate personal protective equipment was established, and the patient was examined. She was able to follow simple commands appropriately. A pulmonary exam was significant for tachypnea. However, no wheezing or crackles were heard. Air movement was appropriate. Her cardiac and abdominal exam was benign.

INTERVENTIONS

The patient was immediately started on a non-rebreather face mask at 15 LPM O_2, which improved the oxygen saturation to 91%. A stat arterial blood gas (ABG) was obtained, which showed pH 7.25, paO_2 56 mmHg, pCO_2 32 mmHg, O_2 sat 89%, lactate 7.2 mmol/L, hemoglobin 6.3 g/dL. Stat chest X-ray was ordered, which showed a new infiltrate in the right lower lobe (Fig. 28.1). Stat blood cultures were obtained, and one dose of piperacillin/tazobactam was started. Then, 2 mg IV morphine was administered for dyspnea. The patient was given etomidate and succinylcholine and intubated at the bedside. The patient was sent for a stat computed tomography (CT) angiogram of the chest to rule out pulmonary embolism and was transferred to the intensive care unit for possible exchange transfusion.

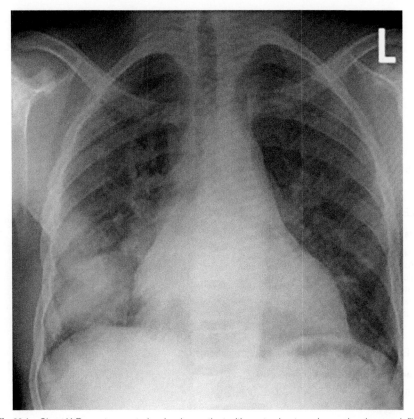

Fig. 28.1   Chest X-Ray anteroposterior view in a patient with acute chest syndrome showing new infiltrate.

FINAL DIAGNOSIS

Acute respiratory failure from acute chest syndrome as a complication of sickle cell disease.

Acute Chest Syndrome

Sickle cell disease is a hemoglobinopathy that occurs in roughly one out of every 365 Black or African American births, per Centers for Disease Control and Prevention (CDC) data. It is caused by a point mutation in the beta-globin allele of the hemoglobin gene that leads to the production of the mutated protein (hemoglobin S). Hemoglobin S is less soluble than normal human hemoglobin (hemoglobin A), leading to its precipitation with the red blood cells (RBCs) in areas of the body with low oxygen tension. This leads to distortion of the shape of the RBC, called "sickling," causing occlusion of the small capillaries, leading to intravascular hemolysis (Fig. 28.2). Sickle cell disease is also associated with splenic sequestration and extravascular hemolysis, which are beyond the scope of this chapter. Vasco-occlusion and subsequent end-organ ischemia are responsible for the significant number of acute complications seen with sickle cell anemia, which include pain crises, stroke, myocardial infarction, acute chest syndrome, venous thromboembolism, renal infarction, dactylitis, and priapism. This chapter will focus on acute chest syndrome, which is most common in the homozygous (SS) disease and carries worse outcomes in adults than children. See Table 28.1 for common causes and triggers of acute chest syndrome.

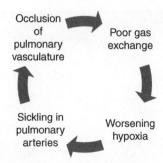

Fig. 28.2 Vicious circle of development of acute chest syndrome.

TABLE 28.1 ■ **Causes of acute chest syndrome**

Causes of acute chest syndrome
• Bone marrow necrosis and fat emboli
• Multi-organ failure syndrome
• Infection
• Asthma
• Inadequate ventilation secondary to oversedation vs. poor respiratory effort from chest pain
• *In situ* pulmonary thrombosis

TABLE 28.2 ■ **Differentials of acute chest syndrome**

Differentials of acute chest syndrome	
Cardiovascular	• Myocardial infarction • Pulmonary embolism
Pulmonary	• Pneumonia • Pulmonary infarct • Asthma exacerbation

DEFINITION AND DIAGNOSIS

Acute chest syndrome is defined as the development of a new pulmonary infiltrate involving at least one pulmonary segment on chest imaging AND one of the following:

- Fever – temperature ≥ 101.3 degrees
- A drop in oxygen saturation of 2% or greater compared to baseline on room air
- Tachypnea
- Increased work of breathing – use of accessory muscles of respiration, intercostal retractions
- Chest pain
- Cough
- Wheezing

Other life-threatening conditions that can present similarly should be ruled out in appropriate clinical settings (Table 28.2).

Suggested Approach to a Patient With Suspected Acute Chest Syndrome

For inpatient scenarios where acute chest syndrome is being suspected, we suggest the following approach based on a thorough literature search and updated guidelines. This can be applied to

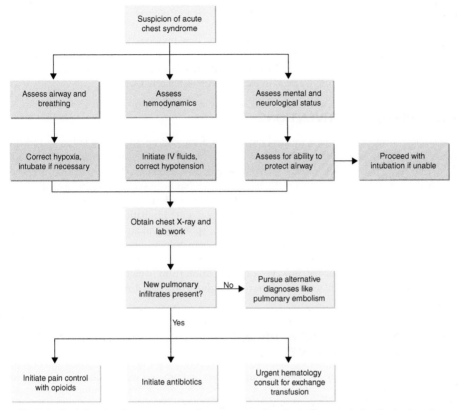

Fig. 28.3 Basic flowchart for assessment and management of a patient with suspected acute chest syndrome.

emergency room scenarios, as the management is universal. See Fig. 28.3 for a basic flow chart for assessment and management of a patient with suspected acute chest syndrome.

FOCUSED HISTORY AND PHYSICAL EXAMINATION

- The acuity of signs and symptoms
- History of acute chest syndrome and respiratory failure
- History of recent use of antiplatelet agents or anticoagulation
- Physical examination should begin with an assessment of airway, breathing, and circulation. Assess for signs of impending respiratory failure and hemodynamic compromise

LABORATORY TESTS

- Complete blood count (CBC) – to assess for the degree of anemia
- ABG, including lactate – to assess for the degree of hypoxia and acidosis
- Troponin, B-type natriuretic peptide, and electrolytes should be obtained if there is suspicion of other etiologies of chest pain and acute respiratory failure
- Type and screen – in anticipation of exchange transfusion

IMAGING STUDIES

- Chest X-ray should be obtained in all cases as new pulmonary infiltrates are one of the criteria for diagnosis of acute chest syndrome
- CT angiogram of the chest can be obtained if there is suspicion of pulmonary embolism, which is a common complication in patients with sickle cell disease

THERAPEUTIC INTERVENTIONS

Acute chest syndrome can be a medical emergency if impending respiratory failure is present. We recommend that all patients be assessed for airway, breathing, and circulation. Hypoxia should be corrected, and the airway should be secured with endotracheal intubation if necessary. A chest X-ray should be obtained once the airway has been secured. It can be challenging to differentiate between the infiltrates from acute chest syndrome and pneumonia; antibiotics should be initiated promptly. In patients who do not require intubation, pain control with opioids should be initiated as soon as possible to reduce splinting and atelectasis. Hypotonic fluids should be initiated to prevent hypovolemia. Urgent hematology consult should be obtained to prepare for exchange transfusion. Simple blood transfusion can be considered if exchange transfusion facilities are not available; however, expert opinion from hematology should be obtained prior. Nebulized bronchodilators and intravenous glucocorticoids have no role in acute chest syndrome.

SUMMARY OF STEPWISE APPROACH A PATIENT WITH SUSPECTED ACUTE CHEST SYNDROME

Step 1: Assess for airway and hemodynamic status and proceed with intubation if indicated. Correct hypotension.

Step 2: Obtain chest X-ray to identify pulmonary infiltrates.

Step 3: Initiate antibiotics, IV fluids, and aggressive pain control.

Step 4: Obtain lab work including CBC, electrolytes, blood gas, troponin, BNP, lactate, and type and screen.

Step 5: Obtain a CT angiogram to rule out pulmonary embolism if there is high clinical suspicion.

Step 6: Obtain urgent hematology consult for exchange transfusion and transfer the patient to intensive care unit for further care.

Suggested Reading

Desai PC, Ataga KI. The acute chest syndrome of sickle cell disease. *Expert Opin Pharmacother.* 2013;14(8):991–999. https://doi.org/10.1517/14656566.2013.783570.

Farooq S, Abu Omar M, Salzman GA. Acute chest syndrome in sickle cell disease. *Hosp Pract.* 2018;46(3):144–151. https://doi.org/10.1080/21548331.2018.1464363.

Joshua J Field, MD, Michael R DeBaun, MD M. Acute chest syndrome in adults with sickle cell disease. UpTo Date.com. https://www.uptodate.com/contents/acute-chest-syndrome-in-adults-with-sickle-cell-disease.

Paul RN, Castro OL, Aggarwal A, Oneal PA. Acute chest syndrome: sickle cell disease. *Eur J Haematol.* 2011;87(3):191–207. https://doi.org/10.1111/j.1600-0609.2011.01647.x.

CHAPTER 29

Hypoxia in a Patient With Massive Pleural Effusion

Rahul R. Bollam ■ Syed Zaidi ■ Mohammad Adrish ■ Firas Abdulmajeed

Case Study

A rapid response event was initiated by the bedside nurse for a patient who developed altered mentation and shallow breathing. On arrival of the condition team, the patient was found to be an 80-year-old female with a history of lung adenocarcinoma who presented a few hours ago for dyspnea on exertion and was found to have a large right-sided pleural effusion. Since admission, she had had progressive difficulty breathing, however, was awake and hemodynamically stable. The patient was planned for a thoracentesis under ultrasound guidance the following day.

VITAL SIGNS

Temperature: 37.4 °F, axillary
Blood Pressure: 130/90 mmHg
Pulse: 120 beats per min – sinus tachycardia on the cardiac monitor
Respiratory Rate: 20 breaths per min
Pulse Oximetry: 75% on room air, 90% on 10 L high-flow nasal cannula

FOCUSED PHYSICAL EXAMINATION

A quick exam showed an elderly cachectic female who appeared somnolent, not responsive to painful stimuli, using accessory muscles of respiration. No air entry was noted on the right lung field with dullness on percussion on auscultation. The remaining physical examination was unremarkable.

INTERVENTIONS

On a quick review of the prior charted data, admission chest radiography, and the history of lung adenocarcinoma, the patient appeared to be in acute hypoxic respiratory failure because of massive pleural effusion. A cardiac monitor and pads were attached for hemodynamic monitoring. Due to hypoxemic respiratory failure, decreased mentation, and inability to protect the airway, the patient was initially ventilated via Ambu-bag and then emergently intubated using the rapid-sequence-intubation technique. Stat chest X-ray and arterial blood gas were obtained. Arterial blood gas showed pH 7.40, pCO_2 40 mmHg, pO_2 60 mmHg, spO_2 90%, which was significant for hypoxemia. Chest X-ray showed an increase in the effusion size compared to admission (Fig. 29.1). Once the patient was stabilized, she was transferred to the intensive care unit for emergent thoracentesis.

FINAL DIAGNOSIS

Massive pleural effusion leading to acute hypoxic respiratory failure.

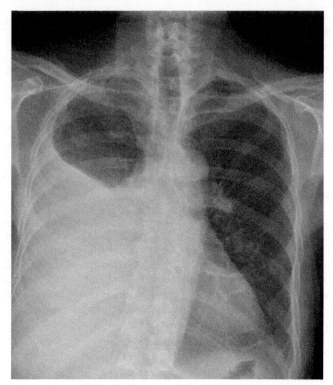

Fig. 29.1   Right-sided pleural effusion.

Massive Pleural Effusion

Pleural effusion is the build-up of excess fluid between the two layers of the pleura. The pleural space usually contains a small amount of pleural fluid, which is formed by pleural capillaries and drained through pleural lymphatics. This fluid helps in lubricating the pleural membranes and sliding motion between the two pleural layers during normal inspiratory and expiratory movements of the lung and chest wall. Pleural effusion accumulates if the pleural fluid formation is more than drainage or if the drainage is impeded in any way (Table 29.1 for different causes of pleural effusion).

- Increased fluid production:
  - Seen with increased intravascular hydrostatic pressure (as seen in heart failure), decreased colloid osmotic pressure (as seen in hypoproteinemia), or increased capillary permeability (seen in pneumonia or hypersensitivity reactions).
- Decreased rate of absorption:
  - Seen in lymphatic obstruction (because of a tumor or decreased venous pressure) or reduced pressure in pleural space (seen in atelectasis)

Pleural fluid can be characterized as either transudate or exudate (Table 29.2).

- Transudative:
  - Results from imbalances in hydrostatic and oncotic pressures.
  - Usually bilateral.
  - In most cases, thoracentesis is not required as a diagnostic tool.

TABLE 29.1 ■ Common causes of large-sized pleural effusions

Cause	Examples
Infectious	• Bacterial – Parapneumonic effusion, spontaneous bacterial empyema, tuberculous empyema • Viral infections – Viral pneumonia including SARS-CoV-2
Malignant	• Local malignancies – lung cancer, breast cancer, mesothelioma, lymphoma • Metastatic malignancies
Pulmonary	• Pulmonary embolism • Asbestos • Sarcoidosis • Trapped lung
Cardiac	• Heart failure • Constrictive pericarditis
Gastrointestinal	• Cirrhosis • Esophageal perforation • Acute pancreatitis • Abdominal surgery
Genitourinary	• Endometriosis • Ovarian hyperstimulation syndrome

- Exudative:
  - Results from pleural/lung inflammation, which increases capillary permeability or decreases lymphatic drainage.
  - Exudative fluid is unilateral in most cases but can be bilateral.
  - Thoracentesis is performed when the pleural fluid is suspected to be exudative.
  - Light's criteria: pleural fluid protein to serum protein ratio >0.5, pleural fluid lactate dehydrogenase (LDH) to serum LDH ratio >0.6, pleural fluid LDH greater than two-thirds times the upper limit of normal for serum LDH. If >1 of these criteria are met, then the pleural fluid is likely exudative.
  - Pleural fluid acidosis (pH <7.30, normal 7.6) can be caused by increased acid production by pleural fluid cells, and bacteria or decreased hydrogen efflux from pleural space can also point toward an exudative effusion.

Pleural effusions produce symptoms based on the acuity of accumulation. When accumulation occurs over time, it allows the lung to adapt, and patients can present with chronically worsening symptoms such as dyspnea on exertion. Rapid accumulation secondary to causes such as empyema and hemorrhage leads to acute onset shortness of breath, chest pain, hypoxia, and respiratory failure in some instances.

Suggested Approach to a Patient With Hypoxic Respiratory Failure From Pleural Effusion

For inpatient scenarios where massive pleural effusion is considered a primary cause of hypoxemic respiratory failure, we suggest the following general approach based on a thorough literature search. This can be expanded and used in emergency room situations as well, as the management is universal. See Fig. 29.2 for a flowchart of steps to evaluate and manage pleural effusion. The usual sequence of history taking, physical exam, investigations, and resuscitative interventions are often not followed during a rapid response; these measures often run parallel to each other in a

TABLE 29.2 ■ Characteristic findings in exudative pleural effusion from common causes as compared to a transudative effusion from cardiac failure

Cause	Appearance of Fluid	Type of Fluid	Predominant Cells In Fluid	White Blood Cell Count (cells/mcL)	Red Blood Cell Count (cells/ mcL)	Glucose	Comments
Cardiac Disease	Serous, straw-colored	Transudate	Few Serosal cells	<10,000	<1000	Equal to serum glucose	Elevated BNP in pleural fluid
Malignancy	Serous, often bloody	Exudate	Lymphocytes (mononuclear predominance)	1000-100,000	100 to several hundred thousand	Equal to serum levels	Positive results on cytologic examination
Uncomplicated Parapneumonic	Clear to turbid	Exudate	Polymorphonuclear cells	5000-25,000	<5000	Equal to serum levels	
Empyema	Turbid/purulent	Exudate	Polymorphonuclear cells	25,000-25,000	<5000	Less than serum levels	Putrid odor suggests anaerobic infection
Tuberculosis	Serous or sero-sanguineous	Exudate	Lymphocytes (mononuclear predominance)	5000-10, 000	<10,000	Equal to serum levels	Positive tuberculin test. Protein >4 g/dL
Rheumatoid	Turbid; greenish yellow	Exudate	Lymphocytes (either polymorphonuclear or mononuclear)	1000-20,000	<1000	<40g/dl	Secondary empyema is common; low complement, high RF are characteristic. Cholesterol in chronic effusions
Pulmonary Infarction	Serous to grossly bloody	Exudate	Red Blood Cells	1000-50,000 (either polymorphonuclear or mononuclear)	100-100,000	Equal to serum levels	
Esophageal Rupture	Turbid to purulent; red-brown	Exudate	No cells predominant	<5000 to >50,000	1000-10,000	Usually low	High amylase levels, effusions are commonly left sided
Pancreatitis	Turbid to sero-sanguinous	Exudate	No cells predominant	1000-50,000	1000-10,000	Equal to serum levels	Usually left sided, high amylase levels

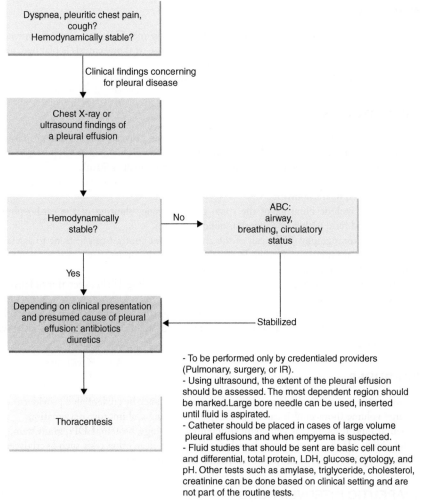

Fig. 29.2 Flowchart for evaluation and management of pleural effusion.

code situation. The following components of the rapid response are discussed in the traditional sequence only to ease understanding.

FOCUSED HISTORY AND PHYSICAL EXAMINATION

- Vital signs, looking for signs of hemodynamic instability like low blood pressure and hypoxemia. This will help decide whether emergent intubation is required
- Assessment of mental status would help determine the ability to protect the airway
- History of acute or chronic illnesses associated with effusion
- History of anticoagulant use as it may affect further management steps
- The physical examination will show dullness on percussion and decreased breath sounds on the affected side
- Signs of volume overload should be assessed

LABORATORY TESTS

- Basic labs such as complete blood count, comprehensive metabolic panel, and B-type natri-uretic peptides (BNP) can be done to look for the cause. If thoracentesis is planned, serum LDH should also be done for Light criteria.
- Blood cultures should be done if an infectious cause is suspected.

IMAGING STUDIES

- Chest X-ray should be done in all patients. The following caveats should be kept in mind:
  - A fluid collection of ≥200 mL is required for it to be visible on an anteroposterior chest X-ray. Lateral chest views can visualize collections as small as 50 mL.
  - Lateral decubitus X-ray can be used to estimate effusion size and determine if the fluid is loculated or free-flowing.
  - Features include blunting of the costo-phrenic angle, blunting of the cardio-phrenic angle, and fluid within horizontal or oblique fissures.
- Computed tomography (CT) scan of the chest without contrast can be done to assess the size of fluid accumulation further. It can also identify the underlying cause, such as pneu-monia, malignancy, infarct, and mediastinitis.
  - The gradient of fluid seen on the CT chest can help distinguish between transudative and exudative effusions
- Bedside lung ultrasound can be done by an intensivist or pulmonary team to detect fluid collections as small as 3-5 mL. It can also detect fluid septations and be used to assist with thoracentesis.

PROCEDURES

- Thoracentesis is routinely done under ultrasound guidance by credentialed providers.
- Large volume thoracentesis can help re-expand the lung and improve oxygenation.
- Pleural fluid tests include cell count differential, cytology, protein, LDH, gram stain, pH, and glucose. If the cause of the pleural effusion is not clear, other tests such as triglyceride, albumin, BNP, cholesterol, adenosine deaminase can be done.

THERAPEUTIC INTERVENTIONS

Patients should be assessed for airway, breathing, and circulation as guided by the airway, breath-ing, circulation approach of resuscitation. In cases where massive pleural effusion is causing sig-nificant respiratory compromise, patients should be intubated with a rapid-sequence intubation technique to improve oxygenation with higher levels of positive end-expiratory pressures. Once an advanced airway is established and the patient is stabilized, large volume aspiration of pleural fluid can relieve symptoms. Emergent thoracentesis (with or without chest tube placement) is done for patients with significant respiratory distress or cardiac decompensation. *Thoracentesis should only be performed by an experienced operator with proper institutional credentialing.*

Thoracentesis can be performed with a large-bore (21 G) needle. Bedside ultrasound improves the success rate and reduces complications. First, the extent of the pleural effusion should be assessed by percussion or imaging modalities. The insertion site should be marked (with the help of ultrasound), cleaned, and infiltrated with lidocaine. The needle should be inserted until the fluid is aspirated. If a catheter is going to be placed, the catheter should be inserted over the needle into the pleural space then the needle can be withdrawn. Vital signs should be monitored continuously, and the procedure should be discontinued if the patient experiences chest discomfort, dyspnea, or

TABLE 29.3 ■ **Possible complications from thoracentesis**

Pain at the needle insertion site	Bleeding: • Hematoma • Hemothorax • Hemoperitoneum
Pneumothorax (12%-30%)	Re-expansion pulmonary edema
Empyema	Soft tissue infection
Spleen or liver puncture	Vasovagal events
Seeding the needle tract with tumor	Retained intrapleural catheter fragments

hypotension. Coughing is normal and represents lung re-expansion. The patient should get a chest X-ray after thoracentesis to assess for any complications. (Refer to Table 29.3 for complications of thoracentesis.)

SUMMARY OF A STEPWISE APPROACH TO A PATIENT WITH MASSIVE PLEURAL EFFUSIO

Step 1: Assess hemodynamic status, mental status, and ability to protect the airway.

Step 2: If unstable, emergently start bag-mask ventilation and then establish an advanced airway for positive pressure ventilation.

Step 3: Once stabilized, patients should be assessed with stat imaging and laboratory tests, including chest X-ray and arterial blood gas. Other life-threatening causes of acute hypoxemia should be ruled out (refer to Chapter 21 for other causes of hypoxia).

Step 4: An experienced operator should perform emergent thoracentesis to relieve the fluid build-up.

Step 5: The patient should be monitored in the intensive care unit till stabilized.

Suggested Reading

He T, Oh S. Diagnostic approach to pleural effusions. *AME Med J.* 2018:23. https://doi.org/10.21037/amj.2018.12.02.

Jany B, Welte T. Pleural effusion in adults- etiology, diagnosis, and treatment. *Dtsch Arztebl Int.* 2019;116(21):377–386. https://doi.org/10.3238/arztebl.2019.0377.

Karkhanis VS, Joshi JM. Pleural effusion: diagnosis, treatment, and management. *Open Access Emerg Med.* 2012;4:31–52. https://doi.org/10.2147/OAEM.S29942.

CHAPTER 30

Hypoxia in a Morbidly Obese Patient

Abdelrhman M. Abo-zed ▦ Syed Arsalan Akhter Zaidi ▦ Firas Abdulmajeed ▦
Mohammad Adrish

Case Study

The bedside nurse initiated a rapid response event for a patient who went to sleep earlier in the evening and was unable to be aroused by verbal commands. The nurse noted his oxygen saturation drop as low as 78% and prolonged episodes of apnea lasting up to 20 s. On prompt arrival of the rapid response team, the patient was given a sternal rub, to which he responded by briefly opening his eyes but promptly went back to sleep. He was a 40-year-old obese male with a known history of heart failure with a preserved ejection fraction, hypertension, coronary artery disease. He was admitted earlier for altered mental status. On admission, it was noted that the patient's arterial blood gas (ABG) showed a pH of 7.28, PCO_2 of 69 mmHg, PO_2 of 72 mmHg, and bicarbonate level of 35 meq/L. He was not on any diuretics.

VITAL SIGNS

Temperature: 98.2 °F, axillary
Blood Pressure: 155/97 mmHg
Heart Rate: 75 beats per min (bpm) – regular rhythm
Respiratory Rate: 12 breaths per min
Pulse Oximetry: 78% on room air, placed on a 15 L/min non-rebreather up to 94%.

FOCUSED PHYSICAL EXAMINATION

A quick exam showed a morbidly obese male with a thick neck who was extremely somnolent. Pertinent findings on the exam included intermittent loud snoring, choking during sleep, apneic episodes, fatigue, and impaired concentration. His heart sounds were normal, and lungs were clear to auscultation with diminished breath sounds bilaterally. His abdomen was distended but had no rigidity or guarding, bowel sounds heard. Of note, his pupils were equal round and reactive.

INTERVENTIONS

A cardiac monitor and pads were attached to the patient. 15 L of oxygen was administered through a non-rebreather mask which improved oxygen saturation to 96%. Stat ABG was ordered, which showed pH 7.18, pO_2 85 mmHg, pCO_2 90 mmHg, lactate 2.9, SpO_2 96% on 15 L non-rebreather. A BMP drawn at the same time showed a bicarbonate level of 26. The patient started to wake up slightly and was protecting his airway appropriately; thus, a decision was made to try non-invasive bi-level positive airway pressure (BiPAP) ventilation for him. BiPAP was started at 16 cm H_2O IPAP, 6 cm H_2O EPAP, and 100% FiO_2 to manage the acute on chronic respiratory acidosis, with a goal to be transitioned to continuous positive airway pressure (CPAP) overnight. Stat chest X-ray was obtained, which was negative for any acute pulmonary pathologic condition.

A pulmonary consult was requested to evaluate the patient for formal sleep testing and further management. The patient was transferred to the intensive care unit (ICU) for closer monitoring and escalation of airway management if needed.

FINAL DIAGNOSIS

Obesity hypoventilation syndrome with acute decompensation.

Obesity Hypoventilation Syndrome

Obesity Hypoventilation Syndrome (OHS) is defined as the presence of daytime alveolar hypoventilation with arterial $paCO_2$ >45 mmHg and paO_2 <70 mmHg in an obese individual with body mass index (BMI) >30 kg/m², which cannot be attributed to any other mechanical, neuromuscular, or metabolic conditions associated with alveolar hypoventilation. OHS is associated with increased cardiovascular morbidity and mortality, which might be secondary to changes in respiratory dynamics and the contribution of obesity to other systemic illnesses. Consequently, early detection and treatment are crucial to minimizing these adverse effects.

PATHOPHYSIOLOGY

Patients with increased body weight (especially with BMI >30 kg/m²) experience increased demands on the respiratory system to maintain adequate ventilation. When considering respiratory dynamics, specific ventilation challenges associated with obese patients include a decrease in total lung capacity (TLC), functional residual capacity (FRC), and vital capacity (VC), as well as increases in pleural pressure and upper and lower airway resistance. There are compensatory mechanisms triggered to maintain adequate ventilation in obesity, but with rising BMI, these mechanisms can fail and give way to OHS. Although 90% of all patients with OHS have some degree of obstructive sleep apnea (OSA), at least 10% of OHS patients have no obstructive symptoms and have pure sleep hypoventilation syndrome.

Although the complete pathophysiology of OHS is not known, several factors are known to produce the symptoms of this disease; some of these are mentioned below:
- Sleep-disordered breathing, including apneic/hypopniec episodes, altered respiratory mechanics, and impaired ventilator control.
- Reduced clearance of carbon dioxide during sleep.
- Hypoxemia during sleep.
- Impaired pulmonary mechanics, including ventilation/perfusion mismatching, especially in lower lobes and decreased respiratory muscle strength.
- Impaired ventilatory control because of reduced neural drive, reduced ventilatory responsiveness, carbon dioxide overproduction, and leptin resistance.

Some risk factors that contribute to the development of OHS are:
- Significant increase in body weight in a small span of time
- Considerable increase in waist to hip ratio (leading to central obesity)
- Reduced lung function because of obesity
- Reduced respiratory muscles strength
- Presence of OSA

Clinical manifestations of OHS are similar to signs and symptoms of OSA, as 90% of patients with OHS have OSA. Clinical manifestations of OSA are given in Table 30.1. Some patients with OHS might present with acute on chronic respiratory failure, which might be triggered by other systemic illnesses leading to excess burden of disease on the body and failure of some compensatory mechanisms which were previously maintaining adequate ventilation.

TABLE 30.1 ■ Clinical features as seen in patients with OHS and OSA

OBESE	Most patients have BMI >30 with central obesity
HYPERSOMNOLENCE	Related to CO_2 retention and CO_2 narcosis
LOUD SNORING	Associated with choking episodes during sleep, fatigue
IMPAIRED CONCENTRATION/MEMORY	Mainly caused by hyper-somnolence
SMALL OROPHARYNX/THICK NECK	Noted on physical exam

TABLE 30.2 ■ Laboratory tests in patients with obesity hypoventilation syndrome

Elevated serum bicarbonate (>27 meq/L)	Secondary to chronic hypercapnia. However, it is important to rule out other causes of elevated serum bicarbonate levels
Daytime hypercapnia (arterial pressure of carbon dioxide [$PaCO_2$] >45 mmHg)	Consistent with hypoventilation, again it is important to rule out other causes
Daytime hypoxemia (PaO_2 <70 mmHg)	• Nocturnal desaturations might be seen as well • Normal A-a gradient. However, mild variation of gradient might be seen in underlying parenchymal or vascular lung disease
Polycythemia	Usually a late manifestation

Many patients with OHS remain undiagnosed and present late in the course of their disease. This leads to presentation with manifestations of end-stage disease, which include:

- **Severe hypoxemic hypercapnic respiratory failure:** Patients may have chronic stable symptoms of chronic hypercapnic respiratory failure. This can be very commonly mistaken with chronic obstructive pulmonary disease (COPD) or asthma despite an absence of obstruction on pulmonary function tests (PFT).
- **Daytime hypoxemia** and significant and sustained reductions in overnight oximetry are noted (peripheral O_2 saturation <80%) – which is rarely seen in OSA or obesity alone (Table 30.2).
- **Right heart failure from pulmonary hypertension** can also be seen as a late complication from OHS/OSA. The findings of right heart failure include dyspnea on exertion, elevated jugular venous pressure, hepatomegaly, and pedal edema, as well as facial plethora from polycythemia.

PULMONARY FUNCTION TESTS

PFTs might be completely normal in these patients or might show restrictive findings because of obesity. These may include reduced FVC and FEV1, but the FEV1/FVC ratio is preserved. Also seen is a decrease in TLC, FRC, and VC. PFTs might not be diagnostic of OHS, but help exclude other obstructive or restrictive diseases in these patients

IMAGING STUDIES

Imaging is not required for the diagnosis of OHS, but echocardiography can evaluate for evidence of right heart failure, which is a late complication of OHS. Chest radiograph might show elevation of both Hemi-diaphragms because of the obese abdomen, and the heart may be enlarged because of right ventricular hypertrophy.

Suggested Approach to a Patient With Suspected OHS With Acute Decompensation

For patients suspected of acute on chronic respiratory failure secondary to OHS/OSA, we suggest the following approach based on a thorough literature review. This approach can be utilized in the emergency department as well since management is universal.

FOCUSED HISTORY AND PHYSICAL EXAM

- Assess for presence of symptoms, the timing of onset, and duration of signs and symptoms.
- Evaluate for risk factors that might contribute to the development of OHS/OSA.
- History findings such as chest pain, fever, lower extremity edema, and palpitations could indicate a concomitant illness or complication.
- Physical exam should begin with an assessment of airway, breathing, and circulation.
- A lung exam would show end-expiratory wheezing if the patient has concomitant COPD exacerbation; refer to Chapter 23 for further reading on COPD exacerbation.
- Evaluate for other systemic diseases which might have contributed to the acute on chronic respiratory failure in OHS.

LABORATORY TESTS

- BMP to evaluate for serum bicarbonate – a level above 27 meq/L is indicative of chronic respiratory failure
- ABG to look at arterial pressure of carbon dioxide and oxygen, daytime levels of $PaCO_2$ >45 mmHg, and PaO_2 <70 mmHg are diagnostic criteria of OHS if seen in obese patients without other causes of respiratory failure.
- CBC to evaluate for polycythemia, which is commonly seen in OHS and OSA.

IMAGING STUDIES

- Chest X-ray – should be obtained in all hypoxic patients to evaluate for pneumonia, pulmonary edema, pleural effusion, pneumothorax
- CT angiogram chest – can be obtained if there is clinical suspicion of pulmonary embolism

EKG

- There is no use of EKG in diagnosing OHS/OSA, but this can be done to rule out cardiac ischemia in patients who cannot provide history.

THERAPEUTIC INTERVENTIONS

Management begins with the assessment of the airway, breathing, and circulation. The capability of the patient to maintain the airway should be assessed. OHS is one of the few conditions with known benefits from non-invasive ventilation (NIV). The assessment for the need for invasive airway via endotracheal intubation should be made as soon as possible. If the patient does not require emergent intubation, a short trial of BiPAP should be initiated after ensuring that the

TABLE 30.3 ■ **Management options of OHS/OSA**

First-line Therapy	Second-line Therapy	Therapies of No Use!
Positive Pressure Ventilation – Continuous positive airway pressure (CPAP) is the typical mode chosen for treatment for OHS plus OSA, while BiPAP, usually in the spontaneous–timed mode, is indicated in those who fail CPAP.	If weight loss efforts fail, **bariatric surgery** might be an option for people who meet the criteria for surgery. Weight loss after bariatric surgery will lead to changes in respiratory mechanics and muscle function to improve ventilation.	**Respiratory stimulants** like Medroxyprogesterone or Acetazolamide have been studied. However, these do not affect the pathogenic contributors to OHS, in particular the recurrent upper airway collapse that occurs during sleep in patients who have coexisting obstructive sleep apnea and thus are of no real use in OHS.
Weight loss directly reverts the mechanisms which initially contributed to the development of OHS. It improves alveolar ventilation, improves nocturnal oxyhemoglobin saturation, decreases the frequency of respiratory events, and improves pulmonary function. Weight loss also reduces the risk of cardiopulmonary complications.	**Tracheostomy**, although rare now since the advent of positive pressure ventilation devices, was previously used for patients to bypass the excessive pressure in the upper airway seen in obese individuals.	**Oxygen alone** is not useful in treating OHS/OSA; although it might treat hypoxemia, it does not affect the altered chemo responsiveness, nocturnal upper airway occlusion, and impaired respiratory mechanics seen in OHS and OSA.

patient has no contraindication to NIV as a bridge to CPAP. Hypoxia should be corrected; oxygen can be delivered via NIV. ABG should be repeated after 1-2 h of BiPAP therapy to assess for CO_2 washout. CPAP is the treatment of choice for patients with OHS/OSA. Patients on NIV should be monitored closely in the first few hours, ideally in an ICU setting or a step-down unit. After the patient has been stabilized, efforts should be directed toward treating the underlying illness such as pneumonia or COPD exacerbation that led to decompensation. See Table 30.3 for further management options for OSH.

STEPWISE APPROACH TO A PATIENT WITH ACUTE RESPIRATORY FAILURE IN THE SETTING OF OHS

Step 1: Assess airway, breathing, and circulation.

Step 2: If no contraindication to NIV, BiPAP should be initiated for respiratory support initially, as a bridge to CPAP.

Step 3: Lab work including CBC, BMP, and ABG should be obtained to assess for leukocytosis, acidosis, hypoxia, CO_2 retention, and electrolyte derangements.

Step 4: A chest X-ray should be obtained to evaluate for concomitant illnesses such as pneumonia, pulmonary edema, and pneumothorax.

Step 5: Electrocardiogram (EKG) should be obtained in tachycardic patients to evaluate for atrial arrhythmias.

Step 6: Patients on NIV should be monitored closely for the first few hours; endotracheal intubation should be pursued if the patient does not show signs of improvement or clinically deteriorates.

Step 7: Once the patient has been stabilized, effort should be directed toward identifying and treating the illness that led to acute decompensation.

Suggested Reading

Ayachi J, Ahmed K, Rahma BJ, et al. Management of acute exacerbations of obesity-hypoventilation syndrome (AE/OHS): toward an early goal-directed therapy algorithm. *Eur Respir J*. 2016;48(Suppl 60):PA2144. https://doi.org/10.1183/13993003.congress-2016.PA2144.

Masa JF, Pépin JL, Borel JC, Mokhlesi B, Murphy PB, Sánchez-Quiroga MÁ. Obesity hypoventilation syndrome. *Eur Respir Rev*. 2019;28(151):1–14. https://doi.org/10.1183/16000617.0097-2018.

Powers MA. The obesity hypoventilation syndrome. *Abdom Surg*. 2008:1723–1730.

CHAPTER 31

Hypoxia in a Patient With Hemoptysis

Rahul R. Bollam ▓ Mohammad Adrish ▓ Firas Abdulmajeed

Case Study

The bedside nurse initiated a rapid response event for a patient who developed large volume hemoptysis along with dyspnea. On arrival of the condition team, the patient was coughing bright red blood and visibly dyspneic, using accessory muscles of respiration. Per report from the nurse, the patient was an 80-year-old male with a history of atrial fibrillation, admitted two days ago for exacerbation of chronic obstructive pulmonary disease. Over the last few minutes, the patient developed hemoptysis and had coughed up approximately 50-100 mL of blood.

VITAL SIGNS

Temperature: 100.4 °F, axillary
Blood Pressure: 90/50 mmHg
Heart Rate: 120 beats per min (bpm) – sinus tachycardia on the monitor
Respiratory Rate: 35 breaths per min
Oxygen Saturation: 70% on room air, 90% on 12 L/min (LPM) high flow nasal cannula

FOCUSED PHYSICAL EXAMINATION

A quick exam showed an older adult who appeared visibly dyspneic and was using accessory muscles of respiration. Crackles were present in the left lower lung field. Heart auscultation was normal except for tachycardia, and his abdomen was soft, non-tender, and non-distended. The remaining examination was unremarkable.

INTERVENTIONS

A cardiac monitor and pads were attached to the patient. Fifteen LPM oxygen was administered through a non-rebreather mask, which improved oxygen saturation to 96%. Due to concerns for airway protection, and the patient's continued hemoptysis, he was intubated by the anesthesiologist on call. He was started on intravenous (IV) fluid resuscitation. Stat arterial blood gas was ordered, which showed pH 7.25, pO_2 92 mmHg, pCO_2 60 mmHg, lactate 4.9 mmol/L. Stat chest X-ray, complete blood count (CBC), prothrombin time, and partial thromboplastin time were done. The patient was on warfarin for his atrial fibrillation, which led to an international normalized ratio of 2.9; this was reversed acutely with 4-factor prothrombin complex concentrate (Kcentra) and 5 mg of IV vitamin K. His chest X-ray revealed multiple opacities in the left lung (Fig. 31.1). The patient was placed in the left lateral position (diseased lung down to prevent the gravity-guided blood pooling in the healthy right lung) and was transferred to the intensive care unit (ICU) for further management and intervention.

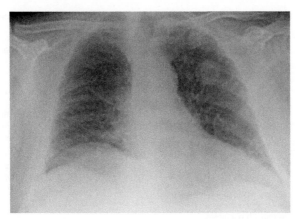

Fig. 31.1   Chest X-ray with multiple left-sided pulmonary mass-like lesions.

FINAL DIAGNOSIS

Acute hypoxic respiratory failure secondary to hemoptysis.

Hemoptysis

Hemoptysis is the spitting up of blood derived from the respiratory system (parenchyma vs. airways) because of pulmonary or bronchial hemorrhage. There are two vascular circulations coursing through the lungs: the pulmonary and the bronchial systems. The low-pressure pulmonary arterial system carries blood from the right ventricle to the lungs. The high-pressure bronchial circulation originates from the aorta and provides arterial blood to the tracheobronchial tree. The bronchial arteries are the site of bleeding in >90% of cases. The components of each of these systems are described in Fig. 31.2.

It is crucial to differentiate hemoptysis from bleeding originating in the nasopharynx, oropharynx, larynx, and gastrointestinal (GI) tract. Factors that suggest an ear, nose, and throat (ENT) or upper-airway source are blood visualized in the nares and the sensation of blood in the posterior pharynx. ENT physicians can perform nasolaryngoscopy at the bedside in patients with concerns for bleeding in these sites. Coffee ground emesis and a history of vomiting/regurgitation suggest GI source of the bleed.

Traditionally, hemoptysis had been categorized based on volume and blood expectorated over 24 h. More than 600 cc blood loss in less than 4 h has been associated with high mortality rates. Complications are associated with hypoxia rather than exsanguination. The classification of hemoptysis is as follows:

1. Non-massive hemoptysis is defined as <100 mL of blood loss and includes blood-streaked sputum
2. Massive hemoptysis (also called life-threatening hemoptysis) is a term used when hemoptysis results in a life-threatening event, including significant airway obstruction, significant abnormal gas exchange, or hemodynamic instability. Although is it difficult to quantify the amount of blood lost in massive hemoptysis, traditionally, the following cut-offs are used:
   a. ≥ 150 ml blood expectorated in a 24 h period, OR
   b. Bleeding at a rate of ≥ = 100 mL/h

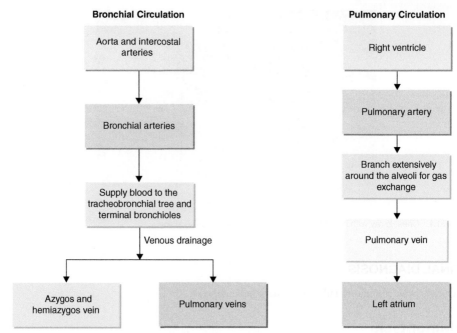

Fig. 31.2 The blood circulation systems in the lungs.

Common causes of hemoptysis include:
1. **Malignancy (most common cause):** Primary lung carcinoma, metastatic carcinoma
2. **Infection:** Bronchiectasis (such as cystic fibrosis), lung abscess, necrotizing pneumonia, aspergilloma, tuberculosis, and septic pulmonary emboli
3. **Vascular:** Granulomatosis with polyangiitis, pulmonary artery aneurysm
4. **Iatrogenic:** Placement of pulmonary artery catheter, transbronchial biopsy, trachea-innominate fistula.

Suggested Approach to a Patient With Massive Hemoptysis

For a patient with life-threatening hemoptysis, we suggest the following approach to evaluate and treat the acute event. The usual sequence of history taking, physical exam, investigations, and resuscitative interventions are often not followed during a rapid response; these measures often run parallel to each other in a code situation. The following components of the rapid response are discussed in the traditional sequence only to ease understanding.

HISTORY AND PHYSICAL EXAMINATION

- Timing of onset and duration of symptoms
- Past medical history, specifically history of lung disease and malignancy
- Medication history, specifically use of anticoagulants
- History of recent procedures

- Physical exam should begin with the evaluation of airway, breathing, and circulation
- The presence of bleeding from other sites could indicate a systemic disorder rather than a focal pulmonary problem, although it is unusual to develop life-threatening hemoptysis from coagulopathy

LABORATORY TESTS

- CBC – to evaluate for the degree of anemia and to evaluate for infections
- Coagulation profile – including fibrinogen to evaluate for coagulopathy and DIC
- Comprehensive metabolic panel, ABG, and lactate – to assess for the degree of acidosis in respiratory failure
- Blood type and screen

IMAGING STUDIES

- Chest radiograph: Initial imaging modality, however, limited utility in these cases. These could help lateralize bleeding.
- Computed tomography (CT) chest with contrast/CT angiography: CT helps identify the bleeding source and underlying etiologies. Angiography can help identify the site of bleeding in case of active bleeding.
- Bronchoscopy: This is the primary method of identifying the bleeding site and examining the airways. Bronchoscopy is pursued after securing the airway with endotracheal intubation and stabilization of the patient.

INTERVENTIONS

Management begins with the assessment of the airway, breathing, and circulation. The capability of the patient to maintain the airway should be assessed. In most patients with life-threatening hemoptysis, intubation is required to protect the airway and reduce the risk of aspirating blood. Indications for intubation are ineffective cough (gurgling, inability to clear blood from airway) or worsening respiratory failure. Preferably, large endotracheal tubes should be used to facilitate bronchoscopy. While the team is preparing for intubation, the patient should be continuously suctioned and pre-oxygenated. If the bleeding site is known, intubation into the non-bleeding lung can minimize further aspiration and provide ventilation. Patients should be positioned to ensure that the suspected bleeding lung is in the dependent position, which can be deduced from history, physical examination, and prior imaging. This is to protect the non-bleeding lung since spillage of blood could impair gas exchange. If the bleeding site is unknown or both lungs are bleeding, the patient should be placed head up. Coagulopathy should be reversed appropriately depending on what anticoagulant the patient is taking. Platelet transfusion should be done in those with platelets <50,000 cells/mm³.

Once the patient has been stabilized appropriately, efforts should be made to evaluate the cause of hemoptysis. For patients who are intubated, bronchoscopy should be done to identify the bleeding source. In patients who are not intubated and clinically stable, the patient can be taken for CT chest with contrast or angiography. If the bleeding source is identified, the patient could undergo interventional embolization before transferring to the ICU for closer monitoring.

For patients in whom definitive management is delayed, nebulized tranexamic acid can be used. Tranexamic acid is an anti-fibrinolytic agent that has shown some benefit in patients with hemoptysis but has not been studied specifically in life-threatening hemoptysis. The dosage for this medication is 500 mg inhaled through a nebulizer. In these patients, non-invasive ventilation is a high risk for aspirating blood. In patients who refuse intubation, high flow nasal oxygen is an option. The management algorithm can be found in Fig. 31.3.

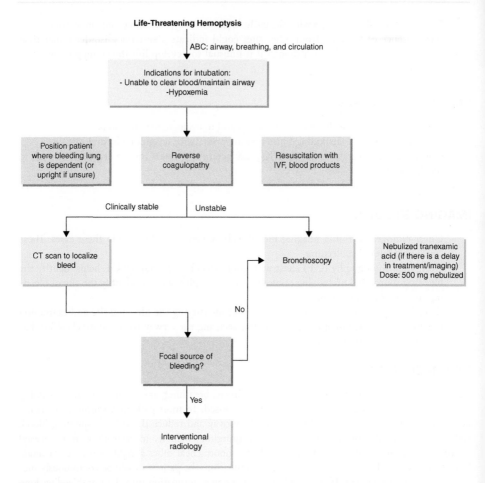

Fig. 31.3 Flowchart of management of a patient with life-threatening hemoptysis.

STEPWISE APPROACH TO THE MANAGEMENT OF A PATIENT WITH MASSIVE HEMOPTYSIS

Step 1: Assess airway, breathing, and circulation.

Step 2: Airway should be secured with endotracheal intubation in patients with hypoxia or inability to protect the airway.

Step 3: Coagulopathy should be reversed with an appropriate agent.

Step 4: Bronchoscopy vs. CT angiogram should be pursued after emergent consultation with pulmonology vs. thoracic surgery vs. interventional radiology.

Suggested Reading

Davidson K, Shojaee S. Managing massive hemoptysis. *Chest.* 2020;157(1):77–88. https://doi.org/10.1016/j.chest.2019.07.012.

Gagnon S, Quigley N, Dutau H, Delage A, Fortin M. Approach to hemoptysis in the modern era. *Can Respir J.* 2017;2017:1565030. https://doi.org/10.1155/2017/1565030.

Ittrich H, Bockhorn M, Klose H, Simon M. The diagnosis and treatment of hemoptysis. *Dtsch Arztebl Int.* 2017;114(21):371–381. https://doi.org/10.3238/arztebl.2017.0371.

CHAPTER 32

Facial Swelling in a Patient After Bronchoscopy

Rahul R. Bollam ■ Syed Arsalan Akhter Zaidi ■ Kainat Saleem

Case Study

A rapid response event was activated for a patient who appeared to be in acute distress. On arrival of the rapid response team, the patient was short of breath with visible swelling of the face. Per the bedside registered nurse, the patient was a 40-year-old male with a history of chronic obstructive pulmonary disease, admitted four days ago for right lower lobe pneumonia with a new right hilar mass. During the hospital course, he was seen by pulmonary and oncology teams, and bronchoscopy with ultrasound-guided biopsy of the mass was performed earlier in the day. In the last 4-5 h, the patient had become increasingly dyspneic and developed progressive swelling of the face, which had not improved with IV antihistamines and a dose of IV methylprednisolone.

VITAL SIGNS

Temperature: 98.5 °F, axillary
Blood Pressure: 140/70 mmHg
Heart Rate: 110 beats per min (bpm)
Respiratory Rate: 30 breaths per min
Oxygen Saturation: 96% on room air

FOCUSED PHYSICAL EXAMINATION

A quick exam showed a middle-aged male lying in bed in apparent distress; he was tachypneic but not using accessory muscles of respiration. Both lung fields were clear with equal air entry bilaterally. Facial swelling was noticed along with pitting with a crackling sensation under the skin. A crackling sensation was detected on the right side of the chest as well. The remaining physical examination was unremarkable.

WORKING DIAGNOSIS

Subcutaneous emphysema, angioedema.

INTERVENTIONS

A cardiac monitor and pads were attached. Stat chest X-ray and arterial blood gas were ordered. Chest X-ray was significant for subcutaneous air in the right chest wall and neck regions (Fig. 32.1). Arterial blood gas was within normal limits. Based on available information, the most likely diagnosis was subcutaneous emphysema in the setting of a recent bronchoscopy procedure. Since the patient was saturating well on room air, did not require supplemental oxygen

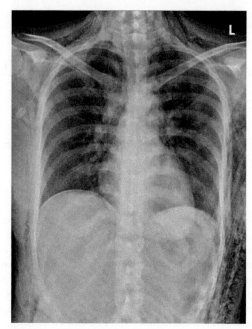

Fig. 32.1   Air in the right chest wall and neck subcutaneous tissue.

therapy, and was protecting his airway, he was retained on the current unit with a low threshold for intensive care unit (ICU) transfer.

FINAL DIAGNOSIS

Subcutaneous emphysema as a complication of bronchoscopic procedure

Subcutaneous Emphysema

Subcutaneous emphysema is the infiltration of air into the subcutaneous tissue under the skin. Skin is comprised of two primary layers, namely the epidermis and dermis. Below the dermal layer lies the subcutaneous tissue, which is composed mainly of fascia and fatty tissue. The air in the subcutaneous tissue may indicate that some air is occupying another deeper area within the body, where it is not physiologically present. Such air/emphysema can expand to other compartments of the body and may lead to pneumomediastinum, pneumoretroperitoneum, and pneumothorax (Fig. 32.2).

These patients can remain asymptomatic or present with sudden, painless soft tissue swelling with a predilection for the upper chest, neck, and face. Difficulty breathing is present occasionally.

Crepitations on skin palpation are pathognomonic of subcutaneous emphysema and are typically painless. If pneumomediastinum is present, then patients can present with precordial chest pain. Another typical finding in pneumomediastinum is the crackling sound with heartbeat (Hamman crunch). Patients with pneumothorax may present with pleuritic chest pain and shortness of breath. A few different causes of subcutaneous emphysema are reviewed in Table 32.1.

Subcutaneous emphysema can also be seen as a component of Boerhaave syndrome, which is characterized by esophageal rupture caused by excessive and forceful vomiting. Symptoms include vomiting followed by chest pain and subcutaneous emphysema; the presence of all three of these forms the Mackler triad.

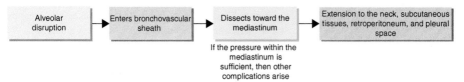

Fig. 32.2 Mechanism underlying spontaneous subcutaneous emphysema.

TABLE 32.1 ■ Categories of subcutaneous emphysema based on cause

Common Causes of Subcutaneous Emphysema		
Traumatic Injury	**Infectious**	**Spontaneous**
The most common cause of subcutaneous emphysema	Commonly seen in necrotizing fasciitis	These are relatively uncommon
Penetrating injury: • Rupture can arise from direct trauma, blunt deceleration forces, or fractures that would allow air to pass through the respiratory tract, gastrointestinal tract, or sinuses. Iatrogenic: • It can be caused by procedures such as chest tube insertion, endotracheal intubation/bronchoscopy, or esophagogastroduodenoscopy. • Following thoracic surgery, the development of subcutaneous emphysema should raise suspicion for a bronchial leak.	• Some soft tissue infections (such as clostridium and Bacteroides species) produce gases that can accumulate in the subcutaneous tissue. • This tends to occur in the extremities, and the area will appear erythematous with warmth/tenderness.	• It is defined as pneumomediastinum without surgical/medical procedures. The accepted explanation is alveolar rupture into the pulmonary vascular sheaths because of an increase in intra-alveolar pressure (refer to Fig. 1)

Suggested Approach to a Patient With Suspected Subcutaneous Emphysema

For a patient who develops subcutaneous emphysema while in the hospital, we suggest the following approach to evaluate and treat the acute event. This can be expanded and used in emergency room situations as well. These suggestions are based on thorough literature research for the management of subcutaneous emphysema (Fig. 32.3 for a flowchart of management).

FOCUSED HISTORY AND PHYSICAL

- Timing of onset and duration of signs and symptoms.
- Progression of symptoms over time.
- Presence of red flags such as chest pain, tenderness on palpation of emphysematous area, erythema, history of protracted vomiting.
- History of recent procedures/trauma/underlying lung disease. History should also be obtained regarding triggers for angioedema which is the main differential.
- Assessment of airway, breathing, circulation.
- Vital signs with particular attention to oxygen saturation and need for supplemental oxygen. Evaluate for hemodynamic instability.
- Signs of infection/sepsis.

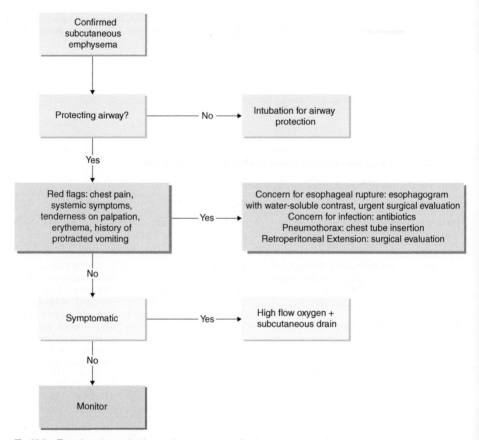

Fig. 32.3 Flowchart for evaluation and management of subcutaneous emphysema.

LABORATORY TESTS

- Laboratory testing is not required to diagnose subcutaneous emphysema.

IMAGING STUDIES

- Chest radiography is the most common initial test; however, CT chest/neck is the most sensitive study. Pockets of gas density within subcutaneous tissue outline facial planes is a typical imaging finding. Air can outline the pectoralis major muscle giving rise to the ginkgo leaf sign. Other possible causes of these radiographic findings are air trapped in clothing, gas associated with soft tissue laceration, or fat density.
- Patients with a history suspicious of Boerhaave syndrome should undergo esophageal – swallow with water-soluble contrast.

THERAPEUTIC INTERVENTIONS

Treatment should always start with securing the airway, breathing, and circulation. In patients with subcutaneous emphysema, treatment is directed at the underlying cause. Symptomatic management should be provided while the body absorbs the subcutaneous gas over time. Emphysema will likely resolve within ten days if the source is controlled. Methods of positive pressure ventilation (such as bi-level positive airway pressure) should be avoided if possible.

In patients who experience discomfort or require expedited resolution, high concentration oxygen can be given to allow for nitrogen washout and diffusion of gas particles. In severe cases of subcutaneous emphysema, subcutaneous catheters can be placed to release the air. Due to the risk of infection and skin scarring, its use is not recommended for longer than 72 h. Some practitioners have used small infra-clavicular incisions (~2 cm, bilaterally) with promising results of improving emphysema resolution time.

The majority of cases are non-fatal. However, massive subcutaneous emphysema can cause compartment syndrome, prevention of thoracic wall expansion, tracheal compression, and tissue necrosis. Without intervention, respiratory and cardiovascular compromise can occur. Patients should be monitored for progression of air leading to various complications.

If the clinical condition continues to worsen, therapeutic intervention might be required; in that case, the cause of emphysema needs to be determined and fixed. For example, if the patient had a recent intubation procedure or bronchoscopy and has evidence of upper airway damage, a tracheostomy tube distal to the damage will prevent leakage. Mucosal repair is another option but is rarely undertaken.

SUMMARY OF STEP-WISE APPROACH FOR EVALUATION AND MANAGEMENT OF SUBCUTANEOUS EMPHYSEMA

Step 1: Assess for airway and hemodynamic status. Attach cardiac monitor and place pacer pads. Secure airway if indicated.

Step 2: Obtain a stat X-ray of the site with emphysema and a chest X-ray to evaluate for the possible cause of emphysema. Compare to prior imaging if hemodynamics allow.

Step 3: If hemodynamically stable, observe conservatively and allow for natural resorption of the subcutaneous air.

Step 4: In unstable patients, after securing the airway, possible surgical decompression should be tried with specialty consultation and in the intensive care setting.

Step 5: Use IV fluids and vasopressors as indicated.

CODING A PATIENT WITH ACUTE HYPOXIC RESPIRATORY FAILURE FROM SUBCUTANEOUS EMPHYSEMA

If a patient with suspected subcutaneous emphysema becomes acutely hypoxic, the first step would be to secure the airway. Intubation can be attempted; however, some patients may require an emergent tracheostomy (will need a difficult airway code to be activated). Once an airway is established, the primary aim is to decompress the thoracic inlet, which can be done with skin incisions (either in supraclavicular or infraclavicular areas) to decompress manually. The surgery team should place a chest tube if pneumothorax is present on the chest X-ray. Once stabilized, the patient should be transferred to the ICU for further care.

Suggested Reading

Aghajanzadeh M, Dehnadi A, Ebrahimi H, et al. Classification and management of subcutaneous emphysema: a 10-year experience. *Indian J Surg.* 2015;77(Suppl 2):673–677. https://doi.org/10.1007/s12262-013-0975-4.

Melhorn J, Davies HE. The management of subcutaneous emphysema in pneumothorax: a literature review. *Curr Pulmonol Reports.* 2021;10(2):92–97. https://doi.org/10.1007/s13665-021-00272-4.

Shan S, Guangming L, Wei L, Xuedong Y. Spontaneous pneumomediastinum, pneumothorax and subcutaneous emphysema in COVID-19: case report and literature review. *Rev Inst Med Trop Sao Paulo.* 2020;62: e76. https://doi.org/10.1590/S1678-9946202062076.

CHAPTER 33

Facial Swelling in a Patient With Penicillin Allergy

Rahul R. Bollam ▪ Mohammad Adrish ▪ Firas Abdulmajeed

Case Study

The bedside nurse initiated a rapid response event after the patient was found to be in acute respiratory distress. Upon the arrival of the rapid response team, the patient was found to be a 34-year-old male with a history of alcohol abuse admitted a few hours ago for suspicion of aspiration pneumonia. He was receiving his first dose of ampicillin-sulbactam when he developed dyspnea and significant facial swelling.

VITAL SIGNS

Temperature: 97.6 °F, axillary
Blood Pressure: 90/60 mmHg
Heart Rate: 110 beats per min (bpm)
Respiratory Rate: 32 breaths per min
Oxygen Saturation: 80% on room air, 96% on 15 L/min non-rebreather mask.

FOCUSED PHYSICAL EXAMINATION

The patient was a young male in severe respiratory distress, tachypneic using accessory muscles of respiration. Appropriate personal protective equipment was established, and the patient was examined. Visible pitting edema was noticed around the eyelids, lips, and throat. There was minimal air entry in bilateral lung fields with inspiratory and expiratory wheezing. The remaining examination was unremarkable.

INTERVENTIONS

A cardiac monitor and defibrillator pads were attached to the patient. He was emergently given epinephrine 0.5 mg intramuscular with methylprednisolone 125 mg IV on suspicion of allergic angioedema and possible anaphylaxis. The patient was emergently intubated via the nasotracheal route and transferred to the intensive care unit (ICU) for further management.

FINAL DIAGNOSIS

Allergic angioedema with anaphylaxis.

TABLE 33.1 ■ Features of angioedema

Features	Mast cell-mediated/Histaminergic angioedema (Allergic)	Bradykinin-mediated angioedema (Non-allergic)
Trigger	Allergic triggers such as medication, food, insects, environmental allergens	Hereditary or acquired; medication induced is a common subtype of acquired such as Angiotensin-converting enzyme inhibitors associated with angioedema
Onset	Fast – may evolve over minutes	Slower - evolves gradually over 24 to 36h
Systemic involvement	Involves other organ systems in the setting of anaphylaxis – hypotension, wheezing, nausea/vomiting, and diarrhea	Usually does not involve other organ systems; sometimes can involve the gastrointestinal tract causing pain, diarrhea, and nausea/vomiting
Treatment	Responds to antihistamines and steroids; 90%-100% will improve	Unresponsive to antihistamines/steroids; 2%-10% may seem to improve

Angioedema

DEFINITION AND DIAGNOSIS

Angioedema is an abrupt onset, transient, localized swelling of deep skin layers or mucous membranes that commonly affects the face, periorbital areas, lips, larynx, and gastrointestinal (GI) tract. Angioedema can have two different underlying mechanisms (Table 33.1). Identification of the predominant mechanism is essential as the treatment of these two entities differs significantly. However, this identification can be challenging given the lack of specific diagnostic tests and overlap of symptoms.

The two main mechanisms of developing angioedema are mast cell mediated and bradykinin mediated. The complete detail of these mechanisms is not in the scope of this text, but a quick schematic is presented in Figs. 33.1 and 33.2, and the main differences between these two are listed in Table 33.1.

Suggested Approach to a Patient With Suspected Angioedema

For inpatient scenarios where angioedema is being considered, we suggest the following approach based on a thorough literature search and updated guidelines. This can be applied to emergency room scenarios, as the management is universal. See Fig. 33.3 for a flowchart of management of angioedema. See Chapter 7 for a short review of anaphylactic shock, among other types of shock.

FOCUSED HISTORY AND PHYSICAL EXAMINATION

- The acuity of signs and symptoms.
- History of prior episodes.
- History of allergies, recent new medications, or new food.
- Physical exam should begin with an assessment of airway, breathing, and circulation. Assess for signs of shock and decreased end-organ perfusion.
- Evaluate the extent of edema, i.e., eyelids, tongue, lips, pharynx, larynx, intestines.
- A brief skin examination should be done for urticaria, erythema.

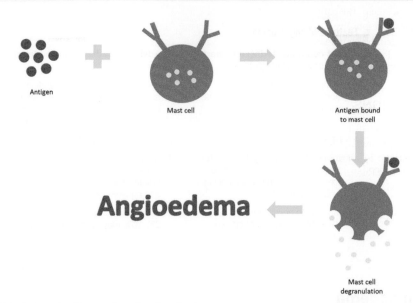

Fig. 33.1   Schematic of mast cell-mediated angioedema.

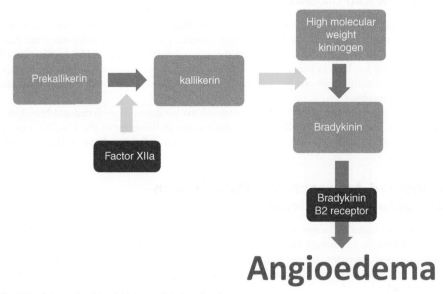

Fig. 33.2   Schematic of bradykinin-mediated angioedema.

- Lung examination should be done to evaluate for wheeze or signs of bronchospasm.
- An abdominal examination can be performed to look for tenderness, guarding, rebound tenderness.

LABORATORY TESTING

- In the acute setting, labs would not affect management. Arterial blood gas can be considered to determine the degree of hypoxia and acidosis in the appropriate setting.

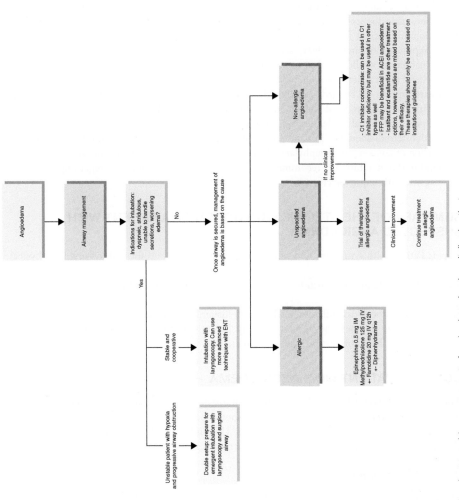

Fig. 33.3 Flowchart to guide management of angioedema in a hospitalized patient.

IMAGING STUDIES

- In the acute setting, imaging would usually not affect the management.

THERAPEUTIC INTERVENTIONS

It is challenging to establish histamine-mediated angioedema vs. bradykinin-mediated angioedema in an emergency setting because of significant crossover between the presenting features. Management of the airway should be the priority. Bradykinin-mediated angioedema can be worsened by trauma and manipulation of the oral and pharyngeal mucosa, and minimal attempts should be made for securing the airway. An experienced provider should attempt nasotracheal intubation. Indications for intubation would include:

1. Significant respiratory distress and stridor.
2. Inability to swallow oral secretions and risk of aspiration.
3. Rapid clinical deterioration and impending respiratory arrest.

An attempt should be made to secure the airway early as intubation tends to get more complicated with the progression of edema. Surgical airway through cricothyroidotomy should be considered per institutional guidelines if the airway cannot be secured via intubation. Antihistamines and corticosteroids should be initiated. Intramuscular epinephrine should be administered if there is suspicion of concomitant anaphylaxis. The use of ecallantide and icatibant in isolated cases can be found in the literature. We recommend following institutional guidelines regarding the use of these agents with unproven efficacy.

SUMMARY OF THE STEPWISE APPROACH OF A PATIENT WITH SUSPECTED ANGIOEDEMA

Step 1: Patient with symptoms and signs of angioedema based on focused history and physical examination.

Step 2: If the patient has impending airway closure, emergent intubation or surgical airway is required.

Step 3: It is difficult to differentiate between histamine-mediated and bradykinin-mediated angioedema in an emergency response setting. Empiric therapy for allergic angioedema should be considered based on institutional guidelines.

CODING A PATIENT WITH ANGIOEDEMA

Anesthesiology should be called to establish an airway either through laryngoscopy or cricothyrotomy. Intravenous or intraosseous access should be obtained. The patient should be given epinephrine 0.5 mg IM with methylprednisolone 125 mg IV for allergic/unspecified angioedema. The patient should be transferred to the ICU for monitoring.

Suggested Reading

Bernstein JA, Cremonesi P, Hoffmann TK, Hollingsworth J. Angioedema in the emergency department: a practical guide to differential diagnosis and management. *Int J Emerg Med.* 2017;10(1):15. https://doi.org/10.1186/s12245-017-0141-z.

Brown AF. Anaphylactic shock: mechanisms and treatment. *J Accid Emerg Med.* 1995;12(2):89–100. https://doi.org/10.1136/emj.12.2.89.

Busse PJ, Christiansen SC. Hereditary angioedema. *N Engl J Med.* 2020;382(12):1136–1148. https://doi.org/10.1056/NEJMra1808012.

Fischer D, Vander Leek TK, Ellis AK, Kim H. Anaphylaxis. *Allergy Asthma Clin Immunol.* 2018;14(Suppl 2). https://doi.org/10.1186/s13223-018-0283-4.

Long BJ, Koyfman A, Gottlieb M. Evaluation and management of angioedema in the emergency department. *West J Emerg Med.* 2019;20(4):587–600. https://doi.org/10.5811/westjem.2019.5.42650.

Misra L, Khurmi N, Trentman TL. Angioedema: classification, management and emerging therapies for the perioperative physician. *Indian J Anaesth.* 2016;60(8):534–541. https://doi.org/10.4103/0019-5049.187776.

Cases With Neurological Pathologies

CHAPTER 34

Altered Mental Status of Unknown Cause

Michael Heslin ■ Kainat Saleem ■ Firas Abdulmajeed

Case Study

The bedside nurse initiated a rapid response event for a patient for acute change in his mental status. The patient's roommate called the nursing staff because he heard the patient thrashing around in his bed for approximately 1 min. Upon the arrival of the rapid response team, the patient's nurse reported that the patient is a 19-year-old male with a history of asthma admitted to the orthopedic trauma service for bilateral ankle fractures sustained in a motor vehicle accident (MVA) awaiting operative management. The bedside nurse reported that the patient was on continuous vitals monitoring and had a brief oxygen desaturation into the mid-'80s that resolved spontaneously before the rapid response team's arrival. The nurse also stated that the patient is usually alert and orientated but confused about the events that brought him into the hospital and is very pleasant and conversant. He has been working with physical therapy and has been able to use a wheelchair without difficulty.

VITAL SIGNS

Temperature: 98.3 °F, axillary
Blood Pressure: 118/68 mmHg
Heart Rate: 68 beats per min (bpm) – normal sinus rhythm on telemetry
Respiratory Rate: 15 breaths per min
Pulse Oximetry: 99% saturation on room air

FOCUSED PHYSICAL EXAMINATION

The patient was a well-developed young adult male lying in his bed who appeared drowsy. He was unable to answer any questions or follow commands. There was a sutured laceration above his left eyebrow with surrounding ecchymosis and significant swelling. There were blood-tinged oral secretions around his lips, but there was no obvious tongue or oral laceration. His pupils were equal in size and reactive to light. His pulmonary and cardiovascular exam was unrevealing. His abdomen was soft and non-tender without any peritoneal signs. He had sugar tong splits to his bilateral lower extremities with soft calf and thigh compartments. Motor testing was unable to be performed. There were no signs of any urinary or bowel incontinence.

INTERVENTIONS

A cardiac monitor was attached. His airway, breathing, and circulation status were assessed and were stable. Given his acute change in mental status, a stat computed tomography (CT) head was ordered to evaluate any possible intracranial pathologic condition, especially since the patient was involved in a significant MVA. A complete blood count (CBC) was ordered to evaluate for a potential infectious process causing the acute mental change. A basic metabolic panel and a magnesium level were ordered to evaluate for any electrolyte abnormality as the cause of the altered mental status (AMS). Prolactin and lactate were ordered to rule out a recent seizure episode. Bedside fingerstick glucose was 82 mg/dL. During the rapid response, the patient was not given any benzodiazepines or other anti-epileptics. The rapid response team followed up on the results, and imaging was unchanged from the previous trauma scans ordered in the emergency room. There were no electrolyte abnormalities. There was mild leukocytosis, and the prolactin and lactate were elevated. Neurology consultation was requested for the need for anti-epileptics and a formal electroencephalogram (EEG) exam.

FINAL DIAGNOSIS

Suspected postictal state from a post-traumatic seizure.

Altered Mental Status

A variety of causes can result in AMS. The underlying cause could either be a primary intracranial pathologic condition such as a tumor or seizure or a systemic cause such as overwhelming sepsis, metabolic, or hormonal derangements. Medications, toxins, and illegal substances of abuse can also induce mental status changes. Strokes and other vascular system disorders and psychogenic causes could also be the culprit (Fig. 34.1, Tables 34.1 and 34.2). Often a combination of any of these broad categories could be at play. During a rapid response, we must quickly and effectively come to the heart of the issue to properly treat the patient.

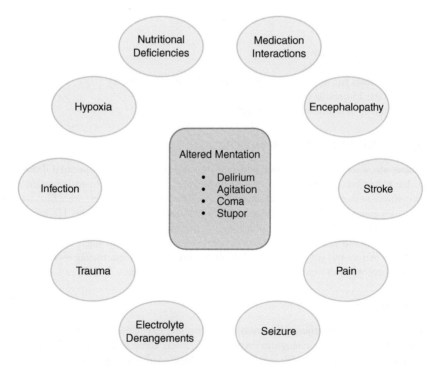

Fig. 34.1 Common causes of altered mental status.

TABLE 34.1 ■ **Life-threatening causes of altered mentation**

Cardiac	Acute coronary syndrome, including myocardial infarction, congestive heart failure, dysrhythmias
Endocrine	Addison disease, Cushing syndrome, diabetic ketoacidosis, hyperosmolar hyperglycemic syndrome, myxedema coma, thyroid storm
Environmental	Heatstroke/exhaustion, hypothermia, high altitude cerebral edema
Infectious	Encephalitis/meningitis, pneumonia, sepsis/septic shock, urinary tract infection
Metabolic	Hypercalcemia, hypo-/hyperglycemia, hypo-/hypernatremia, metabolic acidosis
Neurologic	Acute stroke, concussion, epidural hematoma, non-convulsive status epilepticus, postictal state, subarachnoid hemorrhage, subdural hematoma
Respiratory	Hypercarbia, hypoxia
Toxicological	Alcohol/illicit drug intoxication/withdrawal, medication overdose, polypharmacy

TABLE 34.2 ■ **Common causes of AMS (mnemonic: AEIOU TIPS)**

A	Alcohol, acidosis
E	Electrolytes, endocrine, encephalopathy
I	Infection
O	Overdose, oxygen (hypoxia), other
U	Urea
T	Tumors, trauma
I	Insulin (hypoglycemia)
P	Psychiatric, poisoning
S	Shock, seizure, stroke

The patient's history and demographics can help approach this extensive list of causes. Older age may put items such as stroke, polypharmacy, and delirium higher up on the list of differentials (see Table 34.3 for differences between delirium and dementia). A person with diabetes with AMS could be hypoglycemic or in diabetic ketoacidosis. Younger patients admitted to the detox unit could be withdrawing or could have used illegal drugs while in the hospital.

There are no standard tests to diagnose and treat AMS. The patient's history, labs, imaging should be combined with the provider's experience in dealing with such a situation to reach the underlying cause of the patient's presentation.

Suggested Approach to a Patient With AMS

For a patient with AMS, we suggest the following approach to evaluate and treat the acute event. It should be kept in mind that AMS is a tricky pathologic condition with many underlying causes. It is prudent to start with a comprehensive list of differentials and narrow it down as more information becomes available. A basic flowchart for the evaluation of altered mentation is presented in Fig. 34.2.

TABLE 34.3 ■ **Features of delirium vs. dementia**

Delirium	Dementia
Sudden onset	Gradual onset
Reversible	Chronically progressive
Disorientated at onset	Disorientation occurs later
Waxing and waning	Persistent
Altered mental status early	No alteration in consciousness until later in disease

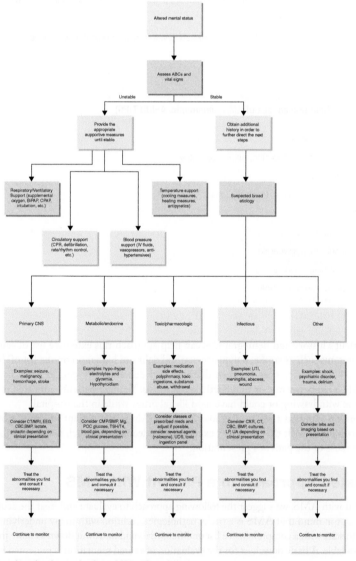

Fig. 34.2 Flowchart for the evaluation of altered mental status.

FOCUSED HISTORY AND PHYSICAL

- The timing of onset and acuity of signs and symptoms, timing and condition of patient's last known well state.
- Past medical history, the reason for admission, hospital course, and baseline mental status.
- History of recent trauma.
- History of home medications and inpatient medications.
- Physical exam should begin with an assessment of airway, breathing, and circulation. A complete, thorough head-to-toe physical exam should be done.
- The patient's AMS may limit the physical exam; thus, subtle clues in the exam should be noted.

LABORATORY TESTS

- Bedside fingerstick glucose testing to quickly rule out hypoglycemia.
- CBC to evaluate for leukocytosis.
- Complete metabolic panel along with a magnesium level to look at possible electrolyte abnormalities, renal impairment, or hepatic impairment.
- Arterial blood gas can help evaluate for hypoxia or CO_2 retention.
- Lactate and prolactin can be drawn, whose elevation can point toward a postictal state in the appropriate clinical setting.
- Serum ammonia level may help with the diagnosis of hepatic encephalopathy (although not needed if clinical suspicion is strong).
- Troponin level may be helpful to see if a cardiac cause is contributing to the patient's clinical status.

EKG

- EKG can manifest conduction and rhythm abnormalities based on certain electrolyte derangements, metabolic disorders, and ischemic abnormalities.

IMAGING STUDIES

- Imaging of the head and brain (CT and/or MRI) will help look for any intracranial pathologic condition such as a mass or stroke. CT head without contrast is the quickest and preferred test to rule out intracranial bleeds.
- A chest X-ray may demonstrate possible pneumonia that could be the infectious source causing the patient's AMS.
- Although rarely utilized in a rapid response event, spot or continuous EEGs can evaluate for seizures or encephalopathy.

THERAPEUTIC INTERVENTIONS

Therapeutic interventions are going to vary depending on what the likely diagnosis is. As always, airway, breathing, and circulation evaluation are of utmost importance. Supplemental oxygen may be needed to correct respiratory pathologies. If CO_2 narcosis is the suspected cause of AMS, positive pressure ventilation will be required to blow off excess CO_2. Non-invasive ventilation is relatively contraindicated in severely altered patients, and endotracheal intubation should be pursued in those unable to protect the airway. Any deranged electrolyte levels should be corrected. Dextrose-containing solutions or glucagon may be needed to correct hypoglycemia. Benzodiazepines and anti-epileptics can be helpful in those who are actively seizing. Infectious causes will need source control and antibiotics per institutional guidelines and local antibiograms. Consultation with a range of specialists may be required in some cases (stroke service, emergent dialysis) based on the underlying cause of AMS.

SUMMARY OF APPROACH TO A PATIENT WITH AMS IN A RAPID RESPONSE EVENT

Step 1: AMS has a broad differential. Management should start with an assessment of the airway, breathing, and circulation.

Step 2: The airway should be secured and hemodynamics stabilized. Temperature abnormalities should be corrected.

Step 3: Once stable, detailed history should be obtained from the nursing staff, chart review, and other available sources. A thorough head-to-toe physical exam should be conducted.

Step 4: Obtain appropriate lab work and imaging based on clinical suspicion.

Step 5: Correct any electrolyte or acid-base abnormalities. Antibiotics should be used in the appropriate clinical setting.

Step 6: Consider making the patient none per oral until mental status improves.

Step 7: Specialist teams such as neurology should be engaged based on the clinical scenario.

CODING A PATIENT WITH AMS

Altered mentation can lead to aspiration, which is one of the leading causes of respiratory arrest in these patients. If such a condition arises, the patient will need emergent endotracheal intubation and broncho-alveolar lavage for washout of aspirations. An altered patient might be in status epilepticus (convulsive or non-convulsive), needing multiple doses of benzodiazepines/anti-epileptics. Such patients may also need intubation for airway protection and continuous EEG monitoring in monitored settings. Neurology consultation is recommended in such a case.

Suggested Reading

Kuzminski JC. Altered mental status. *Nelson Pediatric Symptom-Based Diagnosis*. 2017:543–562. https://doi.org/10.1016/B978-0-323-39956-2.00031-5.

Sanello A, Gausche-Hill M, Mulkerin W, et al. Altered mental status: current evidence-based recommendations for prehospital care. *West J Emerg Med*. 2018;19(3):527–541. https://doi.org/10.5811/westjem.2018.1.36559.

Xiao H-Y, Wang Y-X, Xu T, et al. Evaluation and treatment of altered mental status patients in the emergency department: life in the fast lane. *World J Emerg Med*. 2012;3(4):270–277. https://doi.org/10.5847/wjem.j.issn.1920-8642.2012.04.006.

CHAPTER 35

Altered Mental Status From Medication Adverse Effect

Michael Heslin ▦ Mohammad Adrish ▦ Firas Abdulmajeed

Case Study

The bedside nurse initiated a rapid response event for a patient because of acute onset of confusion in the morning. On arrival of the rapid response team, the patient was found yelling at staff and grabbing at things in the air. The patient's nurse provided a bedside report informing the rapid response team that this was a 72-year-old male with a history of coronary artery disease status post-coronary artery bypass graft, hypertension, hyperlipidemia and diabetes mellitus admitted for chest pain with plans for cardiac catheterization in the afternoon. The nurse reported that the patient was alert and orientated at the initial presentation. She reported that he had trouble falling asleep last night and requested 25 mg diphenhydramine (Benadryl) around 0300 to help him sleep.

VITAL SIGNS

Temperature: 99.4 °F, axillary
Blood Pressure (BP): 158/76 mmHg
Heart Rate: 105 beats per min (bpm) – sinus tachycardia on telemetry
Respiratory Rate: 17 breaths per min
Pulse Oximetry: 98% oxygen saturation on room air

FOCUSED PHYSICAL EXAMINATION

The patient was an elderly male lying in bed yelling at hospital staff. He was agitated, but the rapid response team was able to talk to him and calm him down. He was disorientated to place and time, which was a new finding per his nurse. He was speaking in complete sentences without any respiratory distress. His lungs were clear and without abnormal breath sounds. Upon auscultation of his chest, there was regular tachycardia without any appreciated murmurs. The patient reported some suprapubic tenderness, but the remaining abdominal exam was benign. Cranial nerve testing did not reveal any abnormalities. Strength testing of his extremities was without any focal weakness. During the rapid response, he reached out and attempted to grasp things that were not there.

INTERVENTIONS

Given his acute change in mental status, a stat computed tomography (CT) head was ordered to evaluate for any possible intracranial pathologic condition, especially given that the patient was on multiple antiplatelet medications. A complete blood count (CBC) was ordered to evaluate for a potential infectious process causing the acute mental status change. A basic metabolic panel (BMP) and a magnesium level were ordered to evaluate for any electrolyte abnormality as the cause of the altered mental status (AMS). Prolactin and lactate were ordered to rule out recent seizure episodes. Fingerstick glucose was 94 mg/dL. The rapid response team followed up on the results, and CT of the head did not reveal any acute abnormalities. The CBC and BMP were grossly normal other than potassium of 3.4 meq/L and an increase in the patient's baseline creatinine to 1.3 mg/dL. A bladder scan was performed and demonstrated a volume of 600 cc, for which the nursing staff performed a straight cath. Diphenhydramine was discontinued. Melatonin was added as an as-needed sleep aid.

DIAGNOSIS

Anticholinergic side effects from diphenhydramine

AMS From Medication Adverse Effect

AMS can be a sequela from various disease processes and because of iatrogenic causes. Intoxication or withdrawal from drugs of abuse (i.e., alcohol, illicit drugs) can also produce altered mentation. Both sedating and excitatory drugs contribute to a patient's change in mental status.

Most drugs are excreted either through renal or hepatic mechanisms, so naturally, disease processes that directly or indirectly damage these organs can alter the way drugs are processed. When the kidneys and/or liver are not functioning properly to metabolize drugs, the half-life of the active drug will increase, leading to adverse events. Patients can receive multiple rounds of the same medication, creating a stacking effect of each subsequent dose. Another important mechanism of drug side effects is drug-drug interactions, where drugs potentiate each other's sedative or excitatory properties leading to overstimulation or sedation. Other factors such as older age and subsequently decreased renal function, body fat composition, and nutritional status can also play a role in drug metabolism. Common drugs associated with AMS are discussed in Table 35.1.

TABLE 35.1 ■ **Common drugs associated with altered mental status**

Toxidrome	Drug examples	Effect on vital signs	Physical exam findings
Adrenergic	Amphetamines, cocaine	Increased respiratory rate, heart rate, temperature, and blood pressure (BP)	Agitation, diaphoresis, increased bowel sounds, increased urination, dilated pupils
Anticholinergic	Antihistamines, tricyclic antidepressants, antipsychotics, antispasmodics	Increased temperature and heart rate. BP normal/increased. Respiratory rate unchanged	Dry skin and mucous membranes, decreased urination and bowel sounds, dilated pupils
Cholinergic	Pesticides, Alzheimer drugs	Decreased heart rate. Normal/increased respiratory rate. Temperature and BP unchanged	Diaphoresis, increased bowel sounds, increased urination, constricted pupils
Opioid	Narcotic pain medications, heroin	Decreased respiratory rate. Heart rate, temperature, BP normal/decreased	Constricted pupils, decreased bowel sounds
Sedative-hypnotic	Ethanol, barbiturates	Respiratory rate normal/decreased. Heart rate, temperature, BP normal	Normal bowel sounds, urination, and pupils

Suggested Approach to a Patient With AMS Secondary to Medication Adverse Effect

We suggest the following approach to evaluate and treat the acute event for a patient with AMS from a medication side effect. The differential diagnosis list for AMS can encompass all body systems, even if the AMS is initially suspected to be because of medications, both legal and illegal. Start with a comprehensive list and continuously adjust the most likely diagnosis as more information becomes available (Fig. 35.1).

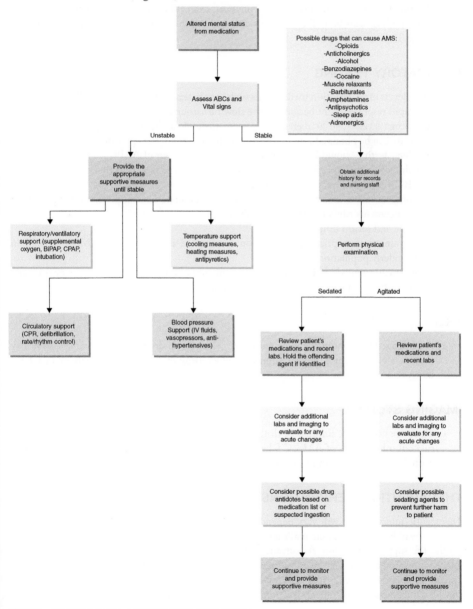

Fig. 35.1 Flowchart for the evaluation of altered mentation.

FOCUSED HISTORY AND PHYSICAL

- Timing of onset and duration of symptoms, timing and condition of patient's last known well state.
- The patient's medical history, admission diagnosis, hospital course, current medications, doses, and time of administration of the medications will help narrow down the AMS differentials.
- Physical exam should begin with an assessment of airway, breathing, and circulation.
- A complete, thorough head-to-toe physical exam should be done. Specific physical exam findings can be pathognomonic for medication toxidromes which are explained in Table 35.1.

LABORATORY TESTING

- Drug levels of prescription medications such as anti-seizure drugs are generally not obtained in a rapid response event because of the slow turnaround time of these tests. However, certain drugs levels such as recreational drugs, toxic alcohols, acetaminophen, ethanol, and salicylate can be obtained rapidly and should be ordered in the appropriate clinical scenario
- Ancillary testing should be pursued to rule out other causes of AMS
  - Point-of-care blood glucose testing – to rule out hypoglycemia as the cause of AMS
  - CBC – to evaluate for ongoing infection
  - Comprehensive metabolic panel (CMP) – to evaluate liver and renal function whose derangements can alter drug metabolism
  - Urine and serum drug screen
  - Cultures as appropriate if an infection is suspected as the source of AMS, especially in the elderly population
  - Serum ammonia level if the patient has a history of underlying liver disease or is on any medication that can cause hyperammonemia

EKG

- A prolonged QTc interval can be associated with certain drugs and drug classes, so it may provide a clue during a rapid response of which drug or drug class the patient may have taken or overdosed on.

IMAGING STUDIES

- There are no specific findings of drug toxicity on head/brain imaging; however, it can help rule out other causes of AMS. CT head, Magnetic resonance imaging brain, and electroencephalogram (EEG) can be pursued per clinician judgment.

THERAPEUTIC INTERVENTIONS

Therapeutic interventions will vary depending on the likely drug causing the presenting symptoms. Airway, breathing, and circulation should be secured in all patients based on the advanced cardiac life support algorithm. An advanced airway may be required for overly sedated patients who cannot protect their airway. Physical restraints may be needed for overly agitated or acutely psychotic patients. Specific drug antidotes (naloxone, flumazenil, N-acetylcysteine) should be considered in appropriate clinical situations per clinician judgment and institutional guidelines.

STEPWISE APPROACH TO A PATIENT WITH AMS BECAUSE OF A MEDICATION SIDE-EFFECT

Step 1: All patients should be assessed for airway, breathing, and circulation.

Step 2: The airway should be secured with endotracheal intubation if necessary. Hypoxia and hypotension should be corrected.

Step 3: Comprehensive physical exam should be conducted to evaluate for findings associated with adverse drug effects.

Step 4: If the patient is stable, the patient's medical history, labs, and medication administration record should be reviewed.

Step 5: Physical or chemical restraints should be employed based on institutional guidelines for acutely agitated or psychotic patients who pose a risk to themselves or others.

Step 6: Head imaging and lab work should be obtained to rule out alternate etiologies of AMS.

Suggested Reading

Alagiakrishnan K, Wiens CA. An approach to drug induced delirium in the elderly. *Postgrad Med J.* 2004;80(945):388–393. https://doi.org/10.1136/pgmj.2003.017236.

Campbell N, Boustani M, Limbil T, et al. The cognitive impact of anticholinergics: a clinical review. *Clin Interv Aging.* 2009;4:225–233. https://doi.org/10.2147/cia.s5358.

Han JH, Wilber ST. Altered mental status in older patients in the emergency department. *Clin Geriatr Med.* 2013;29(1):101–136. https://doi.org/10.1016/j.cger.2012.09.005.

Kuzminski JC. Altered mental status. *Nelson Pediatric Symptom-Based Diagnosis.* 2017:543–562. https://doi.org/10.1016/B978-0-323-39956-2.00031-5.

López-Álvarez J, Zea Sevilla MA, Agüera Ortiz L, Fernández Blázquez MÁ, Valentí Soler M, Martínez-Martín P. Effect of anticholinergic drugs on cognitive impairment in the elderly. *Rev Psiquiatr Salud Ment.* 2015;8(1):35–43. https://doi.org/10.1016/j.rpsm.2013.11.003.

Xiao H-Y, Wang Y-X, Xu T, et al. Evaluation and treatment of altered mental status patients in the emergency department: life in the fast lane. *World J Emerg Med.* 2012;3(4):270–277. https://doi.org/10.5847/wjem.j.issn.1920-8642.2012.04.006.

CHAPTER 36

Altered Mental Status in a Patient With CNS Lymphoma

Kainat Saleem ▪ Firas Abdulmajeed ▪ Mohammad Adrish

Case Study

A rapid response event was initiated by the bedside nurse for acute change in mental status of her patient. On prompt arrival of the rapid response team, it was noted that the patient was a 66-year-old female with a known history of depression, alcohol abuse, and CD20 + diffuse large B-cell lymphoma status post six cycles of rituximab, cyclophosphamide, doxorubicin, vincristine, and prednisone along with intrathecal methotrexate and subsequent isolated central nervous system (CNS) relapse currently being treated with pemetrexed, who was admitted to the hospital earlier in the day for the evaluation of a new fever. The patient had reportedly been feeling fine until 30 min before the rapid response event when she called her nurse to report a new headache and feeling of unwellness. Per the nurse's report, she had found the patient vomiting when she went in for a vitals check, and the patient had promptly become unresponsive after.

VITAL SIGNS

Temperature: 99° F, axillary
Blood Pressure: 210/133 mmHg
Pulse: 95 beats per min (bpm) – sinus rhythm on telemetry
Respiratory Rate: 20 breaths per min
Pulse Oximetry: 82% saturation on room air, improved to 92% with 6L O2 with nasal cannula

FOCUSED PHYSICAL EXAMINATION

The patient was a middle-aged lady lying in bed, snoring. She was unresponsive to voice commands and minimally responsive to sternal rub. She had her arms, legs, and neck extended. No spontaneous movements were observed. Pupils were dilated and minimally responsive to light. Cardiac and pulmonary auscultation was benign. An abdominal exam did not elicit any distress in the patient. The patient was also noted to be incontinent of stool.

INTERVENTIONS

The neurological findings raised concern for a severe intracranial process. The patient was emergently intubated at the bedside to secure the airway. Intravenous mannitol was administered empirically at the bedside after consultation with the neuro-intensivist. Stat computed tomography (CT) head was ordered, and the patient was transported to the neurosurgical intensive care unit (ICU) after the scan. CT of the head was later reported, which showed a new right-sided 2.1 cm subdural hematoma concerning for hyperacute hemorrhage, as seen in Fig. 36.1. A 2 cm leftward subfalcine herniation, a new right uncal herniation, and entrapment of the left lateral

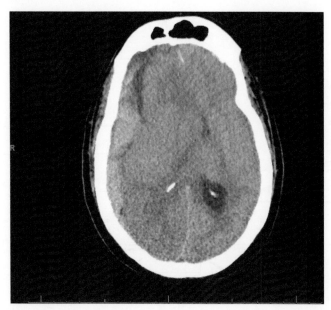

Fig. 36.1 Computed tomography of the axial head section showing right-sided subdural hemorrhage, midline shift, and right lateral ventricle effacement.

ventricle were also seen. Neurosurgery was consulted emergently for surgical evacuation of the hematoma per the family's wishes.

FINAL DIAGNOSIS

Altered mental status secondary to raised intracranial pressure (ICP) from acute intracranial hemorrhage.

Raised Intracranial Pressure

The intracranial compartment in adults is enclosed by the skull, which limits the volume inside this compartment. Brain parenchyma occupies 80% of the intracranial volume, and cerebrospinal fluid (CSF) and blood occupy 10% each. An increase in the volume of any one of these components would lead to a shift in balance and would result in increased ICP and displacement of vital structures.

CSF is produced by the choroid plexus located mainly in the lateral and fourth ventricles of the brain. It is produced at a rate of 0.2–0.35 mL/min or roughly up to 500 mL/d. After production in the lateral ventricles, the CSF flows to the third ventricle through the Foramen of Monroe and then into the fourth ventricle through the cerebral aqueduct of Sylvius. From there, CSF drains into the subarachnoid space and to the subarachnoid granulations through the two lateral foramina of Luschka and one medial Foramen of Magendie (Fig. 36.2). CSF is absorbed through the granulations into the dural sinuses and finally into the venous system. Any disturbance in the CSF pathway from production to absorption can result in the accumulation of CSF in the cranial vault.

Normal ICP in adults ranges at 15 mmHg or less. Pressures in the range of 20 mmHg or above are consistent with pathological intracranial hypertension. Common mechanisms associated with elevated ICP are noted in Table 36.1.

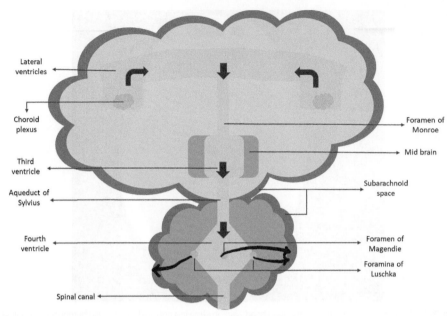

Fig. 36.2   Schema of cerebral spinal fluid flow from production to absorption (indicated by purple arrows).

TABLE 36.1 ▪ Causes of raised intracranial pressure (ICP)

• Intracranial mass lesions	• Increased cerebral spinal fluid (CSF) production
• Tumors	• Choroid plexus papilloma
• Hematomas	• Decreased CSF clearance
• Cerebral edema	• Bacterial meningitis
• Hypoxic encephalopathy	• Obstructive hydrocephalus
• Large infarct	• Venous outflow obstruction
• Severe traumatic brain injury	• Venous sinus thrombosis
• Idiopathic intracranial hypertension	• Jugular vein thrombosis

The signs and symptoms associated with increased ICP are listed in Table 36.2.

It is exceedingly important to identify and treat elevated ICP as early as possible. An increase in ICP can have devastating consequences, such as a reduction in intracranial blood flow that occurs after the intracranial compensatory mechanisms have been exhausted. Elevated ICP can also lead to herniation of the brainstem if left untreated.

Suggested Approach to a Patient With Suspected Raised ICP

For inpatient scenarios where an acute elevation of ICP is being considered the primary cause of altered mental status, we suggest the following approach based on a thorough literature search and updated guidelines. See Fig. 36.3 for a flow-chart of management of such patients and see

TABLE 36.2 ■ Signs and symptoms of raised intracranial pressure (ISP)

Symptoms	• Headache – more prominent in the mornings initially, becomes constant as ICP rises • Neck pain – can represent herniation of cerebellar tonsils • Blurry vision – represents a compression of optic nerves • Confusion – usually reported by family • Falls and feeling of being off-balance • Nausea and vomiting – especially projectile vomiting
Signs	• Progressive cognitive deterioration, including worsening Glasgow coma scale score • Fixed or dilated pupils • Papilledema • Decorticate or decerebrate posturing • Refractory hypertension • Bradycardia • Respiratory depression and arrest

Table 36.3 for common differential diagnosis of raised ICP. The usual sequence of history taking, physical exam, investigations, and resuscitative interventions is often not followed during a rapid response; these measures often run parallel to each other in a code situation. The following components of the rapid response are discussed in the traditional sequence only to ease understanding.

FOCUSED HISTORY AND PHYSICAL EXAMINATION

- The timing of onset and acuity of signs and symptoms, timing and condition of patient's last known well state.
- History of fever, head trauma, meningitis, intracranial tumors, or other known malignancies.
- History of recent use of antiplatelet agents or anticoagulation.
- New change in the neurological examination.
- New change in the pupillary examination.
- Physical examination should begin with an assessment of airway, breathing, and circulation.
- Assess for signs of impending herniation, including unresponsiveness, posturing, bradycardia, and respiratory depression.

LABORATORY TESTS

- No specific lab testing is required for the diagnosis of raised ICP.
- Ancillary testing can be done to evaluate for underlying causes or confounders:
  - Complete blood count and blood cultures can be obtained if there is suspicion of underlying meningitis.
  - Arterial blood gas can be obtained to ensure adequate ventilation.
  - An electrolyte panel can be obtained to ensure there are no sodium derangements.
  - A coagulation profile can be obtained to ensure reversal is not indicated.
  - Flinger-stick glucose to rule out hypoglycemia as the cause of symptoms.
  - Urine and serum toxicology screen to assess for any other co-ingestions.

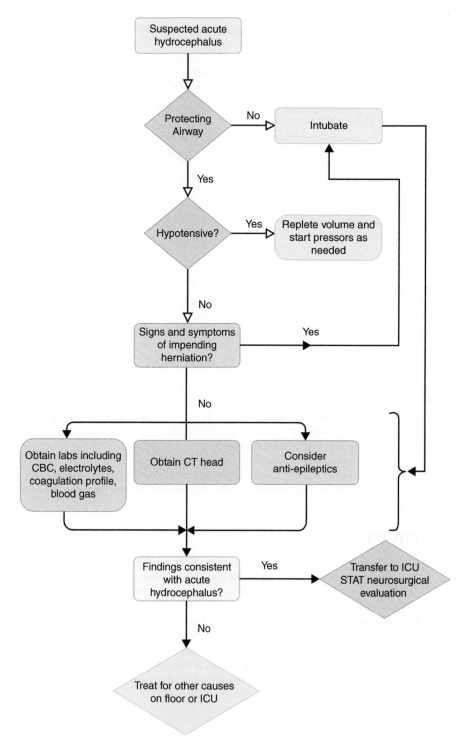

Fig. 36.3 Basic flow-chart for assessment and management of a patient with suspected acute increased intracranial pressure.

TABLE 36.3 ■ Differentials of acute elevated intracranial pressure (ICP)

Diagnoses that mimic elevated ICP	How to differentiate from acute hydrocephalus?
• Toxic/metabolic/hypoxic encephalopathy • Status epilepticus, especially non-convulsive status • Migraine • Catastrophic stroke • Hypoglycemia • Hypothermia	• Hypoglycemia can be ruled out with a fingerstick glucose check during the initial survey • Hypothermia can be ruled out in the initial survey • Computed tomography (CT) of the head is crucial to rule out acute hydrocephalus and catastrophic strokes • Extensive lab workup can be pursued for hypoxic/toxic/metabolic encephalopathy once CT of the head has resulted • Spot vs. continuous electroencephalogram monitoring can be pursued to evaluate for seizure (particularly non-convulsive status epilepticus) once CT of the head has resulted

EKG

- Electrocardiogram (EKG) can be obtained but should not delay other necessary investigations. EKG may show:
  - Sinus bradycardia, part of Cushing's triad and a sign of impending herniation.
  - Deep T waves inversions in all leads.

IMAGING STUDIES

- CT of the head without contrast
  - Most critical study.
  - It can evaluate the size of ventricles, the possible site of obstruction, intracranial bleeding, and abscesses.
  - Drawback: Poor visualization of the posterior fossa.
- Magnetic resonance imaging of the brain with and without contrast
  - Done non-emergently for treatment planning after initial stabilization and interventions.

THERAPEUTIC INTERVENTIONS

Acute elevation of ICP is a medical and surgical emergency. We recommend that all patients be assessed for airway, breathing, circulation. The airway should be secured, intubate if necessary, especially if signs of impending herniation are present. Hypoventilation should be avoided early in intubation. The patient should be placed on a cardiac monitor, and pacer pads should be attached if the patient is bradycardic. Ensure adequate blood pressure and peripheral perfusion. Hypotension should be avoided to allow for adequate cerebral blood flow in the setting of raised ICP. Pressors should be used if indicated. The head of the bed should be elevated to 30 degrees to allow for venous drainage to gravity. Aggressive analgesia and sedation with propofol and fentanyl should be pursued in mechanically ventilated patients; this can help reduce the cerebral blood flow demand. An IV bolus of mannitol or hypertonic saline can be used to reduce ICP based on institutional guidelines. Antiepileptic medications can be used if there is a suspicion of seizures. Once airway and hemodynamics are secured and proper imaging is obtained, immediate neurosurgical consultation should be obtained for further management. The patient should be transferred to the neurosurgical ICU for further management.

SUMMARY OF A STEPWISE APPROACH TO A PATIENT WITH SUSPECTED ACUTE ELEVATION OF ICP

Step 1: The patient should be assessed for signs and symptoms of raised ICP.

Step 2: Assessment should be done for airway and hemodynamic stability. Intubation should be pursued if indicated. Hypotension should be corrected.

Step 3: Mannitol or hypertonic saline can be administered empirically based on institutional guidelines.

Step 4: Baseline ancillary lab work should be obtained. Obtaining lab work should not delay life saving measures or head imaging.

Step 5: Stat CT of the head should be obtained. Head imaging should not wait for the results of lab work.

Step 5: Antiepileptics, antibiotics, reversal of anticoagulation should be done as indicated.

Step 6: Immediate neurosurgical evaluation should be obtained, and the patient should be transferred to neurosurgical ICU.

Suggested Reading

Canac N, Jalaleddini K, Thorpe SG, Thibeault CM, Hamilton RB. Review: pathophysiology of intracranial hypertension and noninvasive intracranial pressure monitoring. *Fluids Barriers CNS.* 2020;17(1):40. https://doi.org/10.1186/s12987-020-00201-8.

Changa AR, Czeisler BM, Lord AS. Management of elevated intracranial pressure: a review. *Curr Neurol Neurosci Rep.* 2019;19(12):99. https://doi.org/10.1007/s11910-019-1010-3.

Ropper AH. Hyperosmolar therapy for raised intracranial pressure. *N Engl J Med.* 2012;367(8):746–752. https://doi.org/10.1056/nejmct1206321.

Tripathy S, Ahmad SR. Raised intracranial pressure syndrome: a stepwise approach. *Indian J Crit Care Med.* 2019;23(Suppl 2):S129–S135. https://doi.org/10.5005/jp-journals-10071-23190.

CHAPTER 37

Altered Mental Status in a Patient With Sepsis

Melissa Chrites ■ Syed Arsalan Akhter Zaidi ■ Firas Abdulmajeed

Case Study

A bedside nurse initiated a rapid response event for a patient with new-onset altered mental status. On prompt arrival of the rapid response team, it was noted that the patient was a 72-year-old female with a history of coronary artery disease, hypertension, chronic kidney disease stage three, hypothyroidism, chronic obstructive pulmonary disease (COPD), tobacco dependence, and prior stroke with residual left-sided weakness. She was admitted a day ago with concern for COPD exacerbation. The nurse reported that the patient was alert and oriented to person, place, time, and situation when she arrived from the emergency department (ED), and prior to hospitalization, she lived at home and has no known history of dementia. She was noted to have had a decreased appetite earlier in the morning during breakfast. Chart review showed that she had received a chest X-ray (CXR) in the ED, which did not show any acute infiltrate. Nursing staff reported her oxygen requirement increased to 4 L/min (LPM) of oxygen instead of 2 LPM that she was on since admission, and she had been more confused and was picking at her intravenous (IV) line when afternoon vital signs were being obtained.

VITAL SIGNS

Temperature: 101 °F, axillary
Blood Pressure: 89/50 mmHg
Heart Rate: 102 beats per min, sinus tachycardia on telemetry
Respiratory Rate: 22 breaths per min
Pulse Oximetry: 94% on 4 LPM O_2 via nasal cannula

FOCUSED PHYSICAL EXAMINATION

A quick exam revealed a lady appearing slightly older than the recorded age. She was trying to remove her IV line during this exam. On orientation questions, she believed she was at home and that she had to get up to get ready for work. She would not follow commands appropriately and could not give thumbs up on either hand. There was no evidence of facial droop, and her pupils appeared equal in size bilaterally. She was moving both arms spontaneously. Her cardiac, pulmonary, and abdominal exams were unremarkable.

INTERVENTIONS

A bedside glucose level was checked, which was 80 mg/dL. A 1 L bolus of lactated ringers was given. Labs including complete blood count (CBC), basic metabolic panel (BMP),

225

thyroid-stimulating hormone (TSH), lactate, arterial blood gas (ABG), and blood cultures were sent. Her blood pressure came up to 95/55 after 500 cc of IV fluids were infused, and she was ordered another 1.5 L of IV fluids to achieve a total of 30 cc/kg of IV fluids. ABG showed a pH of 7.36, $PaCO_2$ of 50, and PaO_2 of 74 with an of O_2 saturation of 94% when the sample was drawn. There was no evidence of hypercarbia or significant discrepancy between the PaO_2 and SpO_2. A TSH was sent because of her history of hypothyroidism; however, the fever, hypotension, and recent cold symptoms made infection higher on the differential. She was started on ceftriaxone IV and continued on azithromycin. She did have a history of stroke, and during episodes of hypotension, recrudescence of old deficits can occur. During the rapid response event, her mental status improved after her IV fluids were administered, likely because of correction of hypotension and improved cerebral perfusion.

FINAL DIAGNOSIS

Septic encephalopathy.

Septic Encephalopathy

Changes in mental status often occur early in sepsis and often before other organ system dysfunction begins. Septic encephalopathy is thought to result from oxidative stress, increased cytokine and pro-inflammatory factor levels, disturbances in cerebral circulation, changes in the blood-brain barrier permeability, and injury to the brain's vascular endothelium. It is important to note that 45% of patients who recover from sepsis will show cognitive dysfunction one year after hospitalization.

Septic encephalopathy can be differentiated from an acute stroke as there is typically a global change in mental status, and examination is typically not consistent with focal weakness. In order to treat the encephalopathy, sepsis itself must be treated (see Table 37.1 for potential causes of sepsis). Sepsis treatment includes circulatory support with IV fluids, typically 30 cc/kg as a bolus, and vasopressor support if needed, as this will help ensure adequate cerebral perfusion. Broad-spectrum antibiotics should be initiated as soon as possible, ideally in less than 60 min. The choice of antibiotics depends on the patient's underlying risk factors, including immunosuppressive status, recent antibiotics use, and prior history of infection with a specific bacteria. If there is a concern for meningitis, then those antibiotics should be chosen that have known penetration through the blood-brain barrier. Renal function should be considered in antibiotic dosing decisions, as kidneys are a common casualty in sepsis and shock. However, this information may not be available at the time, and the regimen can be tailored as lab results become available.

TABLE 37.1 ■ Potential causes of septic encephalopathy

Skin/soft tissue infection	CSF-meningitis, encephalitis, abscess	Intra-abdominal abscess	Pneumonia
Bacteremia, candidemia	Discitis	Ascending cholangitis	Pleural effusion
Endocarditis	Dental or sinus abscess	Acalculous cholecystitis	Empyema
Osteomyelitis	Deep neck space infection	Spontaneous bacterial peritonitis	Urinary and genitourinary tract infections, toxic shock syndrome

DEFINITION

A change in mental status characterized by generalized alternation in brain function (communication, memory, speech, orientation, behavior) caused by the inflammatory response of sepsis.

Suggested Approach to a Patient With Encephalopathy in a Rapid Response Event

For inpatient evaluation of a patient with encephalopathy, we suggest the following approach to evaluate and treat the acute event. This can be expanded and used in emergency room situations as well, as this protocol is based on guidelines for the management of encephalopathy. The differential diagnosis list for altered mental status (AMS) can encompass all body systems, even if the AMS is initially suspected to be because of sepsis. Start with a comprehensive list and continuously adjust the most likely diagnosis as more information becomes available. See Fig. 37.1 for a flowchart of evaluation and management of septic encephalopathy.

FOCUSED HISTORY AND PHYSICAL

- The acuity of signs and symptoms.
- In addition to the general history points, also focus on travel history, exposure to sick contacts, injection drugs, known indwelling hardware, central venous catheters, and pregnancy.
- History of predisposing medical conditions such as lung disease, immunocompromised status because of cancer, or certain medications such as immunosuppressants or chemotherapy.
- System-specific complaints to help guide workup include cough, pleurisy, rashes, joint pain, neck rigidity or headache, changes in vision, dysuria or frequency, abdominal pain or diarrhea, evidence of a new heart murmur.

LABORATORY TESTS

- CBC, BMP, lactate.
- Blood cultures.
- Urinalysis and culture.
- Erythrocyte sedimentation rate.
- Procalcitonin can be considered.
- Lipase to evaluate for pancreatitis.
- TSH to evaluate for severe thyroid dysfunction.
- Cerebrospinal fluid (CSF) studies for bacterial, viral, and fungal pathogens depending on the patient's risk factors.
- Urine antigen testing for legionella, mycoplasma, and streptococcus pneumoniae.

EKG

- EKG is not required for the diagnosis of septic encephalopathy; however it can be considered if there is concern regarding infective endocarditis and its complications.

IMAGING STUDIES

- Imaging should be pursued based upon what is believed to be the underlying source, once the patient has been stabilized:
  - Consider CXR if concern for pneumonia or computed tomography (CT) chest if concern for empyema.

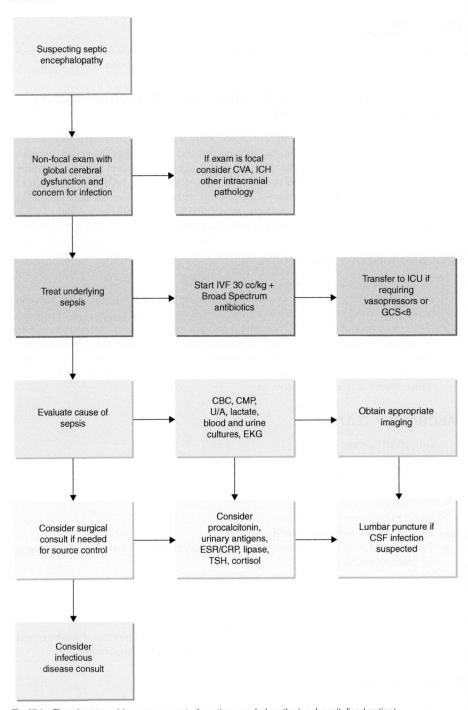

Fig. 37.1 Flowchart to guide management of septic encephalopathy in a hospitalized patient.

- Consider CT scan of extremities if concern for soft tissue abscess.
- Consider CT of the head (required before lumbar puncture [LP]) and CT sinuses to evaluate for potential occult sources.
- CT abdomen and pelvis if concern for acute abdominal pathologic conditions.

THERAPEUTIC INTERVENTIONS

After stabilizing the patient's hemodynamic status with adequate fluid resuscitation as per sepsis protocol, the focus should be on starting broad-spectrum antibiotics and using the history and physical exam findings to guide ordering labs and imaging to identify the underlying cause. Decision-making regarding which antibiotics to start should take into consideration a patient's risk factors for pseudomonas, methicillin-resistant staphylococcus aureus, or atypical infections. Antibiotic therapy should be directed toward the most probable source of infection.

If there is suspicion of meningitis, antibiotic therapy should not be postponed until an LP is performed. Institutional guidelines should be considered here. If pneumococcal meningitis is suspected, it would be appropriate to administer dexamethasone. Antibiotics that have good CSF penetration include vancomycin, ceftriaxone, cefotaxime, cefepime, meropenem, and ampicillin. Ampicillin should be used when Listeria monocytogenes is suspected (typically patient > age 50). If there is a concern for allergy to cephalosporins, consider the use of trimethoprimsulfamethoxazole to cover for Listeria and aztreonam to cover for gram negatives. Institutional antibiotic stewardship programs should be consulted before using unconventional or off-label antibiotics.

Source control is of paramount importance in the treatment of sepsis and its complications. However, the source of sepsis is not always immediately apparent in the setting of a rapid response event. Immediate surgical consultation should be obtained if source control requires surgical intervention, such as necrotizing fasciitis, toxic megacolon, empyema, or occult abscesses. Depending on the patient's history, consultation with an infectious disease specialist may be appropriate.

Patients with circulatory collapse or inability to protect their airway will require transfer to an intensive care unit for vasopressor support and possibly ventilatory support.

SUMMARY OF STEPS TO MANAGE ENCEPHALOPATHY IN HOSPITAL

Step 1: Ensure that the patient's exam is not concerning for stroke, intracranial bleed, intracranial hypertension, or other intracranial pathologic condition. If this is the case, consider emergent CT of the head.

Step 2: If there is global cerebral dysfunction with concern for infection, ensure adequate cerebral perfusion by providing an IV fluid bolus. Start broad-spectrum antibiotics and assess if there is any history to guide antibiotic choice if available.

Step 3: Obtain labs, EKG, and appropriate imaging. This may include X-rays, CT, or magnetic resonance imaging depending upon the area requiring imaging and the suspected source.

Step 4: If meningitis is suspected, a CT of the head might be required to rule out elevated intracranial pressure before obtaining an LP to avoid brainstem herniation.

Step 5: Consultation with the appropriate specialist for source control (surgery, neurosurgery).

Step 6: Involvement of infectious disease may be appropriate depending on the situation.

CODING A PATIENT WITH SEPTIC ENCEPHALOPATHY

We recommend that all patients be assessed for airway, breathing, circulation. If a vasopressor is started for hypotension and the patient remains hypotensive, stress steroids can be considered based on institutional guidelines. Risk factors for adrenal insufficiency should be reviewed in refractory hypotension (detailed discussion can be found in Chapter 56). Acidemia should be addressed to prevent myocardial suppression. If a patient with septic encephalopathy has a cardiac arrest, we suggest following the advanced cardiac life support protocol to ensure proper securement of the airway and initiation of effective cardiopulmonary resuscitation per guidelines. Post-cardiac arrest care should be instituted once the return of spontaneous circulation is achieved.

Suggested Reading

Chaudhry N, Duggal AK. Sepsis associated encephalopathy. *Adv Med*. 2014;2014:762320. https://doi.org/10.1155/2014/762320.

Ren C, Yao RQ, Zhang H, Feng YW, Yao YM. Sepsis-associated encephalopathy: a vicious cycle of immunosuppression. *J Neuroinflammation*. 2020;17(1):1–15. https://doi.org/10.1186/s12974-020-1701-3.

Ziaja M. Septic encephalopathy. *Curr Neurol Neurosci Rep*. 2013;13(10):383. https://doi.org/10.1007/s11910-013-0383-y.

CHAPTER 38

Altered Mental Status in a Patient With Substance Use Disorder

Michael Heslin ▧ Kainat Saleem

Case Study

The bedside nurse initiated a rapid response event for a patient because of acute onset of unresponsiveness. The registered nurse (RN) was doing his morning medication rounds and found the patient unresponsive. The patient was also taking infrequent shallow breaths. On arrival of the rapid response team, the bedside RN informed that the patient is a 23-year-old male with a history of heroin abuse and anxiety, admitted two days ago for suspected infective endocarditis. He was started on antibiotics via a peripherally inserted central catheter (PICC) line for tricuspid endocarditis. The only other medication he was receiving was sertraline. While performing a fingerstick glucose check, the nursing staff found a needle and syringe by the patient's side. Additionally, two small plastic bags with a white powder residue were found on the floor.

VITAL SIGNS

Temperature: 98.9 °F, axillary.
Blood Pressure: 118/60 mmHg
Heart Rate: 74 beats per min – normal sinus rhythm on telemetry
Respiratory Rate: 6 breaths per min
Pulse Oximetry: 84% on room air

PHYSICAL EXAMINATION

A quick exam revealed a young adult male with a Glasgow Coma Scale (GCS) score of ten (E3 V3 M4) with pinpoint pupils. He was initially noted to have cyanosis of his lips and agonal breathing. His heart rate was regular without an appreciable murmur. His extremities were warm with good distal pulses.

INTERVENTIONS

Initially, the cause for the patient's respiratory depression was unknown, so a bag-valve mask with high flow supplemental oxygen was placed on the patient for ventilatory support. While the nursing staff was obtaining a fingerstick glucose level, drug paraphernalia was found. The patient was immediately given 0.5 mg of IV naloxone. His GCS and respiratory rate improved slightly. He ultimately received a total of 1.0 mg of naloxone. His GCS improved to 15, and he maintained oxygen saturations above 97% on room air with a normal respiratory rate. The patient admitted to using heroin via his PICC line. An EKG was performed and demonstrated normal sinus rhythm with normal intervals. Due to the patient's rapid return to baseline after naloxone administration and the patient admitting to heroin use, it was suspected that this was an accidental opioid overdose. The patient remained on the floor with a 1:1 sitter.

231

FINAL DIAGNOSIS

Heroin overdose.

Opioid Overdose

Heroin is a derivative of the opioid morphine and shares a similar drug profile to opioid-based pain medications. According to the Centers for Disease Control and Prevention data, with the initial opioid epidemic and subsequent tightening of prescribing opioid pain medications, heroin use has dramatically increased over the last several years. Heroin tends to be more readily available and cheaper than prescription opioid drugs. Heroin can be snorted, smoked, or injected subcutaneously, intramuscularly, or intravenously. Purified heroin is typically a white or brownish powder that is often mixed with other substances, such as baking soda, powdered milk, fentanyl, to dilute the heroin, so more is available to sell. Black tar heroin is an impure form of heroin and typically has a sticky, hard consistency.

Since heroin and narcotic pain medications share similar biochemical characteristics, the signs and symptoms of overdose, along with their mechanism of action, are practically identical. Both heroin and narcotic pain medications act on opioid receptors found in the central and peripheral nervous systems. Depending on the administration route, the amount of drug used and length of abuse history can both play a role in the clinical manifestations of overdose. The telltale sign of heroin or opioid overdose is respiratory depression in the setting of other vital signs being relatively normal. Another clue on physical exam of acute opioid overdose is pinpoint pupils (miosis).

Naloxone (Narcan) is the antidote for acute opioid or heroin overdose. Naloxone works by competing and displacing opioids at their specific opioid receptors in the central and peripheral nervous systems. The most common routes of administration are intravenous and intranasal. Typically, multiple doses of naloxone are needed in an acute overdose setting because the duration of action for naloxone is shorter than the duration of action for opioids. Initial dosing, frequency of administration, and maximum dosing will be discussed later in the "Therapeutic Interventions" section. If too much naloxone is used quickly, it can precipitate symptoms of acute withdrawal; therefore, it is essential to remember that naloxone therapy aims to restore the respiratory status and not mental status.

Suggested Approach to a Patient With an Opioid Overdose in a Rapid Response Event

For a patient with a suspected opioid overdose, we suggest the following approach to evaluate and treat the acute event. The ultimate management decisions are based on the treating clinician's discretion and institutional guidelines. See Fig. 38.1 for a flowchart of management of such patients. The usual sequence of history taking, physical exam, investigations, and resuscitative interventions is often not followed during a rapid response; these measures often run parallel to each other in a code situation. The following components of the rapid response are discussed in the traditional sequence only to ease understanding.

FOCUSED HISTORY AND PHYSICAL

- The acuity of signs and symptoms, time and condition of patient's last known well state.
- Past medical history, the reason for admission, hospital course, and baseline mental status (endocarditis in an otherwise young, healthy individual should put a history of intravenous drug abuse as a possible setting).
- History of home medications and inpatient medications.

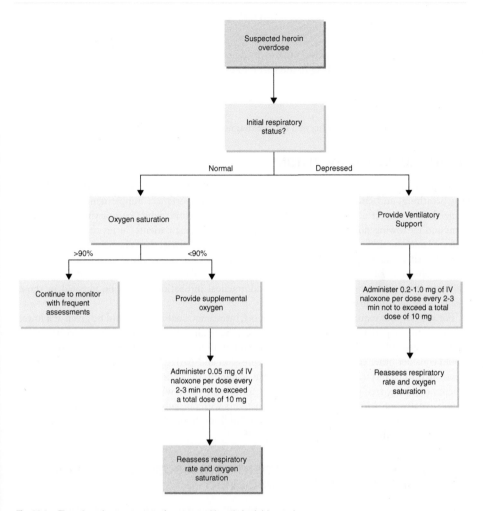

Fig. 38.1 Flowchart for treatment of suspected heroin/opioid overdose.

- Physical exam should begin with an assessment of airway, breathing, and circulation. A complete, thorough head-to-toe physical exam should be done after establishing adequate airway and circulation. Pinpoint pupils are usually a telltale sign of opioid overdose.
- The patient's altered mental status (AMS) may limit the physical exam; thus, subtle clues in the exam should be noted.
- It should be made sure that the scene is safe, especially if drug paraphernalia is found. Avoid a possible needle stick from unseen sharps.

LABORATORY TESTS

- No emergent labs are needed for the diagnosis of opioid overdose. However, if the diagnosis is not clear, labs can be done to evaluate for altered mentation (see Chapter 34).
- Arterial blood gas should be obtained in patients with persistent hypoxia and AMS despite naloxone administration.

EKG

- No acute changes in the EKG are usually demonstrated, but it is good practice to obtain an EKG to evaluate the QT/QTc interval for any possible overdose.

IMAGING STUDIES

- No emergent imaging is needed for the diagnosis of opioid overdose.

THERAPEUTIC INTERVENTIONS

Interventions in opioid overdose are based on the overall clinical status of the patient. The airway, breathing, and circulation evaluation is of utmost importance. Supplemental oxygen may be needed to correct acute hypoxia because of opioid overdose while completing the physical exam and narrowing down differentials. For apneic/hypopneic patients, intravenous naloxone is preferred and should be given at a higher initial dose (0.2-1.0 mg). Non-invasive techniques like bi-level positive airway pressure are relatively contraindicated in severely altered patients because of the inability to protect the airway. Thus bag-valve ventilation should be pursued for patients while awaiting treatment with naloxone. Endotracheal intubation should be pursued in those unable to protect the airway.

For patients not requiring ventilatory support, intravenous naloxone should be given at a lower dose than apneic patients (0.05 mg). Naloxone can be readministered every 2-3 min with a maximum total dose of 10 mg. If there is no improvement after administering 10 mg of naloxone, one should consider other causes of respiratory depression and AMS. The goal of naloxone therapy is to restore normal respiratory status rather than obtaining the patient's baseline mental status. For patients requiring frequent naloxone administrations or those with an overdose on long-acting opioids, a naloxone drip might be needed. In patients with polysubstance abuse (cocaine, amphetamines, acetaminophen, or another substance in addition to opioids), other toxidromes could be present and should be addressed (see Chapter 35).

STEPWISE APPROACH TO A PATIENT WITH A SUSPECTED HEROIN OVERDOSE IN A RAPID RESPONSE EVENT

Step 1: Management should start with an assessment of airway, breathing, and circulation.

Step 2: The airway should be secured and hemodynamics stabilized. Temperature abnormalities should be corrected.

Step 3: Evaluate patient for signs and symptoms of a possible heroin/opioid overdose (respiratory depression in the setting of other vital signs being relatively normal, pinpoint pupils, AMS, fresh track marks).

Step 4: Naloxone should be administered. The patient's respiratory status, IV access, and history of drug use will determine the route and dosing of naloxone.

Step 5: The patient should be re-evaluated after naloxone administration. Did the respiratory status and mentation improve?

Step 6: If no clinical improvement, naloxone can be administered every 2-3 min to achieve a normal respiratory rate.

Step 7: If no clinical improvement after receiving a total dose of 5-10 mg of naloxone, other causes for the patient's respiratory depression and AMS should be evaluated.

Suggested Readings

Boyer EW. Management of opioid analgesic overdose. *N Engl J Med*. 2012;367(2):146–155. https://doi.org/10.1056/NEJMra1202561.

Clarke SFJ, Dargan PI, Jones AL. Naloxone in opioid poisoning: walking the tightrope. *Emerg Med J*. 2005;22(9):612–616. https://doi.org/10.1136/emj.2003.009613.

Danovitch I, Vanle B, Van Groningen N, Ishak W, Nuckols T. Opioid overdose in the hospital setting: a systematic review. *J Addict Med*. 2020;14(1).

Hendley TM, Hersh EV, Moore PA, Stahl B, Saraghi M. Treatment of opioid overdose: a brief review of naloxone pharmacology and delivery. *Gen Dent*. 2017;65(3):18–21.

Lewis C, Vo H, Fishman M. Intranasal naloxone and related strategies for opioid overdose intervention by nonmedical personnel: a review. *Subst Abuse Rehabil*. 2017;8:79–95. https://doi.org/10.2147/sar.s101700.

Shaw LV, Moe J, Purssell R, et al. Naloxone interventions in opioid overdoses: a systematic review protocol. *Syst Rev*. 2019;8(1):138. https://doi.org/10.1186/s13643-019-1048-y.

Wermeling DP. Review of naloxone safety for opioid overdose: practical considerations for new technology and expanded public access. *Ther Adv Drug Saf*. 2015;6(1):20–31. https://doi.org/10.1177/2042098614564776.

CHAPTER 39

Altered Mental Status in a Patient Transferred From ICU

Ali Uddin ▪ Kainat Saleem ▪ Firas Abdulmajeed ▪ Mohammad Adrish

Case Study

A rapid response event was initiated by a nurse for a patient with altered mental status (AMS). On the arrival of first responders, the patient was agitated and disoriented. The bedside nurse stated that the patient has not been responding to questions appropriately and has been trying to take out her intravenous (IV) catheters and climbing out of bed despite frequent reorientation. Per the report, the patient was an 86-year-old female with a past medical history of chronic obstructive pulmonary disease (COPD), type 2 diabetes mellitus, hypertension (HTN), hyperlipidemia, and hearing loss who was recently transferred to the medical floor following a one-week intensive care unit (ICU) stay for acute on chronic hypercapnic respiratory failure secondary to COPD exacerbation that required intubation. The patient had finished a five-day course of steroids and antibiotics. She was extubated one day prior and had been saturating well on 4 L/min (LPM) O_2 via nasal cannula. The nurse stated that the patient was transferred from the ICU 1 h prior and was drowsy on arrival; the nurse did not witness any seizure-like activity.

VITAL SIGNS

Temperature: 98.3°F, axillary
Blood Pressure: 134/87 mmHg
Heart Rate: 94 beats per min (bpm)
Respiratory Rate: 16 breaths per min
Pulse Oximetry: 95% oxygen saturation on 4 LPM O_2 via Nasal cannula

FOCUSED PHYSICAL EXAMINATION

A quick exam revealed an elderly female who was agitated and speaking loudly intermittently. She was unable to answer any questions or follow commands. Her pupils were equal in size and reactive to light. Her pulmonary and cardiovascular exam was unrevealing. Her abdomen was soft and non-tender without any peritoneal signs. Motor testing was unable to be performed. There were no signs of any urinary or bowel incontinence.

INTERVENTIONS

Due to suspected acute change in mental status, a stat computed tomography (CT) scan of the head was ordered to evaluate for acute intracranial pathologic conditions. Basic laboratory tests were drawn, including bedside blood glucose, basic metabolic profile, and urinalysis. Due to a history of COPD and recent respiratory failure, an arterial blood gas was drawn. All lab results were within expected parameters. CT of the head was negative for any acute pathologic conditions that could explain the patient's AMS. Due to the low likelihood of seizures (no prior history of seizure, no witnessed seizure activity) or stroke (no focal deficits on the exam), and no other abnormalities found on laboratory or radiological examinations, the most likely diagnosis was hyperactive delirium secondary to a prolonged ICU stay. Due to her agitation being a potential barrier to recovery and her attempts at climbing out of bed posing a fall risk, she was given a small dose of haloperidol.

FINAL DIAGNOSIS

Mixed delirium, secondary to a prolonged ICU stay.

Delirium

Delirium is an acute change in cognitive function which waxes and wanes throughout the day. According to the *Diagnostic and Statistical Manual of Mental Disorders (DSM)-5*, delirium is characterized by:

- Disturbance in attention from baseline.
- Which develops over a short period of time and fluctuates throughout the day.
- With an additional disturbance in cognition.
- The disturbances cannot be explained better by another cause.
- There is evidence that the disturbance is caused by a medical condition, substance intoxication/withdrawal, or medication side effect.

Delirium can be classified as hyperactive, hypoactive, or mixed, as described in Fig. 39.1. Risk factors for delirium are discussed in Table 39.1.

There are no standard tests for the diagnosis of delirium. It is important to note that delirium is a diagnosis of exclusion, and other causes of AMS should be ruled out before attributing the symptoms to delirium.

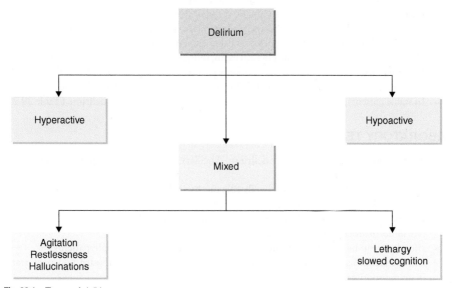

Fig. 39.1 Types of delirium.

TABLE 39.1 ■ **Common risk factors for delirium**

Conditions associated with delirium	
• Advanced age	• Hypoxia and hypercapnia
• Hearing impairment	• Central nervous system infections
• Inadequate pain control	• Hospitalization, especially intensive care unit stay
• Sepsis	• Alcohol use
• High-grade fever	• Medications
• Electrolyte imbalance, especially sodium and calcium	• Opioids
	• Sedatives
• Thyroid disorders	• Antihistamines
• Blood glucose derangement	• Skeletal muscle relaxants
• Liver disease	• Corticosteroids
• Renal failure	• Substance abuse

Suggested Approach to a Patient With AMS due to Delirium

For a patient with AMS, we suggest the following approach to evaluate and treat the acute event. It should be kept in mind that AMS is a tricky pathologic condition with a wide variety of underlying etiologies which need to be ruled out before a diagnosis of delirium can be made. It is prudent to start with a comprehensive list of differentials which can be narrowed down as more information becomes available. See Fig. 39.2 for a flowchart for evaluation and management of delirium.

FOCUSED HISTORY AND PHYSICAL

- The acuity of signs and symptoms, time of patient's last known well state.
- Past medical history, the reason for admission, hospital course, and baseline mental status.
- History of home medications and inpatient medications.
- Physical exam should begin with an assessment of airway, breathing, and circulation. A complete, thorough head-to-toe physical exam should be done.
- The patient's AMS may limit the physical exam; thus, subtle clues in the exam should be noted.
- Particular attention should be paid to motor power to assess for focal deficits. Due to limited participation from the patient, spontaneous movements should also be noted.
- In stable patients, the confusion assessment method can help diagnose delirium (Table 39.2).

LABORATORY TESTS

- There is no specific blood test for delirium. Ancillary testing should be pursued to rule out other causes of AMS.
- Point-of-care glucose testing to quickly rule out hypoglycemia.
- Complete blood count to evaluate for leukocytosis.
- Comprehensive metabolic panel along with a magnesium level to look at possible electrolyte abnormalities, renal impairment, or hepatic impairment.
- Blood gas can help evaluate for hypoxia or CO_2 retention in appropriate patients.
- Lactate and prolactin levels can be drawn, whose elevation can point toward a postictal state in an appropriate clinical setting.
- Urinalysis can give clue towards a urinary tract infection.

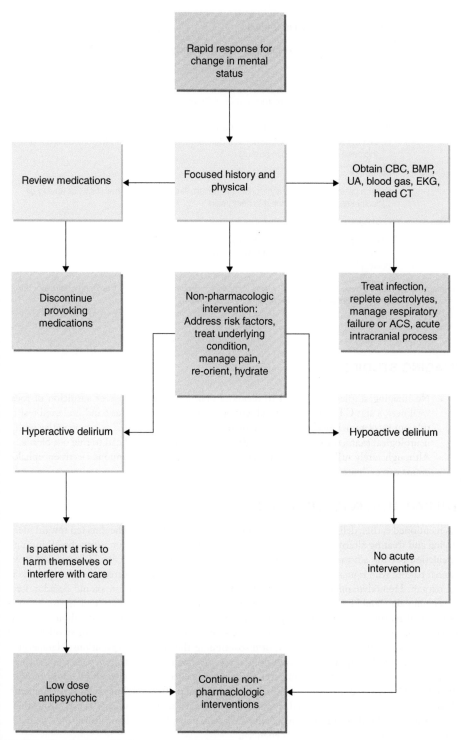

Fig. 39.2 Flowchart to guide the management of delirium.

TABLE 39.2 ■ **Confusion Assessment Method**

A standardized, evidence-based tool for recognition of delirium. Diagnosis requires features one AND two plus three OR four

Feature 1	Acute onset or Fluctuating course
	History obtained from family member or nurse and is shown by a positive response to the following questions: A) Is there evidence of an acute change in mental status from the patient's baseline? B) Did the abnormal behavior fluctuate during the day, that is, tend to come and go, or increase and decrease in severity?
Feature 2	Inattention
	Did the patient have difficulty focusing attention, illustrated by distractibility, or having difficulty keeping track of what is being said?
Feature 3	Disorganized Thinking
	Was the patient's thinking disorganized or incoherent, such as rambling or irrelevant conversation, unclear or illogical flow of ideas, or unpredictable switching from subject to subject?

Reference for CAM: Inouye S, van Dyck C, Alessi C, Balkin S, Siegal A, Horwitz R. Clarifying confusion: the confusion assessment method. Ann Int Med 1990;113(12):941–948.

IMAGING STUDIES

- No imaging studies are needed to diagnose delirium. Still, in case of suspicion of focal weakness, a stat CT scan of the head without contrast is the quickest and preferred test to rule out intracranial bleeds. In cases of delirium where the patient is not cooperative with a neurological exam, some providers prefer to do a CT scan of the head to rule out bleeds.
- Although rarely utilized in a rapid response event, spot or continuous electroencephalograms can evaluate for seizures or encephalopathy

THERAPEUTIC INTERVENTIONS

As mentioned earlier, delirium is a diagnosis of exclusion. Efforts should be directed toward identifying and treating alternate diagnoses. All patients should be assessed for airway, breathing, and circulation per the advanced cardiac life support algorithm. The airway should be secured in an altered patient who is unable to protect the airway. Hypoxia should be corrected with supplemental oxygen. Hemodynamics should be stabilized, and severe hypertension should be addressed. Fever and pain should be addressed. For hyperactive delirium, non-pharmacologic measures, such as frequent reorientation, maintaining sleep/wake cycle, and avoiding restraints, should be used where possible. However, in an acute situation of severe agitation, low-dose antipsychotics can be used to prevent self-harm and the risk of discontinuing therapeutic interventions. Haloperidol, risperidone, and olanzapine were found to be similarly effective in treating hyperactive delirium. It should be kept in mind that antipsychotics are associated with increased all-cause mortality in the elderly. These medications should be administered after weighing risks versus benefits. Benzodiazepines should be avoided in patients with delirium, if possible, as these medications tend to worsen the delirium. For hypoactive delirium, non-pharmacological measures, as mentioned above, have been shown to be beneficial.

STEPWISE APPROACH TO A PATIENT WITH AMS BECAUSE OF DELIRIUM IN A RAPID RESPONSE EVENT

Step 1: Management should start with an assessment of airway, breathing, and circulation.

Step 2: The airway should be secured and hemodynamics stabilized. Temperature abnormalities should be corrected.

Step 3: Once stable, detailed history should be obtained from the nursing staff, chart review, and any other available sources. A thorough head-to-toe physical exam should be conducted.

Step 4: Obtain appropriate lab work and imaging to rule out common causes of AMS.

Step 5: Try to reorient the patient, treat any underlying acute medical conditions, manage pain, and hydrate if appropriate.

Step 6: If the patient continues to be agitated, low-dose antipsychotics (haloperidol, olanzapine, or risperidone) can be administered.

Step 7: Continue non-pharmacologic interventions and frequent reorientation.

Suggested Readings

Arumugam S, El-Menyar A, Al-Hassani A, et al. Delirium in the intensive care unit. *J Emerg Trauma Shock.* 2017;10(1):37–46. https://doi.org/10.4103/0974-2700.199520.

Divatia JV. Delirium in the ICU. *Indian J Crit Care Med.* 2006;10(4):215–218. https://doi.org/10.4103/0972-5229.29838.

Grover S, Avasthi A. Clinical practice guidelines for management of delirium in elderly. *Indian J Psychiatry.* 2018;60(Suppl 3):S329–S340. https://doi.org/10.4103/0019-5545.224473.

Hayhurst CJ, Pandharipande PP, Hughes CG. Intensive care unit delirium: a review of diagnosis, prevention, and treatment. *Anesthesiol.* 2016;125(6):1229–1241. https://doi.org/10.1097/ALN.0000000000001378.

Marcantonio ER. Delirium in hospitalized older adults. *N Engl J Med.* 2017;377(15):1456–1466. https://doi.org/10.1056/nejmcp1605501.

Thom RP, Levy-Carrick NC, Bui M, Silbersweig D. Delirium. *Am J Psychiatry.* 2019;176(10):785–793. https://doi.org/10.1176/appi.ajp.2018.18070893.

CHAPTER 40

Acute Vision Loss in a Patient With Eye Pain

Ali Uddin ▪ Kainat Saleem ▪ Firas Abdulmajeed ▪ Mohammad Adrish

Case Study

A rapid response event was initiated by a bedside nurse for a patient with acute vision loss. On arrival of first responders, the patient was lying in bed in severe pain, stating she could not see out of her right eye. Per the bedside nurse report, the patient was a 64-year-old female with a history of hypertension, heart failure, gastroesophageal reflux disease (GERD), and allergic rhinitis. She was admitted for heart failure exacerbation. A few minutes before initiating this code, the patient endorsed a sudden loss of vision in the right eye, which did not improve in the past 10 min. Upon medication review, the patient was currently being treated with furosemide for heart failure, and her home medications of lisinopril, carvedilol, and insulin were continued. She was also being given her home dose of loratadine for chronic allergic rhinitis. Her home medication of hydrochlorothiazide (HCTZ) was held inpatient while she was getting furosemide. The nurse stated the patient has been nauseous and has thrown up a few times since the pain started. The patient reported halos in her visual field and severe headache.

VITAL SIGNS

Temperature: 98.3 °F, axillary
Blood Pressure: 145/97 mmHg
Heart Rate: 102 beats per min (bpm) – sinus tachycardia on telemetry
Respiratory Rate: 17 breaths per min
Pulse Oximetry: 97% on room air

PHYSICAL EXAMINATION

The patient was an overweight adult female lying upright in bed in acute distress. She was alert and oriented and endorsed a 10/10 right eye pain. Her eye exam showed conjunctival injection, non-reactive mid-dilated pupil on the right eye, clouded cornea, photophobia, tenderness to palpation over the right eye, and increased rigidity of the right eye ball compared to the left. A cardiovascular exam revealed tachycardia without a murmur. A quick motor and sensory exam did not reveal any acute abnormalities except for the findings in the right eye.

INTERVENTIONS

The patient showed characteristic features such as acute vision loss associated with headache, nausea, conjunctival injection, photophobia, and a non-reactive mid-dilated pupil consistent with acute angle-closure glaucoma. Computed tomography (CT) scan of the head was ordered to rule out intracranial ischemic stroke/bleed. A stat ophthalmology consult was called, and recommendations were taken over the phone while waiting for them to evaluate the patient physically. Per expert recommendations, pressure-lowering eye drops were administered. Timolol maleate, apraclonidine, and pilocarpine were given 1 min apart. CT of the head was done and was normal. On arrival of ophthalmology team, tonometry was done, revealing intraocular pressure (IOP) of 40 mmHg. Once the diagnosis was confirmed by ophthalmology, acetazolamide 500 mg oral was given. The patient was retained on the floor.

FINAL DIAGNOSIS

Acute angle-closure glaucoma.

Acute Angle-Closure Glaucoma

Acute angle-closure glaucoma (AACG) is defined as an acute narrowing of the anterior chamber of the eye, preventing adequate aqueous flow. This results in increased IOP. AACG is considered an ophthalmologic emergency requiring prompt identification and treatment. Characteristic findings include decreased visual acuity associated with severe eye pain, conjunctival injection, headache, nausea, vomiting, presence of halos around lights, and a pathognomonic non-reactive mid-dilated pupil. A conjunctival injection (or 'red eye') can be seen in various other ophthalmological pathologies, which are discussed in Table 40.1.

At-risk populations include those aged >60 years, females, Asian descent, positive family history, and use of certain medications such as loratadine and HCTZ. Delayed treatment can result in blindness which is caused by increased pressure behind the iris because of blockage of aqueous humor flow through the anterior chamber. Prolonged pressure build-up results in optic nerve damage, which causes visual disturbances shown in AACG. Angle-closure glaucoma can be classified into two main types, primary angle-closure glaucoma and secondary angle-closure glaucoma (Table 40.2).

Normal intraocular pressure IOP ranges from 8 to 21 mmHg. Patients with AACG have pressures >30 mmHg. Once AACG is suspected, a stat ophthalmology evaluation should be requested. Gonioscopy confirms the diagnosis. However, if an ophthalmologist cannot be at the bedside within 1 h, treatment to lower IOP should be initiated. There are various classes of drugs

TABLE 40.1 ▣ Differentiating features of various causes of red eye

Diagnosis	Clinical features
Iritis	Aversion to light in the affected and unaffected eye Red ring around iris = ciliary flush
Hyphema	Visible blood in the anterior chamber
Infectious keratitis	Contact lens wearer White over anterior chamber from a layer of white blood cells
Bacterial keratitis	Foreign body sensation, inflamed conjunctiva, purulent discharge
Viral keratitis	Foreign body sensation, watery discharge
Episcleritis	No pain, benign
Scleritis	Severe constant pain radiates to the face. Worse in the morning and night
Subconjunctival hemorrhage	No pain, benign, clears on its own

TABLE 40.2 ■ **Classification of angle-closure glaucoma**

Primary angle-closure		Secondary angle-closure	
Primary Angle-closure Suspect (PACS)	Normal intraocular pressure (IOP) and optic disc, but occludable angles in at least two quadrants	Caused by impairment of aqueous outflow secondary to apposition between peripheral iris and the trabeculum. There are two main mechanisms for this:	
Primary angle-closure (PAC)	Occludable drainage angles, increased IOP, and/or evidence of synechial closure, but no evidence of optic nerve damage	Pushing of the iris from behind	Seen in pupillary block, plateau iris syndrome, malignant glaucoma, and dislocated lens
Primary Angle-closure Glaucoma (PACG)	PAC with optic nerve damage because of glaucoma and/or visual field loss	Pulling of the iris forward	Seen in iris incarceration after trauma, migration of corneal endothelium, epithelium down-growth

TABLE 40.3 ■ **Drugs used for the treatment of angle-closure glaucoma**

Medication	Route	Class	Mechanism
Timolol 0.5%	Topical	Beta-blocker	Blocks production of aqueous humor
Apraclonidine 1%	Topical	Alpha-2 agonist	Blocks production of aqueous humor
Brimonidine 0.15%	Topical	Alpha-2 agonist	Blocks production of aqueous humor
Dorzolamide 2%	Topical	Carbonic anhydrase inhibitor	Blocks production of aqueous humor
Latanoprost 0.005%	Topical	Prostaglandin	Increases aqueous humor drainage
Pilocarpine 1%-2%	Topical	Muscarinic agonist	Facilitates aqueous humor drainage from the anterior chamber
Prednisolone Acetate 1%	Topical	Steroid	Reduce inflammation and corneal hazing
Acetazolamide	Systemic	Carbonic anhydrase inhibitor	Blocks production of aqueous humor
Mannitol	Systemic	Osmotic diuretic	Decreases volume of vitreous humor

used to lower the IOP; some of them work by decreasing the production of aqueous humor, while some improve the drainage of aqueous humor from the anterior chamber. Steroids can reduce inflammation and corneal hazing and are used concurrently with other drugs. These drugs are discussed in Table 40.3. If pressure is unrelieved, the patient will need emergent surgery to decompress the chamber, relieving aqueous flow.

Suggested Approach to a Patient With AACG in a Rapid Response Event

For a patient with sudden visual disturbance or loss of vision, and symptoms consistent with AACG, the following approach can be used for immediate risk assessment and management (Fig. 40.1). This should be done with stat consultation with ophthalmology:

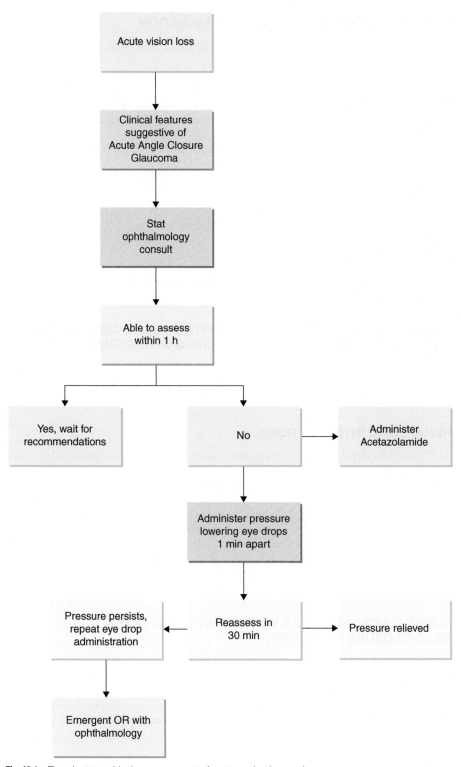

Fig. 40.1 Flowchart to guide the management of acute angle-closure glaucoma.

FOCUSED HISTORY AND PHYSICAL EXAMINATION

- The acuity of signs and symptoms, time and condition of patient's last known well state.
- Description of symptoms.
- Past medical history, the reason for admission, hospital course, and baseline mental status.
- History of home medications and inpatient medications.
- A quick neuro exam should be done to see if any other neurological signs are present; if any are found, the patient should be worked up for stroke as well (see Chapter 41 for detailed workup of stroke).
- A focused eye exam by an ophthalmologist to assess IOP.
- Rule out other common causes of red eye (Table 40.1).

LABORATORY TESTS

- There are no specific blood tests for diagnosis of AACG.

IMAGING STUDIES

- No specific imaging is recommended in the setting of acute angle-closure, as that can delay treatment leading to permanent loss of vision.

SPECIAL TESTS (TO BE DONE BY AN OPHTHALMOLOGIST ON-CALL OR EMERGENCY DEPARTMENT PHYSICIANS WITH APPROPRIATE TRAINING

- Tonometry: a pressure of >30 mmHg is usually seen in angle-closure glaucoma.
- Gonioscopy is the gold standard test – done by an ophthalmologist.

THERAPEUTIC INTERVENTIONS

AACG should be suspected when characteristic findings are present. An ophthalmologist will most likely not be readily available at the time of the rapid response, and tonometry will also be challenging to obtain. A general eye exam and history can lead a clinician to the likely diagnosis. Once the diagnosis is suspected, ophthalmology should be consulted stat, and the case should be discussed. If the patient cannot be seen within 1 h of the consult, timolol maleate, apraclonidine, and pilocarpine should be given 1 min apart to relieve IOP (with approval from teleophthalmology). It is also suggested to administer acetazolamide, either oral or intravenous (IV). Following administration, eye pressures should be checked in 30 min, and eye drops should be re-administered if still elevated. If the increased pressure and symptoms persist, the patient will likely need emergent surgery for decompression.

STEPWISE APPROACH TO A PATIENT WITH SUSPECTED ANGLE-CLOSURE GLAUCOMA

Step 1: Evaluate and identify the patient with sudden vision loss and characteristic findings of AACG. Evaluate for any concomitant neurological deficits that could point toward a stroke.

Step 2: Stat consult ophthalmology.

Step 3: If the consult takes >1 h since symptom onset, start therapeutic intervention with recommendations from the teleophthalmology consult team. A common approach is to administer pressure-lowering eye drops; timolol, apraclonidine, and pilocarpine 1 min apart and acetazolamide 500 mg PO or IV.

Step 4: Reassess the patient in 30 min, monitor IOPs every 30 min.

Step 5: If pressure persists, re-administer eye drops.

Step 6: If symptoms fail to resolve, the patient will need surgical intervention by ophthalmology.

Suggested Readings

Petsas A, Chapman G, Stewart R. Acute angle closure glaucoma – A potential blind spot in critical care. *J Intensive Care Soc.* 2017;18(3):244–246. https://doi.org/10.1177/1751143717701946.

See JLS, Aquino MCD, Aduan J, Chew PTK. Management of angle closure glaucoma. *Indian J Ophthalmol.* 2011;59(Suppl 1).

CHAPTER 41

Acute Vision Loss in a Patient With Atrial Fibrillation

Ali Uddin ▪ Mohammad Adrish ▪ Firas Abdulmajeed

Case Study

A rapid response event was initiated for a patient for acute onset change in vision. On prompt arrival of first responders, the patient was found to be a 64-year-old female with a known history of atrial fibrillation, anticoagulated with apixaban, type 2 diabetes mellitus, hypertension, and coronary artery disease for which she had received coronary artery bypass graft one year before. She was admitted to the hospital two days before for management of alcohol-induced pancreatitis and was still not feeling well enough to tolerate any oral intake, including any oral medications. The patient had been doing well neurologically until 30 min before the rapid response was initiated, which was when she had developed an acute onset change in vision.

VITAL SIGNS

Temperature: 98.5 °F, axillary
Blood Pressure: 148/89 mmHg
Heart Rate: 115 beats per min – telemetry showed atrial fibrillation
Respiratory Rate: 14 breaths per min
Pulse Oximetry: 98% oxygen saturation on room air

FOCUSED PHYSICAL EXAMINATION

A quick exam showed a thin elderly appearing female in mild distress. Cranial nerve exam showed pupils were equal and reactive to light and accommodation. Bilateral visual field defects were present, which were consistent with homonymous hemianopia with macular sparing. Other cranial nerves were intact. Gross sensations, strength, and coordination were intact. Cognition was intact on a focused exam. A cardiovascular exam revealed tachycardia with an irregularly irregular rhythm; no carotid bruits were present on auscultation.

INTERVENTIONS

A cardiac monitor and pacer pads were attached immediately. Bedside blood glucose was done which showed a capillary glucose level of 154 mg/dL. The National Institutes of Health Stroke Scale (NIHSS) was administered, and the patient scored three based on complete bilateral hemianopia. Stat complete blood count (CBC), electrolyte panel, and coagulation profile were ordered. Electrocardiogram (EKG) was obtained and showed atrial fibrillation. Computed tomography (CT) of the head was ordered and obtained emergently, which did not show any acute intracranial bleed. CT angiogram of the head and neck were negative for any major vascular occlusions.

An emergent consult was obtained from stroke neurology, and it was decided to administer tPA given the patient's disabling persistent neurological deficit. The patient was transferred to the intensive care unit for systemic thrombolysis and subsequent monitoring.

FINAL DIAGNOSIS

Embolic posterior cerebral artery ischemic stroke secondary to atrial fibrillation.

Ischemic Stroke

Stroke is the sudden onset of focal neurologic deficits associated with dysfunction of the central nervous system (brain, retina, or spinal cord) because of either ischemia or hemorrhages. It is associated with clinical or radiological findings of permanent injury to neurological tissues. It can be broadly defined as either ischemic or hemorrhagic. Ischemic stroke is the more common subtype and accounts for 80% of the cases (see Table 41.1 for causes of stroke). It is caused by reduced blood flow to cerebral parenchyma resulting in an infarct of neural tissue. Hemorrhagic stroke, in contrast, is caused by the extravasation of blood into the brain parenchyma or the subarachnoid space because of the rupture of a blood vessel. Hemorrhagic strokes constitute approximately

TABLE 41.1 ■ **Causes of ischemic stroke**

Cause	Mechanism

Thrombosis	• Large vessel diseases
	  • Atherosclerosis – affects extracranial and intracranial vessels
	  • Arterial dissection – affects extracranial and intracranial vessels
	  • Vasculitis – affects extracranial and intracranial vessels
	  • Fibromuscular dysplasia – affects extracranial vessels
	  • Moyamoya syndrome – affects intracranial vessels
	• Small vessel diseases
	  • Lipohyalinosis and fibrinoid degeneration
	  • Atheroma formation

Embolism	• Cardiac source
	  • Atrial fibrillation, sustained atrial flutter
	  • Mechanical heart valve
	  • Atrial or ventricular thrombus
	  • Infective endocarditis
	  • Non-infective endocarditis (lupus, marantic endocarditis)
	  • Atrial myxoma
	  • Atrial or left ventricular aneurysm
	  • Patent foramen ovale
	• Arterial source
	  • Aortic atheroma
	  • Aortic root aneurysm
	• Cryptogenic – unknown source of embolism

Systemic hypoperfusion	• Shock – any cause, but more commonly with cardiogenic shock • Severe anemia
Hypercoagulability	• Sickle cell disease • Polycythemia vera • Essential thrombocytosis • Hypercoagulable disorders – prothrombin gene mutation, APLS, protein C/S deficiency, Factor V Leiden, antithrombin III deficiency • Heparin-induced thrombocytopenia

TABLE 41.2 ▓ **Inclusion and exclusion criteria for the use of tPA in acute ischemic stroke**

Inclusion criteria	• Diagnosis of ischemic stroke causing measurable neurological deficit • Symptom onset within 4.5 h
Exclusion criteria	Absolute contraindications • Ischemic stroke or severe head trauma in the last three months • Intracranial or intraspinal surgery in the past three months • Previous or current intracranial hemorrhage • Subarachnoid hemorrhage • GI malignancy • GI hemorrhage in the past three weeks • Active bleeding • Infective endocarditis • Bleeding diathesis • Current severe uncontrolled hypertension • Platelet count <100,000 • Current anticoagulant use with an international normalized ratio (INR) >1.7 or PT >15 s or aPTT >40 s • Oral anticoagulant use (excluding warfarin) with the last dose within 48 h or therapeutic low molecular weight heparin use with the last dose within 24 h
	Additional absolute contraindications between 3 and 4.5 h • Age >80 years • NIHSS >25 • History of diabetes AND prior stroke • Active use of oral anticoagulation, regardless of INR
	Relative contraindications • Low NIHSS with rapid improvement of symptoms • Hypoglycemia (serum glucose <50 mg/dL) • Major surgery in the last two weeks • Serious trauma in the last two weeks • History of gastrointestinal or genitourinary bleeding • Seizures with postictal neurological deficits • Large unruptured, untreated intracranial aneurysm • Untreated intravascular malformation • Pregnancy

20% of all strokes. Transient ischemic attacks are a separate entity and constitute transient, focal neurological deficits without clinical or radiological evidence of infarction.

The diagnosis of stroke is clinical, based on clinical exam and neurological findings, and supported by neuroimaging. Prompt recognition is of utmost importance as systemic thrombolysis can be administered within 4.5 h of the patient's last known well state (Table 41.2). Mechanical thrombectomy of large vessel occlusions can be done only within 24 h of symptom onset. NIH SS is an excellent tool that is validated for bedside assessment of the degree of neurological deficits and helps guide therapy. However, it lacks sensitivity for posterior circulation strokes, which should be kept in mind during the interpretation of the results.

Suggested Approach to a Patient With Suspected Acute Stroke

For a patient with sudden focal neurologic deficits consistent with stroke, we suggest the following for immediate risk assessment. See Fig. 41.1 for a flowchart of management of such patients; this should be done in consultation with stroke service. The usual sequence of history taking,

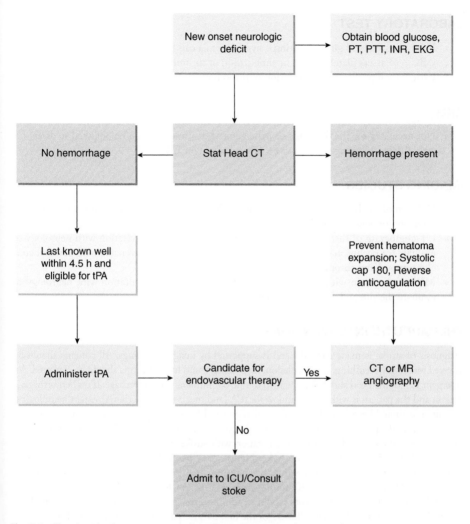

Fig. 41.1 Flowchart for the management of a patient with suspected acute stroke.

physical exam, investigations, and resuscitative interventions is often not followed during a rapid response; these measures often run parallel to each other in a code situation. The following components of the rapid response are discussed in the traditional sequence only to ease understanding.

FOCUSED HISTORY AND PHYSICAL EXAM

- The acuity of signs and symptoms – time and condition of patient's last known well state.
- History of similar symptoms in the past or any baseline neurological deficits.
- History of predisposing conditions.
- Medication history, including antiplatelet agents and anticoagulants.
- Presence of contraindications to tPA use.
- Physical exam should start with an assessment of airway, breathing, and circulation.
- Detailed neurological exam, including NIHSS.

LABORATORY TEST

- Point of care blood glucose testing – hypoglycemia can mimic stroke.
- CBC – to assess platelet count in anticipation of thrombolysis.
- Coagulation profile – in anticipation of thrombolysis.

EKG

- Not necessary for the diagnosis or management of stroke but can be obtained to assess for arrhythmias. Imaging should not be delayed to obtain EKG.

IMAGING STUDIES

- CT scan of the head without contrast should be obtained on an emergent basis to evaluate for acute intracranial bleed.
- CT angiogram of the head and neck can be obtained after consultation with neurology to evaluate for occlusion of any major vessels, which might be intervenable with percutaneous clot removal and thrombectomy.
- MRI of the brain without contrast can be obtained after consultation with neurology to evaluate the site and extent of ischemic injury.

THERAPEUTIC INTERVENTIONS

Diagnosis of stroke is made clinically and is supported by imaging findings. All patients should be assessed for airway, breathing, and circulation. Hypotension and hypoglycemia should be corrected. An emergent CT of the head should be obtained to rule out intracranial hemorrhage. If no hemorrhage is present and the patient is within the window for tPA (and meets all other criteria), expert neurological consultation should be obtained per institutional protocol for systemic thrombolysis. Aspirin should not be given to the patient who is planned to undergo systemic thrombolysis. A decision for mechanical thrombectomy should be made in consultation with stroke neurology. Blood pressure should be lowered below 185/110 mmHg before tPA administration per institutional guidelines. The patient should be monitored in a step-down or intensive care unit after tPA administration. The patient's blood pressure should be kept below 180/105 mmHg after tPA therapy for at least 24 h. If the patient is not a candidate for tPA, antiplatelet agents should be administered in consultation with stroke neurology. Permissive hypertension should be allowed for the first 24 h for patients who do not get tPA.

STEPWISE APPROACH TO A PATIENT WITH SUSPECTED ACUTE STROKE

Step 1: Secure the airway and stabilize hemodynamics – determine the time and condition of patient's last known well state.
Step 2: Administer the NIHSS.
Step 3: Obtain point of care blood glucose. Correct hypoglycemia and hypotension.
Step 4: CBC and coagulation profile should be obtained.
Step 5: Obtain stat head CT to rule out hemorrhage.
Step 6A: If hemorrhage is present, blood pressure control should be initiated, and stat consultation to neurosurgery should be obtained.
Step 6B: If no hemorrhage is present, candidacy for tPA should be determined in consultation with neurology.
Step 7: Antiplatelet agents and anticoagulation should be decided in consultation with neurology.

Suggested Readings

Hurford R, Sekhar A, Hughes TAT, Muir KW. Diagnosis and management of acute ischaemic stroke. *Pract Neurol*. 2020;20(4):306–318. https://doi.org/10.1136/practneurol-2020-002557.

Petty K, Lemkuil BP, Gierl B. Acute ischemic stroke. *Anesthesiol Clin*. 2021;39(1):113–125. https://doi.org/10.1016/j.anclin.2020.11.002.

CHAPTER 42

Acute Onset Facial Droop

Michael Heslin ▧ Syed Zaidi ▧ Firas Abdulmajeed

Case Study

The bedside nurse initiated a rapid response event for a patient because of acute onset left-sided facial droop that was noted by the physical therapist, who was evaluating the patient for his morning therapy session. On arrival of the rapid response team, the patient's nurse informed the team that the patient is a 63-year-old male with a history of hypertension and gout that is postoperative day one of a right total knee replacement. The patient's nurse reported that he did not have a facial droop when she saw him 2 h ago.

VITAL SIGNS

Temperature: 98.3 °F, axillary
Blood Pressure: 132/76 mmHg
Heart Rate: 81 beats per min – normal sinus rhythm on telemetry
Respiratory Rate: 11 breaths per min
Pulse Oximetry: O_2 saturation of 99% on room air

FOCUSED PHYSICAL EXAMINATION

A quick exam revealed a well-built middle-aged man in no acute distress resting comfortably in his bed. Upon auscultation, his lungs were clear, and his heart sounds were regular. There was a pronounced left-sided facial droop. The patient was not able to raise his left eyebrow. The left eye did not fully close when the patient was instructed to close his eyes tightly. There was an absence of wrinkles noted on the left side of the forehead. The remaining cranial nerve testing did not reveal any abnormalities. He was alert and orientated, had full strength in his upper extremities and left lower extremity. His right lower extremity demonstrated 4/5 strength that was limited secondary to pain. Finger-nose-finger testing was intact. He denied any headaches, vision problems, or dizziness. He reported that he had some eye dryness and irritation over the last two days, but he attributed this to being in the hospital and undergoing his knee replacement. His National Institutes of Health (NIH) score was three.

INTERVENTIONS

Given the neurological exam findings, a stroke alert was called, and expert stroke team consultation was sought. A stat computed tomography (CT) of the head was done, which did not show any acute hemorrhage. Stat magnetic resonance imaging (MRI) of the brain was obtained and was negative for any acute infarcts. A presumptive diagnosis of Bell palsy was made, and the patient was started on 60 mg of oral prednisone; he received his first dose after the imaging had been reported. Due to the patient being unable to close his left eye fully, artificial tears and an eye patch were ordered to prevent ocular injury.

FINAL DIAGNOSIS

Bell palsy.

Bell Palsy

The facial nerve (cranial nerve VII) has a complex anatomy and a wide distribution. It has four broad functions: somatic motor, somatic sensory, visceral motor, and visceral sensory.

The motor portions of the facial nerve arise from the facial nerve nucleus located in the pons. The facial nerve's sensory portions are derived from the superior salivatory nuclei and the solitary nucleus in the pons. The motor and sensory nerves travel individually through the temporal bone, where they come together as a single nerve in the geniculate ganglion. While in the temporal bone, the facial nerve gives off the greater petrosal nerve, which will provide parasympathetic innervation to the lacrimal glands, the nerve to the stapedius, which is a motor nerve that innervates the stapedius muscle of the inner ear, and the chorda tympani, which provides sensory fibers to the anterior two-thirds of the tongue, and the submandibular and sublingual glands.

The extracranial portion of the facial nerve begins just posterior to the mastoid process, where it quickly distributes three branches. The first branch is the posterior auricular nerve, and it supplies motor control to some of the muscles around the ear. The nerve to the digastric muscle and the nerve to the stylohyoid are the other two branches. The facial nerve then travels to the level of the parotid gland and branches into its five terminal branches (temporal, zygomatic, buccal, marginal mandibular, and cervical), which innervate the muscles of facial expression around the forehead, cheek, mouth, and neck (platysma) (Fig. 42.1).

Having a sound understanding of neuroanatomy can help understand Bell palsy's pathogenesis. The forehead musculature is supplied by motor neurons from both the left and right temporal branches, which ultimately are derived from each side of the pons. At their origin, a portion of these motor fibers ultimately crosses sides to provide bilateral innervation to the forehead musculature. Because of this crossing over, an upper motor lesion, such as a stroke, will not completely eliminate the motor fibers from the unaffected pons allowing the patient to raise his eyebrows and causing wrinkles of the forehead. However, since Bell palsy is a lower motor lesion, motor innervation of the forehead musculature from both temporal branches is affected. This causes the patient to have paralysis of the forehead muscles, resulting in the inability to raise his eyebrow and loss of the forehead's wrinkles. See Table 42.1 for differences between upper versus lower motor neuron lesions of the facial nerve.

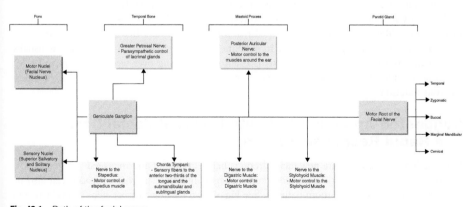

Fig. 42.1   Path of the facial nerve.

TABLE 42.1 ■ Features of upper vs. lower motor neuron lesions of the facial nerve

Upper motor neuron lesions	Lower motor neuron lesions
• Spastic paralysis	• Flaccid paralysis
• No muscle atrophy	• Muscle atrophy present
• Increased deep tendon reflexes	• Absent deep tendon reflexes
• No muscle fasciculation	• Possible muscle fasciculation
• Examples: stroke, trauma, neoplasm, central nervous system infections, amyotrophic lateral sclerosis	• Examples: Bell palsy, polio, muscular dystrophies, myasthenia gravis

TABLE 42.2 ■ How to differentiate between Bell palsy and stroke

Symptom/characteristics	Bell palsy	Stroke
Upper face paralysis	Present	Possible
Lower face paralysis	Present	Possible
Extremity weakness/numbness	Not present	Possible
Speech/swallowing problems	Not present	Possible
Balance problems	Not present	Possible
Confusion/AMS	Not present	Possible
Age	Usually 20s-50s	Usually >60
Onset	Hours to days	Seconds to minutes
Risk factors	Diabetes, pregnancy	Hypertension, atrial fibrillation, tobacco use, diabetes mellitus

DEFINITION AND DIAGNOSIS

Bell palsy is a lower motor neuron lesion of the facial nerve causing sudden weakness or paralysis of facial muscles on one side of the face. Common physical exam findings include the inability to close the affected eye, the loss of wrinkles above the forehead on the affected side, and facial droop on the affected side. Less common findings (dryness of the eye on the affected side, hearing difficulties, and altered taste) are occasionally seen as the presenting feature. Physical exam findings for a patient with Bell palsy can closely resemble findings associated with an acute stroke. A detailed neurological exam can help lead one to the correct diagnosis (Table 42.2).

Bell palsy is thought to be idiopathic. However, recent viral infections may play a role in the pathogenesis. Men and women are at equal risk for being affected. Bell palsy can occur in any age group, but there is a peak incidence in patients in their 40s. Bell palsy symptoms are usually gradual in onset (days), and the paralysis is often self-resolving over weeks to months. Quick initiation of steroid therapy with or without antiviral therapy can help lessen the facial nerve paralysis duration.

Suggested Approach to Acute Onset of Facial Droop in a Rapid Response Setting

For inpatient scenarios where new facial droop is being evaluated and managed, we suggest the following for immediate risk assessment and management; this stepwise approach can also be used to evaluate emergency room patients. See Fig. 42.2 for a flowchart of steps to evaluate and manage a patient with facial droop.

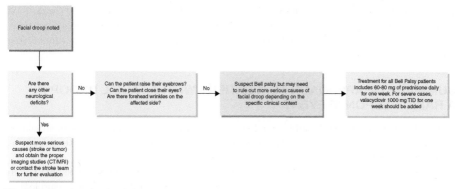

Fig. 42.2 Flowchart for the evaluation of a facial droop.

FOCUSED HISTORY AND PHYSICAL

- The acuity of signs and symptoms – time and condition of patient's last known well.
- History of suspected or known recent viral infection.
- Detailed neurological exam with particular attention to facial nerve deficits.
- NIH scale should be administered by certified staff.

LABORATORY TESTS

- No emergent labs are needed for the diagnosis of Bell palsy.
- Point-of-care testing glucose should be obtained as presentation of hypoglycemia can mimic neurological deficits.
- Ancillary testing, including complete blood count, comprehensive metabolic panel, and coagulation profile, can be done for treatment planning as stroke is a major differential diagnosis.

EKG

- There are no acute electrocardiogram (EKG) changes associated with Bell palsy.

IMAGING STUDIES

- As stroke is in the differential, the following studies should be obtained on an emergent basis, especially if the patient is within the window for thrombolysis. These studies would be negative in Bell palsy.
  - CT of the head without contrast – to evaluate for acute intracranial bleed.
  - CT angiogram of the head and neck – to evaluate for occlusion of any major vessels, which might be intervenable with percutaneous clot removal and thrombectomy.
  - MRI of the brain without contrast – to evaluate the site and extent of ischemic injury.

THERAPEUTIC INTERVENTIONS

All patients should be assessed for airway, breathing, and circulation. Hypotension and hypoglycemia should be corrected. Stroke is high in the list of differentials of Bell palsy, and expert consultation from stroke neurology should be obtained per institutional guidelines. After consultation with the stroke team, any considerations for systemic thrombolysis should be made. If the decision is made to treat as Bell palsy, high-dose steroids should be initiated to shorten the recovery period. Eye patches and artificial tears should be ordered to protect the cornea if the patient cannot close the eye.

SUMMARY OF APPROACH TO A PATIENT WITH A FACIAL DROOP IN A RAPID RESPONSE EVENT

Step 1: Evaluate for airway, breathing, and circulation. A detailed neurological exam should be done to evaluate other neurological deficits such as sensory deficits, extremity weakness, confusion, dysarthria, dysphagia.

Step 2: Emergent brain imaging should be done to rule out stroke. Lab tests can be obtained to plan for the next steps in management if an ischemic stroke is ruled in. Expert neurological consultation should be sought based on institutional guidelines.

Step 3: Steroids can be initiated once an ischemic/hemorrhagic stroke is ruled out.

Suggested Readings

Eviston TJ, Croxson GR, Kennedy PGE, Hadlock T, Krishnan AV. Bell's palsy: aetiology, clinical features and multidisciplinary care. *J Neurol Neurosurg Psychiatry*. 2015;86(12):1356–1361. https://doi.org/10.1136/jnnp-2014-309563.

Somasundara D, Sullivan F. Management of Bell's palsy. *Aust Prescr*. 2017;40(3):94–97. https://doi.org/10.18773/austprescr.2017.030.

CHAPTER 43

Loss of Consciousness in a Patient With Viral Gastroenteritis

Michael Heslin ▪ Mohammad Adrish ▪ Firas Abdulmajeed

Case Study

A rapid response event was initiated by the bedside nurse for a patient with a brief loss of consciousness. The rapid response team quickly arrived to find the patient resting comfortably in bed. The patient was a 57-year-old female with a history of rheumatoid arthritis on methotrexate admitted for severe dehydration secondary to vomiting and diarrhea and was being treated with intravenous (IV) fluids. Prior to her hospitalization, she was taking care of her three grandchildren, who had similar symptoms of nausea and vomiting. The patient was attempting to ambulate to the bathroom with her nurse's help. The patient had stood up from bed quickly and subsequently fell back into the bed. She was unresponsive for a few minutes and then regained consciousness without any intervention. After regaining consciousness, she was confused initially but recovered to her baseline within a few minutes. Per the nurse, there was no evidence of any urinary or bowel incontinence or any jerking motions after falling back onto the bed.

VITAL SIGNS

Temperature: 98.1 °F, axillary
Blood Pressure: 102/58 mmHg
Heart Rate: 118 beats per min (bpm) – sinus tachycardia on telemetry
Respiratory Rate: 16 breaths per min
Pulse Oximetry: 100% on room air

FOCUSED PHYSICAL EXAMINATION

A quick exam revealed a middle-aged female lying in bed in no acute distress. She was alert and orientated. Pupils were equal, round, and reactive, and there was no nystagmus noted. Her mucous membranes were dry and tacky. Her lungs were clear to auscultation. Her heart sounds demonstrated regular tachycardia without any appreciable murmur, and her radial pulses were strong and bounding. Her abdomen was soft, with mild diffuse tenderness and hyperactive bowel signs but without peritoneal signs. There was no calf tenderness or pedal edema on the examination of her extremities. She was able to recall the events before and shortly after falling back onto the bed. She reports she stood up, felt her vision dimming, and then woke up on her bed with her nurse standing over her. She denied any chest pain before this episode.

INTERVENTIONS

A cardiac monitor was attached to the patient immediately. Then, 1 L of IV fluid bolus was initiated, given concern for volume depletion. Complete blood count (CBC), comprehensive metabolic panel (CMP), and serum lactate level were obtained, which were concerning for potassium level of 3 meq/L. Stat electrocardiogram (EKG) was obtained, which showed sinus tachycardia. No acute ST changes were seen. Computed tomography (CT) of the head was deferred given the lack of focal neurological signs on exam. The patient was retained on the floor for further rehydration.

FINAL DIAGNOSIS

Syncope secondary to orthostatic hypotension in the setting of volume depletion.

Syncope

Syncope is a brief and abrupt loss of consciousness with a return to the patient's mental baseline after the episode.

Syncope can be broken down into four main categories based on the underlying pathologic condition. Having a general understanding of each main type can help direct the proper next steps in evaluation, especially during a rapid response. The four main syncope categories are cardiac, orthostatic, neurally mediated (reflex), and neurologic/other (Table 43.1). The most common type of syncope is vasovagal syncope, which is a subset of the reflex category. Vasovagal syncope is induced by anxiety, painful stimuli, or fear.

Various other conditions can mimic the clinical presentation of syncope, and special attention should be paid to these conditions to make sure they are not missed. These are listed in Table 43.2.

Suggested Approach to a Patient With Suspected Syncope

For a patient with syncope, we suggest the following approach to evaluate and treat the acute event. As defined above, syncope is a temporary, transient loss in consciousness with a return back

TABLE 43.1 ■ Classification of syncope

Classification	Examples	History/associated features
Cardiac	Arrhythmias, obstructive cardiomyopathy, structural heart/valvular disease, acute cardiovascular pathologies (pulmonary embolism, aortic dissection, myocardial infarction)	Risk factors for cardiac disease, family history of sudden death, heart murmur on exam, hypercoagulable states
Orthostatic	Volume depletion, autonomic dysfunction, drug induced (Table 43.3)	Poor intake, vomiting, diarrhea, spinal cord injury, Parkinson disease, alcohol use. Drugs: anti-diabetic, antihypertensives, vasodilators
Neurally mediated (reflex)	Situational, vasovagal, carotid sinus syndrome	Phobias, stressful situations, head rotation/shaving/tight collars cause symptoms, preceding nausea
Neurologic/other	Vascular steal syndromes, cerebrovascular accident risk factors, basilar artery disease, psychogenic	Somatization disorders, abnormal neuro exam, use of arms causing syncope

TABLE 43.2 ■ **Conditions that mimic syncope**

• Intoxication	• Cataplexy
• Epilepsy	• Psychogenic
• Hypoglycemia	• Hypoxia
• Transient ischemic attack	• Drop attacks

to the patient's mental baseline. If these criteria are not met, look for other causes of the patient's symptoms. It should be kept in mind that syncope is a tricky pathologic condition with various underlying causes. It is prudent to start with a comprehensive list of differentials which can be narrowed down as more information becomes available. The usual sequence of history taking, physical exam, investigations, and resuscitative interventions is often not followed during a rapid response; these measures often run parallel to each other in a code situation. The following components of the rapid response are discussed in the traditional sequence only to ease understanding. See Fig. 43.1 for a flowchart of steps to evaluate syncope.

FOCUSED HISTORY AND PHYSICAL

- The timing of onset and acuity of signs and symptoms, the time and condition of patient's last known well state.
- Past medical history, the reason for admission, hospital course, and baseline mental status.
- History of home medications and inpatient medications.
- Physical exam should begin with an assessment of airway, breathing, and circulation. A complete, thorough head-to-toe physical exam should be done. Particular attention should be paid to a thorough cardiac exam for possible murmurs and arrhythmias.
- A neurological exam should be done to rule out any new focal neurological deficits.
- Evaluate for any injuries in case of trauma associated with syncope.
- Examine the patient's volume status. Physical exam findings of being volume depleted (tachycardia, dry mucous membranes, decreased skin turgor, positive orthostatic vital signs).
- Although not generally done in a rapid response condition, a quick review of the chart can tell if there is any family history of young family members dying from sudden cardiac events – this hints toward possible cardiomyopathy.
- Orthostatic vital signs can also provide further insight into the patient's syncope.
- Tilt table testing can be done to look for dysautonomia (not usually done in a rapid response setting).

LABORATORY TESTS

- CBC – to determine if acute symptomatic anemia may be contributing to the patient's presentation.
- Electrolyte panel including magnesium – to see if an electrolyte abnormality may be contributing to a possible arrhythmia that may be contributing to the patient's syncope.
- Troponin level – to evaluate for cardiac ischemia if a cardiac cause is suspected.

EKG

- EKG should be obtained in all patients unless it is deferred based on clinician judgment. It is done to evaluate for any acute ischemic changes, arrhythmias, conduction problems

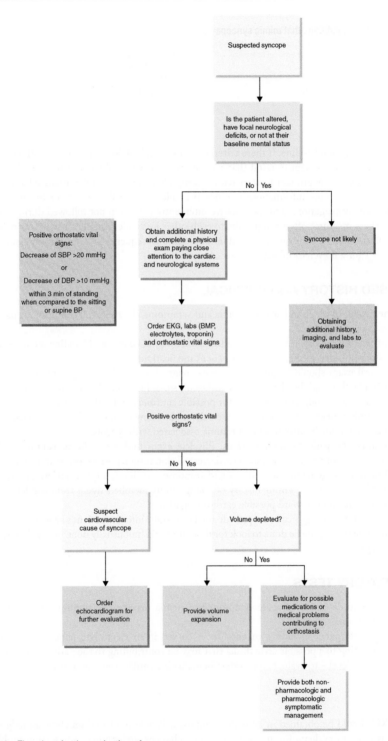

Fig. 43.1   Flowchart for the evaluation of syncope.

TABLE 43.3 ■ **Drugs associated with orthostatic hypotension and syncope**

• Alcohol	• Muscle relaxants
• Alpha-blockers	• Narcotic pain medications
• Selective serotonin reuptake inhibitors	• Calcium channel blockers
• Monoamine oxidase inhibitors	• Nitroglycerin
• Tricyclic antidepressants	• Phosphodiesterase inhibitors
• Sympathetic blockers	• Benzodiazepines
• Antipsychotics	• Diuretics
• Beta-blockers	

(heart block), and may point to specific electrolyte abnormalities. The EKG can also be helpful to evaluate for possible signs of structural heart disease, although these findings are often non-specific (ventricular hypertrophy, atrial enlargement).

IMAGING STUDIES

- A head CT can be obtained in a rapid response setting based on the clinical scenario; however, it is likely to be of little value in a patient without focal neurological deficits and whose mental status returns to baseline. Persistent altered mental status is a red flag, and head imaging should be considered strongly in that scenario.

THERAPEUTIC INTERVENTIONS

- Therapeutic interventions should be directed toward the underlying cause of syncope.
- Airway, breathing, and circulation evaluation is of utmost importance.
- In patients that are volume depleted, repletion with IV fluids and electrolyte repletion should be done.
- If a specific drug is suspected to be the culprit, it should be discontinued (Table 43.3).

STEPWISE APPROACH TO A PATIENT WITH SYNCOPE IN A RAPID RESPONSE EVENT

Step 1: Assess airway, breathing, and circulation. Secure airway if necessary, correct hypoxia, and treat hypotension as indicated. Fever should be treated.

Step 2: Assess the patient's mental status. A return to baseline favors syncope over more sinister differentials of loss of consciousness. Evaluate for alternate causes such as seizures which can mimic syncope.

Step 3: Detailed neurological exam should be done to evaluate for focal neurological deficits.

Step 4: Assess for any injuries if syncope was associated with trauma.

Step 5: Labs (CBC, metabolic panel, troponin), EKG, and cardiac monitoring should be ordered for further evaluation. Head imaging should be obtained based on the clinician's suspicion of alternate causes.

Step 6: Fluid resuscitation should be pursued for patients suspected of orthostatic syncope. Any culprit medications should be discontinued.

Step 7: Care can be escalated to a higher acuity unit based on the patient's stability.

Suggested Readings

Shen WK, Sheldon RS, Benditt DG, et al. ACC/AHA/HRS guideline for the evaluation and management of patients with syncope: a report of the American College of Cardiology/American Heart Association Task Force on Clinical Practice Guidelines and the Heart Rhythm Society. *Circulation*. 2017;136(5):e60–e122. https://doi.org/10.1161/CIR.0000000000000499.

Waytz J, Cifu AS, Stern SDC. Evaluation and management of patients with syncope. *JAMA*. 2018;319(21): 2227–2228. https://doi.org/10.1001/jama.2017.21992.

CHAPTER 44

Loss of Consciousness in a Patient With Seizure Disorder

Michael Heslin ▪ Syed Arsalan Akhter Zaidi ▪ Firas Abdulmajeed ▪
Mohammad Adrish

Case Study

A rapid response event was initiated by the bedside nurse for a patient because of seizure-like activity. A phlebotomist was preparing to draw labs from the patient when she began to shake uncontrollably and lost consciousness. The phlebotomist promptly alerted the patient's nurse. The nurse checked on the patient, and the rapid response was called. Per the bedside nurse, the patient was a 42-year-old female with a history of anxiety, depression, fibromyalgia, GERD, and seizure disorder on levetiracetam; she was admitted for lower extremity chemical burns that she had sustained at her job.

VITAL SIGNS

Temperature: 98.4 °F, axillary
Blood Pressure: 126/72 mmHg
Heart Rate: 87 beats per min (bpm) – normal sinus rhythm on telemetry
Respiratory Rate: 16 breaths per min
Pulse Oximetry: 98% on room air

FOCUSED PHYSICAL EXAMINATION

A quick exam revealed a young woman lying in bed slumped to the side. The patient would not open her eyes on command and resisted passive eye-opening by the rapid response resident. There were no frothy or bloody secretions around her mouth. There was no tongue laceration or other oral trauma noted. Her heart sounds demonstrated a regular rate and rhythm without any murmurs. Her distal pulses were intact. Her bilateral lower extremities were wrapped in bandages. Auscultation of the lungs did not reveal any abnormalities. Her abdomen was soft and non-tender. After the abdominal exam, the patient began to have twitching of her legs, arms, and side to side movement of her head. She would not answer questions. Her hand was lifted above her face and dropped to avoid hitting her face. A sternal rub made the jerking movements stop; the patient opened her eyes immediately and started answering questions appropriately. No postictal confusion was noticed. Her cranial nerve testing did not demonstrate any abnormalities. Her oxygen saturation did not drop during this event.

INTERVENTIONS

Given the presentation of seizure-like activity in the setting of a known seizure disorder, there was initially a significant concern for an epileptic seizure. A bedside glucose level was checked and found to be 99 mg/dL. A complete blood count (CBC) and a basal metabolic panel were drawn to evaluate for possible infectious or metabolic abnormalities causing her symptoms. Lactate and prolactin levels were also drawn to assess for signs that the patient may have had an epileptic seizure. Additional head imaging was not ordered as the patient quickly returned to her baseline, with no postictal focal neurological deficits and stable vital signs during her witnessed episode. A routine electroencephalogram (EEG) was ordered for further evaluation. Lab test results were available shortly after the rapid response, and all were within normal limits. Given the strong suspicion of non-convulsive seizures, a neuro-psychiatry consult was placed for further evaluation.

FINAL DIAGNOSIS

Non-epileptiform seizure episode.

Non-Epileptiform Seizures

Seizures can be either epileptiform or non-epileptiform. The pathophysiology of epileptiform seizures is an abnormal firing of neurons in the brain. In contrast, the true underlying cause of non-epileptiform seizures (NES) is unknown. However, it is believed that psychogenic factors such as traumatic events, abuse, or other sudden significant changes in one's life play a role in developing this disorder. NES can also be triggered by systemic disorders like low glucose levels or cardiac arrhythmias. Both types of seizures can present with similar physical characteristics of falling, shaking, decreased responsiveness, and staring into space. The most common type of NES is a dissociative seizure.

The physical examination can help distinguish non-epileptiform from epileptiform seizures. NES tend to be longer in duration than epileptiform seizures (>2 min vs. 1–2 min, respectively). Eye closure during the episode, especially if the practitioner is met with resistance, suggests non-epileptiform activity. The motor movements of NES tend to wax and wane and can include pelvic thrusting, head-turning, and the patient rolling over from side to side. Variations in vital signs such as tachycardia and hypoxia usually are not present in NES (Table 44.1).

As NES carries some similarities with true epileptiform seizures, we will provide a brief review of various types of generalized epileptiform seizures to help distinguish NES from true seizure activity. The various sub-types of generalized epileptiform seizures are described in Table 44.2.

Suggested Approach to a Patient With NES in a Rapid Response Event

For a patient with seizure-like activity consistent with NES, the following approach can be used for immediate risk assessment and management. Fig. 44.1 gives a simple flowchart for the evaluation and management of NES.

TABLE 44.1 ■ Comparison of epileptiform vs. non-epileptiform seizures

Epileptic seizures	Non-epileptic seizures
• Can have an aura	• Not associated with an aura
• Synchronous, rhythmic movements of the extremities	• Asynchronous movement of extremities, bizarre movements (head shaking, whole-body shaking, rolling motions)
• Incomprehensible vocalizations	
• Associated with tongue biting	
• Non-combative during the episode	• Rare to see oral injuries, but if they occur, usually to just the tip of the tongue
• Usually, a single episode at a time	

TABLE 44.2 ■ Types of generalized seizures

Type	Synonyms	Clinical features
Absence Seizures	Petit Mal Seizures	• Associated with brief staring episodes, it typically does not involve jerking of extremities • Commonly seen in children, less common in adults
Myoclonic Seizures	None	• Associated with a sudden jerking of the extremities, it often occurs bilaterally • Often a cluster of jerks is seen
Tonic and Atonic Seizures	Drop Attacks	• Associated with sudden stiffness or loss of tone of the limbs leading to falls • Seen in patients with brain injuries and intellectual disabilities
Tonic-Clonic	Grand Mal Seizures	• The most common type of generalized epileptiform seizures • Associated with stiffening of the body/limbs followed by jerking motion

FOCUSED HISTORY AND PHYSICAL EXAMINATION

- Timing of onset and duration of symptoms can be an essential clue in differentiating epileptiform seizures from NES. Description of the patient's seizure is also important.
- The patient's seizure history, such as baseline seizure frequency, last seizure, and seizure medication, is beneficial.
- The patient's medical history, admission diagnosis, hospital course, and current medications can help with the differential diagnosis during a rapid response. A history of psychological stressors is common in NES.
- Physical exam should always begin with the patient's airway, breathing, and circulation status during a rapid response, especially if it is initially unclear if the seizure activity is epileptiform or non-epileptiform.
- Epileptiform or NES can present similarly, so look for other clues such as oxygenation desaturation, urinary/bowel incontinence, tongue/cheek biting, and any postictal confusion or neurological deficits.

LABORATORY TESTS

- Hypoglycemia can put the body under stress, and it may manifest as a seizure, so a good first-line test in someone with a loss of consciousness is obtaining a fingerstick glucose level.
- If the patient has a history of seizures and is on anti epileptic medications, a drug level can help determine non-compliance and therapeutic dosing. However, the turnaround time of these labs is generally not in the scope of a rapid response event.
- A CBC can help determine if an infectious cause may be contributing to lowering a patient's seizure threshold. After an epileptiform seizure, a reactive leukocytosis may also be seen. If there is a high suspicion of a CNS infection causing the seizure, a lumbar puncture should be ordered once the patient is stable (this is not within scope for a rapid response event).
- A basic metabolic panel is crucial for evaluating a possible electrolyte abnormality, specifically hyponatremia or hypocalcemia, that can precipitate a seizure.
- Drug panels such as urine drug screens and ethanol levels can help evaluate if toxic ingestion may be contributing to the decreased seizure threshold.
- If drawn shortly after the seizure-like activity, lactate and prolactin may indicate the type of seizure the patient had. Elevated lactate and prolactin are associated with epileptiform seizures.

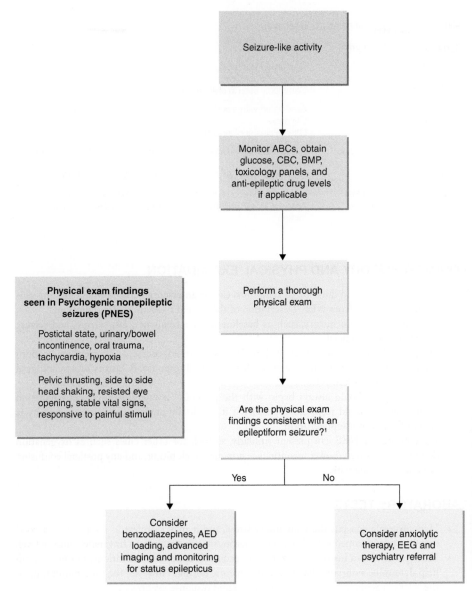

Fig. 44.1 Flowchart for evaluation of a non-epileptiform seizure.

EKG

- EKG is of no utility in diagnosing an epileptic or NES. In addition, it will be challenging to obtain an EKG if the patient is having convulsions. An EKG can be considered for QTc evaluation after the patient has been stabilized, if there is concern for drug intoxication/overdose.

IMAGING STUDIES

- If a NES is suspected and the patient does not have any focal neurological deficits, imaging of the head will be of little utility.
- If there are neurological deficits or a change in mental status, imaging of the head and brain may need to be obtained via CT, CTA, or MRI, depending on the clinical picture.
- A spot or continuous EEG is a crucial study to evaluate if the patient is actively having seizures. This is not routinely done in a rapid response situation but can be ordered once the patient is stable. An ideal diagnostic situation would be to have the patient have an episode of convulsions without any epileptiform discharges noted on EEG.

THERAPEUTIC INTERVENTIONS

As the diagnosis of NES is mainly based on an EEG, a clinician will rely heavily on focused history and physical exam to make the diagnosis during a rapid response event. If the typical symptoms of NES resolve spontaneously, no immediate interventions are usually required. If there is suspicion of epileptiform seizures, then immediate treatment should be initiated. We suggest always starting with the airway, breathing, and circulation. Maintaining an appropriate airway is the first step. IV access is crucial for administering medications. The management protocol for status epilepticus has been discussed in more detail in Chapter 45. For actively seizing patients, benzodiazepines are first-line treatment; lorazepam is the drug of choice because of its quick onset and long half-life. It should preferably be given intravenously but can be given intramuscularly if unable to obtain IV access. For patients who are not seizing anymore, benzodiazepines and other anxiolytics can also help treat the acute physiological stressors contributing to the patient's NES. A consult to the neuro-psychiatry team is suggested for patients with NES. Continuous EEG monitoring can be considered in challenging clinical cases to determine the underlying cause of convulsions.

STEPWISE APPROACH TO A PATIENT WITH NES

Step 1: The most critical step in a rapid response event for seizure-like activity is to ensure that the patient is maintaining the airway, breathing, and circulation. If any part of this vital chain is disrupted, quick correction is needed.

Step 2: Physical exam should be performed with the focus on distinguishing between epileptiform vs. NES.

Step 3: If the exam is more consistent with epileptiform seizures, benzodiazepines should be considered, followed by loading with antiepileptic drugs and additional imaging. If the exam is more consistent with NES, consider anxiolytics, EEG (spot or continuous), and psychiatry consultation.

Step 4: Lab work should be obtained to evaluate possible causes of the patient's seizure-like activity. Electrolyte abnormalities or hypoglycemia can precipitate seizures. Hypoglycemia can precipitate NES as well. It should be corrected.

Suggested Reading

Lanzillotti AI, Sarudiansky M, Lombardi NR, Korman GP, et al. Updated review on the diagnosis and primary management of psychogenic nonepileptic seizure disorders. *Neuropsychiatr Dis Treat.* 2021;17:1825–1838. doi:10.2147/NDT.S286710.

Perez DL, LaFrance Jr WC. Nonepileptic seizures: an updated review. *CNS Spectr.* 2016;21(3):239–246. https://doi.org/10.1017/S109285291600002X.

Reuber M, Elger C. Psychogenic nonepileptic seizures: review and update. *Epilepsy Behav.* 2003;4:205–216. https://doi.org/10.1016/S1525-5050(03)00104-5.

CHAPTER 45

Seizures in a Patient With Medication Non-Compliance

Ali Uddin ▪ Mohammad Adrish

Case Study

A rapid response event was initiated by a floor nurse for a patient having persistent seizure-like activity. On arrival of first responders, the patient was non-arousable and was having generalized tonic-clonic movements. Per the bedside nurse, she had just administered 2 mg of IV lorazepam to no effect. Per the report, the patient was a 24-year-old male with a past medical history of seizure disorder and type 2 diabetes. He was admitted one day prior to the surgical service for small bowel obstruction. The patient had been *nil per os* (NPO) with a nasogastric (NG) tube placed for bowel decompression. Upon medication review, it was noted that his home medications had been held, including his oral levetiracetam. He was only receiving a low dose sliding scale insulin while NPO with Q6h glucose checks. The nurse reported continuous tonic-clonic jerking movements for approximately 4 min.

VITAL SIGNS

Temperature: 98.4 °F, axillary
Blood Pressure: 115/86 mmHg
Heart Rate: 104 beats per min (bpm) – sinus tachycardia on telemetry
Respiratory Rate: 18 breaths per min
Pulse Oximetry: 94% oxygen saturation on room air

FOCUSED PHYSICAL EXAMINATION

A quick exam showed a well-developed young male lying in bed with generalized tonic-clonic movements of all four extremities and rapid eye twitching. He was non-arousable to tactile or vocal stimuli. The rest of his physical exam was not conducted because of active seizures.

INTERVENTIONS

Due to persistent seizure-like activity approaching 5 min, the most likely diagnosis was status epilepticus, secondary to not receiving his antiepileptic medications. After securing the airway by placing an oral airway, the patient was turned to his lateral side (to prevent aspiration). A pulse oximetry probe was placed on his finger to monitor oxygen saturation. Capillary blood glucose was checked to rule out hypoglycemia, which revealed a glucose level of 130 mg/dL. A basal metabolic panel (BMP) was drawn to rule out electrolyte abnormalities. The patient was given an additional dose of lorazepam (4 mg IV) followed by a loading dose of 1500 mg levetiracetam. The patient's seizure failed to resolve by benzodiazepines and levetiracetam, and he started to get hypoxic; thus, he was intubated for airway protection and started on a propofol drip. This stopped the seizures, and the patient was transferred to the intensive care unit (ICU) for further monitoring and management.

FINAL DIAGNOSIS

Status epilepticus secondary to sudden discontinuation of antiepileptic therapy.

Status Epilepticus

Generalized convulsive status epilepticus is defined as >5 min of continuous seizure episode or more than two seizures for which in-between there is incomplete recovery to baseline mentation.

The classification of status epilepticus per the International League Against Epilepsy is given in Table 45.1.

Common etiologies that predispose patients to status epilepticus are: structural brain injury (both acute and chronic), metabolic abnormalities, toxic ingestions of substances that lower seizure threshold, alcohol and benzodiazepine withdrawal, antiepileptic non-adherence, or discontinuation. Status epilepticus is a medical emergency that needs prompt evaluation and treatment. Delay in treatment can have grave consequences, such as neuronal injury leading to neuronal death and permanent neurological sequelae.

For any patient with status epilepticus, the initial approach is to administer benzodiazepines, followed by an acceptable second-line anti-seizure medication (Table 45.2). If seizures do not respond to an adequate initial benzodiazepine dose and a second antiepileptic agent loading dose, they are further classified as "refractory status epilepticus." This can be either a clinical or electrographic diagnosis.

TABLE 45.1 ■ Classification of status epilepticus (SE)

Convulsive	
Generalized	**Focal**
Generalized convulsive SE	Focal motor SE
• Primary generalized convulsive SE	
• Generalized convulsive with focal onset	

Non-convulsive	
• Typical absence SE	• Complex partial SE, with prolonged or repeated
• Other primarily generalized non-convulsive	focal seizures (i.e., focal onset seizures with
status epilepticus (NCSE)	impaired or altered awareness)
• Atypical absence SE	• Other focal SE with non-motor features (i.e.,
• Other generalized NCSE, with focal onset	focal onset seizures with dyscognitive features)
	(e.g., aphasic or sensory)

TABLE 45.2 ■ Common anti-seizure medications

Medication	Loading dose*
Lorazepam	0.1 mg/kg IV Q 3-5 min
Diazepam	0.15 mg/kg IV
Midazolam	10 mg IM
Levetiracetam	60 mg/kg
Fosphenytoin	20 mg/kg
Phenytoin	20 mg/kg
Valproic acid	30 mg/kg

*Please consult dosing guidelines for specific medications per institutional guidelines, expert consultation from clinical pharmacists can also be obtained.

Rarely, seizure episodes might continue for more than 24 h, even after general anesthetics have been administered, which is then classified as "super refractory status epilepticus." These terms of refractory and super refractory status epilepticus can be applied to both convulsive and non-convulsive seizures.

Status epilepticus should be differentiated from acute repetitive seizures, which occur when a patient develops three or more seizures within a period of 24 h where the patient's chronic seizure frequency is less than three episodes per day. Patients with acute repetitive seizures also maintain their mental status and cognitive abilities during seizure episodes, which is not true for status epilepticus.

Suggested Approach to a Patient With Status Epilepticus in a Rapid Response Event

For a patient with prolonged seizure-like activity consistent with status epilepticus, the following approach can be used for immediate risk assessment and management:

FOCUSED HISTORY AND PHYSICAL EXAMINATION

- The timing of onset and acuity of signs and symptoms, the timing and condition of patient's last known well state.
- Past medical history, the reason for admission, hospital course, and baseline mental status.
- History of home medications and inpatient medications.
- Physical exam should begin with an assessment of airway, breathing, and circulation.
- The patient's seizures may limit the physical exam; a full physical exam can be completed after the seizure episode has resolved.

LABORATORY TESTS

- Blood glucose level to rule out hypoglycemia.
- BMP for electrolyte derangements, specifically hyponatremia and hypocalcemia.
- Lactate level is generally elevated because of tonic-clonic muscle activity and rapidly resolves once the seizure episode terminates.

IMAGING STUDIES

- CT of the head can be done after seizure resolves to assess for any acute intracranial abnormality such as hemorrhage.
- Magnetic resonance imaging of the brain can be pursued if there is suspicion of seizure activity being secondary to a new stroke.

THERAPEUTIC INTERVENTIONS

As status epilepticus is an electro-clinical diagnosis, a clinician will rely heavily on focused history and physical exam to make the diagnosis during a rapid response event. Airway, breathing, and circulation should be secured per advanced cardiac life support guidelines. IV access is crucial for administering medications; therefore, two IVs should be placed. It is not always possible to obtain IV access in actively seizing patients, and this should not delay therapy as intramuscular route can be used. Once an IV is placed, Benzodiazepines are the first-line treatment. Lorazepam is the drug of choice because of its quick onset and long half-life; it should preferably be given intravenously but can be given intramuscularly if unable to obtain IV access. If seizures remain refractory to the first dose of lorazepam, the airway should be reassessed, and another round of lorazepam should be administered, being mindful of hemodynamic instability. If the seizure remains refractory, a loading dose of a non-benzodiazepine anti-seizure drug such as levetiracetam, valproate, or fosphenytoin should be administered. The established status epilepticus treatment trial showed all three medications to be equally effective. If the seizure persists, the patient should be intubated for airway protection and started on a general anesthetic such as propofol or midazolam infusion and transferred to an ICU setting. Refer to (Fig. 45.1) for a flowchart of management of status epilepticus.

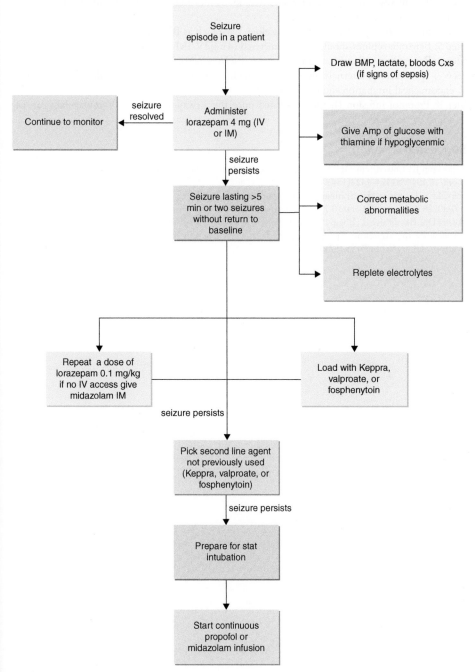

Fig. 45.1   Flowchart for the management of status epilepticus.

STEPWISE APPROACH TO GUIDE MANAGEMENT OF STATUS EPILEPTICUS

Step 1: Management should start with an assessment of airway, breathing, and circulation.

Step 2: The airway should be secured and hemodynamics stabilized. Temperature abnormalities should be corrected. Obtain IV access.

Step 3: Finger-stick glucose should be checked. Labs such as BMP, lactate should be drawn.

Step 5: Benzodiazepines should be administered (4 mg IV/IM lorazepam).

Step 6: Repeat benzodiazepine administration if seizure persists >3-5 min.

Step 7: If refractory, alternate non-benzodiazepine seizure medication should be loaded, and endotracheal intubation should be pursued.

Step 8: Propofol infusion should be started once the airway is secured. IV midazolam can be added based on response.

Suggested Reading

Betjemann JP, Lowenstein DH. Status epilepticus in adults. *Lancet Neurol*. 2015;14(6):615–624. https://doi.org/10.1016/S1474-4422(15)00042-3.

Seinfeld S, Goodkin HP, Shinnar S. Status epilepticus. *Cold Spring Harb Perspect Med*. 2016;6(3):a022830-a022830. https://doi.org/10.1101/cshperspect.a022830.

Vossler DG, Bainbridge JL, Boggs JG, et al. Treatment of refractory convulsive status epilepticus: a comprehensive review by the American Epilepsy Society Treatments Committee. *Epilepsy Curr*. 2020;20(5):245–264. https://doi.org/10.1177/1535759720928269.

CHAPTER 46

Seizures in a Patient With Hyponatremia

Ali Uddin ▪ Kainat Saleem ▪ Firas Abdulmajeed ▪ Mohammad Adrish

Case Study

A rapid response event is initiated by a bedside nurse for a patient having seizure-like activity. On arrival of first responders, the patient was confused, however, not actively seizing. Per the bedside nurse, the patient was a 37-year-old male with a past medical history of alcohol use disorder admitted to the hospital a few hours earlier with confusion, headaches, and nausea. The nurse described right-sided jerky movements lasting 1 min, during which the patient was non-arousable. It was noted that a recent basal metabolic panel showed a sodium of 110 meq/L and an alcohol level of 350 mg/dL. His social history was notable for significant alcohol use, almost 24 beers daily. He was placed on an alcohol withdrawal assessment score; the highest he had scored was five, and he had not required any lorazepam till this time. His hyponatremia was being worked up, and he was noted to have a urine osmolality of <100. During chart review, the patient had another episode of a right-sided focal seizure lasting ~1 min.

VITAL SIGNS

Temperature: 97.9 °F, axillary
Blood Pressure: 128/97 mmHg
Heart Rate: 96 beats per min (bpm), sinus rhythm on telemetry
Respiratory Rate: 22 breaths per min
Pulse Oximetry: 98% oxygen saturation on room air

FOCUSED PHYSICAL EXAMINATION

A quick exam revealed a thin male lying on his back in bed. He was arousable to vocal stimuli. He was not alert or oriented and was very drowsy. A cardiovascular exam revealed a regular rate and rhythm without murmurs. His respiratory exam was notable for tachypnea, equal breath sounds, and no rhonchi or wheezes. The neurologic exam was limited because of the patient's mental status. His right upper extremity was noted to be contracted, spontaneous movements of the left arm and both legs were seen. His skin turgor was decreased.

INTERVENTIONS

A cardiac monitor was attached, and because of multiple seizures within 5 min, the patient was given 4 mg IV lorazepam, which terminated the seizures. A stat computed tomography (CT) of the head was done to rule out intracranial pathologies, and it was unremarkable. The likely differential was seizures because of hyponatremia and less likely an acute intracranial process, infection, or alcohol withdrawal. This presumptive diagnosis was based on his history, blood tests, vitals, and alcohol withdrawal assessment score. Considering this presumptive diagnosis, a stat consult was obtained from nephrology regarding hyponatremia. The patient was given a 100 mL bolus of hypertonic saline over 10 min with a goal sodium increase of 4-6 meq/L. The patient was transferred to the intensive care unit for closer monitoring of his neurological status and electrolyte levels.

FINAL DIAGNOSIS

Seizures secondary to severe hyponatremia caused by beer potomania.

Symptomatic Hyponatremia

Hyponatremia is defined as a serum sodium level of less than 135 meq/L.

Hyponatremia has many causes including syndrome of inappropriate antidiuretic hormone secretion (SIADH), low effective arterial blood volume, glucocorticoid deficiency, psychogenic polydipsia, cerebral salt wasting, medication-induced hyponatremia, and beer potomania. This disorder can be classified as hypervolemic, euvolemic, and hypovolemic (Fig. 46.1); the diagnostic features of these sub-classes are outside the scope of this text.

Hyponatremia can manifest as being completely asymptomatic in one patient to causing coma in another patient. The neurologic symptoms seen in hyponatremia are because of cerebral swelling from osmotic fluid shifts into cells because of decreased tonicity outside of cells. The severity of symptoms correlates with the degree of hyponatremia. Mild symptoms are seen in sodium concentrations below 125-130 meq/L. This manifests as nausea and malaise. Severe symptoms such as lethargy, headache, seizures, coma, and respiratory arrest can result with sodium levels below 115-120.

In a rapid response event for severe symptoms of hyponatremia, the main aim is to terminate acute symptoms and start gradual correction of sodium levels. Alternate differentials of new-onset seizures should be considered, such as toxic ingestion/withdrawal, intracranial process, infection, and metabolic abnormalities.

Suggested Approach to a Patient With Hyponatremia in a Rapid Response Event

For a patient with severe neurologic manifestations in the setting of hyponatremia, the following approach can be utilized for immediate risk assessment and management. The usual sequence of history taking, physical exam, investigations, and resuscitative interventions is often not followed during a rapid response; these measures often run parallel to each other in a code situation. The following components of the rapid response are discussed in the traditional sequence only to ease understanding.

FOCUSED HISTORY AND PHYSICAL EXAMINATION

- The time of onset and acuity of signs and symptoms, the timing and condition of patient's last known well state.
- Past medical history, the reason for admission, hospital course, and baseline mental status.
- History of home medications and inpatient medications.
- Last alcohol intake in a patient with a history of heavy alcohol use.
- Physical exam should begin with an assessment of airway, breathing, and circulation.
- The patient's seizures may limit the physical exam; a full physical exam can be completed after the seizure episode has resolved.

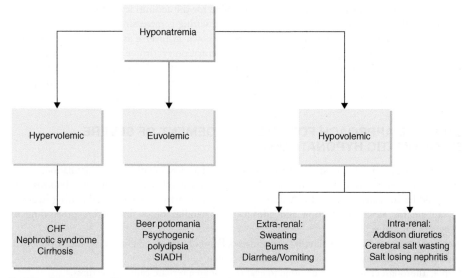

Fig. 46.1   Classification of hyponatremia based on volume status.

LABORATORY TESTS

- Blood glucose to rule out hypoglycemia.
- Basal metabolic panel for electrolyte derangements, especially sodium level, should be checked stat and compared with the baseline sodium level if it is known.
- Blood cultures if any suspicion of infection is present.

IMAGING STUDIES

- CT of the head can be done after seizure resolves to assess for any acute intracranial pathologic condition.
- MRI of the brain can be considered in patients with a high suspicion of alternate differentials such as new-onset stroke as the cause of the seizure.

THERAPEUTIC INTERVENTIONS

Management should begin with the assessment of the airway, breathing, and circulation. Maintaining an appropriate airway is the first step. IV access is crucial for administering medications. Seizures in the setting of hyponatremia are a sign of cerebral swelling which should be treated promptly to avoid further complications, including death. In a rapid response event, the cause of hyponatremia is less important than correcting it, especially when it is manifesting with neurologic symptoms. Whether acute or chronic hyponatremia, if the patient has severe symptoms, the management is identical. An emergent consult with nephrology or critical care should be requested. A common approach to management is to administer a 100 mL bolus of 3% saline over 10 min and repeat this up to two more times if symptoms persist. However, if the patient seizes for over 5 min or has multiple seizures without returning to baseline mentation, using benzodiazepine such as lorazepam 2 mg IV is appropriate to abate seizure (see Chapter 45 for how to manage status epilepticus). Some physicians prefer giving benzodiazepines first to break the seizures and then give the hypertonic saline for the sodium level; this approach is also reasonable. The goal of sodium correction in the acute setting is increasing it by 4-6 meq/L in 6 h or less. Even the most severe symptoms have been shown to reverse at this level of correction. Overcorrection, however, can result in osmotic demyelination syndrome. Patients with persistent seizures should be treated as status epileptics (refer to Chapter 45 for definition and management). Patients should be monitored in a critical care setting if manifesting neurologic complications of severe hyponatremia.

STEPWISE APPROACH FOR THE MANAGEMENT OF SEVERE SYMPTOMATIC HYPONATREMIA

Step 1: Management should start with an assessment of airway, breathing, and circulation.

Step 2: The airway should be secured and hemodynamics stabilized. Temperature abnormalities should be corrected. Obtain IV Access. If the patient is actively seizing, and getting hypoxic, intubate for airway protection and administer benzodiazepines first before proceeding to hypertonic saline.

Step 3: Alternative diagnoses should be considered. Point of care blood glucose should be obtained. Electrolytes and infectious workup should be drawn.

Step 4: Thorough chart should be done to evaluate for an alternate cause of seizures.

Step 5: A stat consult should be obtained with nephrology.

Step 6: 100 mL of 3% saline should be administered. 3% saline can be repeated with a goal increase of 4-6 meq in 6 h or per nephrology recommendations.

Suggested Reading

Braun MM, Barstow CH, Pyzocha NJ. Diagnosis and management of sodium disorders: hyponatremia and hypernatremia. *Am Fam Physician*. 2015;91(5):299–307.

Hoorn EJ, Zietse R. Diagnosis and treatment of hyponatremia: compilation of the guidelines. *J Am Soc Nephrol*. 2017;28(5):1340–1349. https://doi.org/10.1681/ASN.2016101139.

Tandukar S, Rondon-Berrios H. Treatment of severe symptomatic hyponatremia. *Physiol Rep*. 2019;7(21): e14265. https://doi.org/10.14814/phy2.14265.

Weismann D, Schneider A, Höybye C. Clinical aspects of symptomatic hyponatremia. *Endocr Connect*. 2016;5(5):R35–R43. https://doi.org/10.1530/EC-16-0046.

CHAPTER 47

Seizures in a Patient With New Hemodialysis

Ali Uddin ▪ Syed Arsalan Akhter Zaidi ▪ Firas Abdulmajeed ▪ Mohammad Adrish

Case Study

A rapid response event was initiated for a patient in the dialysis unit. On arrival of first responders, the patient was non-arousable and having generalized shaking of extremities. Per the dialysis nurse, the patient started having seizure-like activity 3 min prior. He was also reporting nausea and headache earlier. On chart review, the patient was a 58-year-old male with a past medical history of diabetes mellitus-2, hypertension, and recently diagnosed end-stage renal disease. The patient was admitted 2 h prior for altered mental status and was found to be uremic, for which he was receiving urgent hemodialysis. This was his first hemodialysis session. Two hours into the dialysis session, he had sudden onset of seizure-like activity. Due to this, his dialysis session was stopped, and a rapid response was called.

VITAL SIGNS

Temperature: 100.7 °F, axillary
Blood Pressure: 139/96 mmHg
Heart Rate: 96 beats per min (bpm), sinus rhythm on telemetry
Respiratory Rate: 17 breaths per min
Pulse Oximetry: 96% oxygen saturation on room air

FOCUSED PHYSICAL EXAMINATION

A quick exam revealed a middle-aged male lying in bed with generalized tonic-clonic movements. He was unresponsive to stimuli and did not withdraw from a painful stimulus. An arteriovenous fistula was visible in the antecubital fossa of his left arm. His cardiac and respiratory exams were not performed because of active seizures.

INTERVENTIONS

After securing the airway by placing an oral airway, the patient was turned to his lateral side (to prevent aspiration), and pulse oximetry was placed to monitor oxygen saturation. Capillary blood glucose was checked to rule out hypoglycemia, which revealed a glucose level of 108 mg/dL. A basal metabolic panel (BMP) was drawn to rule out electrolyte abnormalities. The patient was given a dose of lorazepam (4 mg IV), which broke his seizure episode. Due to seizure-like activity lasting almost 5 min, in the setting of uremia and first-time hemodialysis, with no prior history of seizures, the most likely diagnosis was dialysis disequilibrium syndrome (DDS). Nephrology attending was present at the bedside, and further dialysis was stopped. The patient was transferred to the intensive care unit for closer monitoring.

FINAL DIAGNOSIS

Seizures in the setting of dialysis disequilibrium syndrome (DDS).

Dialysis Disequilibrium Syndrome

Neurologic symptoms ranging from confusion to coma, which are mostly seen in patients on first-time hemodialysis or non-adherence to HD.

Risk factors for DDS included BUN >175, older age, previous head trauma, seizure disorder, stroke, conditions that increase blood-brain barrier permeability, and conditions associated with cerebral edema. While poorly understood, it is thought to be caused by the presence of increased urea which quickly declines from the bloodstream during hemodialysis resulting in an osmotic shift toward the urea that has built up into tissues, which results in cerebral edema.

Patients can present with a wide variety of symptomatology. Mild symptoms include nausea, headache, confusion, and disorientation. Severe symptoms include seizures, coma, and death. DDS remains a clinical diagnosis based on symptoms and typical history. While most of the mild symptoms usually self-resolve, for severe symptoms, the diagnosis will be one of exclusion and will require workup of alternate causes of altered mental status. Various causes of seizures and altered mental status in a patient on hemodialysis are discussed in Table 47.1.

Treatment for DDS regardless of symptoms requires sodium modeling; this works by making the blood more hypertonic to lessen the degree of osmotic shift, thereby mitigating the effect on cerebral edema. However, this can take up to 30 min to come into effect. If a patient continues to seize, hypertonic saline or mannitol can be given after consultation with nephrology and neuro-critical care physicians. Severe symptomatology should be managed when possible to prevent neuronal injury, as in the case of prolonged seizures.

TABLE 47.1 ■ Causes of Seizures in Patients on Hemodialysis

Cause of Seizure	Features
Dialysis disequilibrium syndrome	Neurologic symptoms ranging from confusion to coma, which are mostly seen in patients on first-time hemodialysis or non-adherence to hemodialysis
Uremic encephalopathy	Seen in patients with severe uremia. Patients exhibit similar symptoms as dialysis disequilibrium syndrome. Seizures tend to occur before dialysis
Erythropoiesis-stimulating agent related seizures	Uncommon, however, can be seen following the administration of erythropoiesis-stimulating agents. Caused by hypertensive encephalopathy, which can result in seizures
Medication toxicity of drugs cleared by the renal system	Medications include metoclopramide, theophylline, L-dopa, lithium, meperidine acyclovir, penicillin, carbapenem, ertapenem, and cephalosporins
Dialysis dementia	Caused by exposure to aluminum. Uncommon because of modern water treatment and non-aluminum phosphate binders
Electrolyte abnormalities	Hemodialysis patients are susceptible to hypo/hypernatremia, hypocalcemia, and hypoglycemia

Suggested Approach to a Patient With DDS in a Rapid Response Event

For a patient with new-onset seizure activity in the setting of a new hemodialysis session, the following approach can be used for immediate risk assessment, evaluation, and management:

FOCUSED HISTORY AND PHYSICAL EXAMINATION

- The timing of onset and acuity of signs and symptoms and the timing and condition of patient's last known well state.
- Patient's dialysis history, including the history of compliance to treatment.
- Past medical history, the reason for admission, hospital course, and baseline mental status.
- History of home medications and inpatient medications with a focus on medications that can precipitate seizures or lower seizure threshold.
- History of alcohol use and illicit drug use.
- Physical exam should begin with an assessment of airway, breathing, and circulation.
- The patient's seizures may limit the physical exam; a full physical exam can be completed after the seizure episode has resolved.

LABORATORY TESTS

- Blood glucose level to rule out hypoglycemia.
- BMP to rule out electrolyte abnormalities.
- Blood cultures and urinalysis/urine culture if an infection is suspected.

IMAGING STUDIES

- Since the diagnosis of DDS is one of exclusion, CT of the head can be done after seizure resolves to assess for any acute intracranial abnormality such as hemorrhage.
- MRI of the brain can be pursued if there is suspicion of seizure activity being secondary to a new stroke

THERAPEUTIC INTERVENTIONS

The initial management of a patient with new-onset seizures in the setting of DDS will be similar to that of the general population with regards to seizures. Severe symptomatic DDS will be a diagnosis of exclusion. Discontinuation of dialysis should be done in consultation with the nephrology team, as sodium modeling can be done through dialysis. Sodium modeling should be initiated only in consultation with nephrology or neuro-critical care. The job of the rapid response team will be to assess if the patient is maintaining an appropriate airway; if not, stat intubation will need to be called. If the airway is patent and the patient continues to seize, IV benzodiazepines should be administered as would be in status epilepticus (see Chapter 45). Electrolytes should be repleted if deficient. If seizure persists, the algorithm would be consistent with that for the management of status epilepticus.

STEPWISE APPROACH TO A PATIENT WITH SEIZURES IN THE SETTING OF DDS

Step 1: New-onset seizures should be identified in a patient undergoing first-time hemodialysis to diagnose DDS in an appropriate clinical setting.

Step 2: Management should start with an assessment of airway, breathing, and circulation.

Step 3: The airway should be secured and hemodynamics stabilized. Temperature abnormalities should be corrected. Obtain IV access.

Step 4: Finger-stick glucose should be checked. Labs such as BMP, lactate should be drawn.

Step 5: If seizures persist, benzodiazepines can be administered. Hypertonic saline or mannitol can be considered in consultation with nephrology and critical care teams.

Step 6: Sodium modeling to be done by a nephrologist or neuro-critical care.

Step 7: If seizures persist despite the above therapy, the patient should be treated as status epilepticus (algorithm given in Chapter 45).

Suggested Reading

Mistry K. Dialysis disequilibrium syndrome prevention and management. *Int J Nephrol Renovasc Dis.* 2019;12:69–77. https://doi.org/10.2147/IJNRD.S165925.

Agarwal MR. Dialysis disequilibrium syndrome. UpToDate.com. 2021. Available at: www.uptodate.com/contents/dialysis-disequilibrium-syndrome

CHAPTER 48

Severe Headache in a Patient With Migraines

Michael Heslin ▪ Syed Arsalan Akhter Zaidi ▪ Firas Abdulmajeed ▪
Mohammad Adrish

Case Study

A rapid response event was initiated by the bedside nurse for a patient because of a severe head-ache and multiple episodes of vomiting. The patient paged her nurse to inform her that she had an intense, pounding right-sided headache for the past 2 h and that the lights were making her headache worse. The patient had an episode of vomiting just before her nurse arrived. Upon prompt arrival of the rapid response team, the nurse informed that the patient was a 42-year-old female with a history of hypothyroidism; she was post-operative day zero after laparoscopic cholecystectomy.

VITAL SIGNS

Temperature: 98.2 °F, axillary
Blood Pressure: 138/68 mmHg
Heart Rate: 87 beats per min (bpm) – normal sinus rhythm on telemetry
Respiratory Rate: 14 breaths per min
Pulse Oximetry: 99% saturation on room air

FOCUSED PHYSICAL EXAMINATION

A quick exam revealed a middle-aged female sitting in bed with a pair of sunglasses on. She was in moderate distress secondary to pain. The patient's cranial nerve testing did not demonstrate any abnormalities, but the penlight used for the exam worsened her distress. She did not have any temple tenderness. She was alert and orientated. She demonstrated full strength of all extremities. Heel-shin testing was within normal limits. Her cardiac and pulmonary exams were benign. Her abdominal exam revealed several clean, dry, and intact bandages. Bowel sounds were present in all four quadrants. She denied any numbness, tingling, double vision, and blurry vision. She endorsed some mild abdominal discomfort from her recent surgery. The patient reported that she has a history of occasionally getting migraines that would require her to come to the emergency room for treatment. She stated that her current headache felt similar to her previous migraine episodes.

INTERVENTIONS

Since there were no focal neurological deficits on the physical exam, vital signs were stable, and the headache was similar in presentation to her previous migraines, it was determined that the patient was experiencing her typical migraine. No emergent imaging or labs were obtained. She was given a 1 L bolus of lactated ringers, ketorolac 30 mg IV, ondansetron 4 mg IV, and diphenhydramine 25 mg IV. Then, 2 h later, the patient's nurse contacted the intern on the rapid response team to let her know that the patient's headache had completely resolved.

FINAL DIAGNOSIS

Severe headache because of intractable migraine.

Migraine

Despite being one of the top five most prevalent diseases globally and accounting for over one million visits to emergency rooms in the United States each year, the pathogenesis behind migraines remains a mystery. Although initially thought to be related to vasodilation and vasoconstriction of cerebral blood vessels, current research points toward the trigeminal nerve and its surrounding vasculature being influenced by inflammatory compounds may be the true source of migraines. There tends to be a strong familial component to migraines. However, despite the current advances in genomics, no specific gene(s) have been identified that predispose individuals to migraines.

Migraine is typically described as a unilateral headache that tends to be pounding or pulsatile. The headache can last from hours to several days and is usually associated with nausea and/or vomiting. Photophobia and phonophobia are also commonly associated symptoms. Some migraine sufferers will also have a preceding aura, which can either be visual, sensory, or less commonly motor. Common visual auras include blurry vision, partial vision loss, or even complete vision loss. Unilateral extremity or facial numbness/tingling are seen with sensory auras. Motor auras, the rarest form of migraine auras, can manifest with extremity or facial weakness.

It can occasionally be challenging to distinguish migraine from other forms of headaches, especially in the setting of a rapid response called for severe headache, despite the distinct characteristics of each type of headache. It is important that characteristics of other types and etiologies of headaches be kept in mind. Table 48.1 presents a brief comparison of various types of headaches.

Occasionally it can also be challenging to distinguish migraine from other more sinister neurological pathologies such as an acute stroke or subarachnoid hemorrhage. Migraine with motor aura can be especially difficult to distinguish clinically from a more serious neurological pathologic condition. It is essential to obtain detailed neurological history and physical exam in patients suspected of migraine. Findings such as focal neurological deficits should raise suspicion of an alternate pathologic condition and prompt further investigation (Table 48.2).

First-line treatment for a migraine typically includes non-steroidal anti-inflammatory drugs (NSAIDs), intravenous fluids, anti-emetics, and diphenhydramine. For most migraine sufferers, this treatment or a slight variation tends to be abortive. See the section on "Therapeutic interventions" and flowchart for additional details for second- and third-line therapies.

TABLE 48.1 ■ **Common types of headaches**

	Migraine	Cluster	Sinus	Tension
Characteristics	Unilateral, pounding, or pulsatile, associated with nausea/vomiting	Severe pain around the eye with eye tearing, runny nose, eye redness, or drooping eyelid	Forehead pain, runny nose/congestion, ear pain	Dull, pressure across the forehead, "band-like pain," most common type of headache
Acute Treatment	IV fluids, non-steroidal anti-inflammatory drugs (NSAIDs), anti-emetic, diphenhydramine	High flow oxygen (12-15 L/min via non-rebreather), triptan therapy	Decongestants, nasal sprays	NSAIDs, acetaminophen, caffeine

TABLE 48.2 ■ Migraine mimics with red flag signs

Presentation feature	Differential diagnosis other than migraine
Rapid onset of symptoms	Migraine headache is usually a slower onset type headache. In the setting of a rapid onset headache, consider arterial dissection, transient ischemic attack, subarachnoid hemorrhage, hypoglycemia, seizures, venous sinus thrombosis
Thunderclap headache	Such headache reaches maximum pain intensity in less than 1 min and may allude to subarachnoid hemorrhage, hemorrhagic stroke, or pituitary apoplexy
Presence of other neurologic signs and symptoms	Can be present in arterial dissection, stroke, temporal arteritis, or glaucoma
Prominent neck pain with or without fever	Consider meningitis
Age of onset >50 years	Consider temporal arteritis, intracranial tumors, or uncontrolled hypertension
Worsening with position changes	Idiopathic intracranial hypertension, venous sinus thrombosis, intracranial mass, or cerebral spinal fluid leak
New or worsening headache in a patient with h/o migraines	Medication overuse headache, hypertension, intracranial mass, or medication side effects

Suggested Approach to a Patient With a Severe Headache Due to Migraine in a Rapid Response Event

For a patient with a suspected migraine headache, the following approach can be used to evaluate and treat the acute event. See Fig. 48.1 for a flowchart of evaluation and management of a migraine attack.

FOCUSED HISTORY AND PHYSICAL EXAMINATION

- The timing of onset and acuity of signs and symptoms, the time and condition of patient's last known well state.
- A detailed history of prior headaches with a special focus on pattern and similarity with previous episodes.
- The presence of red flag symptoms should be evaluated.
- Past medical history, the reason for admission, hospital course, and baseline mental status.
- History of home medications and inpatient medications.
- Physical exam should begin with an assessment of airway, breathing, and circulation.
- Perform a detailed neurological exam to evaluate for any deficits. Cerebellar testing should also be performed.

LABORATORY TESTS

- No emergent labs are needed for the diagnosis of a migraine.

IMAGING STUDIES

- CT of the head, CT angiogram of the head and neck, and MRI of the brain should be considered for evaluation of a more sinister cause based on history, physical exam, and suspicion of alternate cause.

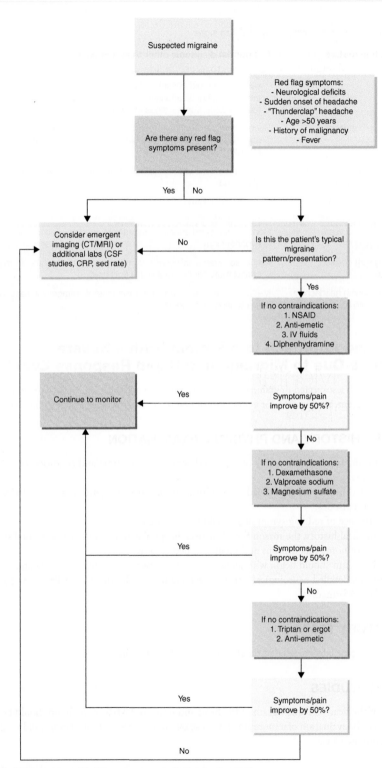

Fig. 48.1 Flowchart to guide the management of migraine headache.

THERAPEUTIC INTERVENTIONS

As a migraine headache is a clinical diagnosis, a clinician will rely heavily on focused history and physical exam to diagnose this during a rapid response event. Airway, breathing, and circulation should be secured per the advanced cardiac life support guidelines. The first-line treatment for migraines includes NSAIDs (typically ketorolac), anti-emetics (typically ondansetron), diphenhydramine, and IV fluids. If the first-line treatment does not reduce the symptom intensity by half, the next line of therapy should be pursued. The next step includes administration of dexamethasone, valproate sodium, and magnesium sulfate. If the second-line fails to reduce symptoms by half, triptan therapy or ergot can be used combined with an anti-emetic to help resolve the headache. Opioids should be avoided in the setting of a migraine. Neurology consultation should be requested for further management. A migraine headache that fails to resolve for more than 72 h is labeled status migrainous, which is beyond the scope of this text.

STEPWISE APPROACH TO A PATIENT WITH MIGRAINE HEADACHE IN A RAPID RESPONSE EVENT

Step 1: Management should start with an assessment of airway, breathing, and circulation.

Step 2: The airway should be secured and hemodynamics stabilized. Temperature abnormalities should be corrected. Obtain IV access.

Step 3: Detailed neurological history and physical exam should be obtained, focusing on the history of prior headaches and similarity of the current episode to previous episodes. Red flags for more sinister neurological pathologies should also be considered.

Step 4: Neurological imaging should be obtained if there are any neurological deficits or clinical suspicion of an alternate cause of headache based on clinician judgment.

Step 5: Treatment should be initiated, following the recommended lines of therapy discussed in the "therapeutic interventions" section.

Step 6: If the patient is still experiencing a migraine after the third-line of medications, additional imaging and labs should be considered to determine the cause.

Suggested Reading

Gilmore B, Michael M. Treatment of acute migraine headache. *Am Fam Physician*. 2011;83(3):271–280.

Smith JH, Schwedt TJ, van Garza M. Acute treatment of migraine in adults. UpToDate.com. 2021. Available at: https://www.uptodate.com/contents/acute-treatment-of-migraine-in-adults.

Vargas BB. Acute treatment of migraine. *Contin Lifelong Learn Neurol*. 2018;24(4). https://doi.org/10.1212/CON.0000000000000639.

CHAPTER 49

Severe Headache in a Patient After Lumbar Puncture

Michael Heslin ▧ Kainat Saleem ▧ Firas Abdulmajeed ▧ Mohammad Adrish

Case Study

A rapid response event was initiated by a nurse for a patient with a severe headache and nausea. The patient was found walking around the unit by the unit coordinator, trying to find a snack machine after coming up from the emergency room (ER) about 30 min before. She was brought back to her room, where she reported noticing a severe headache when she was walking around. Her pain had improved when she was back in bed and lying down. The bedside nurse informed the rapid response team that the patient was a 20-year-old female college student without any significant past medical history admitted for suspicion of meningitis.

VITAL SIGNS

Temperature: 101.6 °F, axillary
Blood Pressure: 142/70 mmHg
Heart Rate: 92 beats per min (bpm) - normal sinus rhythm on telemetry
Respiratory Rate: 16 breaths per min
Pulse Oximetry: 98% saturation on room air

FOCUSED PHYSICAL EXAMINATION

A focused exam revealed a young female lying completely flat and still in her bed. She was awake, alert, and appropriately oriented. Her cranial nerve testing was unremarkable. Finger-nose-finger testing did not demonstrate any dysmetria. Sensations were equal and intact to all of her extremities. There was no gross motor weakness noted. The patient was cooperative with the physical exam, but she was confused regarding recent events. She was warm to the touch. There was positive nuchal rigidity and Brudzinski's sign. Her cardiac exam demonstrated regular rhythm and rate. Her lungs were clear. She did not have any abdominal tenderness. She stated that any movement whatsoever makes her headache worse, but her pain does not seem as bad if she lays still. She reported that she did not have any vision problems but would like the rapid response team to shut off the lights if possible.

INTERVENTIONS

The rapid response team reviewed the ER notes, laboratory test reports, and imaging studies. The patient had an elevated white blood cell count of 14.2 K/uL with the rest of the complete blood count without any significant abnormalities. Her basal metabolic panel was normal. She had a computed tomography (CT) scan of her head, which was also normal. She had a lumbar puncture in the ER, and her cerebr ospinal fluid (CSF) studies were consistent with bacterial meningitis.

There was a large number of red blood cells in the first CSF tube but an almost negligible number in the last CSF tube. The CSF gram stain and culture were still pending at the time of the rapid response. The rapid response team did not order any additional labs or imaging, but interventional radiology was contacted to perform an epidural blood patch urgently. After returning from the radiology department, the patient reported that her headache was gone, and she could move around in bed without having any distress.

FINAL DIAGNOSIS

Post lumbar Puncture Headache (PLPH)

Post Lumbar Puncture Headache

A lumbar puncture is usually a safe and effective procedure that is performed to obtain CSF for lab testing and to deliver drugs for anesthesia or chemotherapy. As with any invasive procedure, there are always risks and possible complications. PLPH is the most common side effect for lumbar punctures, occurring in up to one-third of patients.

As a lumbar puncture is performed, a needle is driven through the skin, subcutaneous tissues, and back musculature. It passes through the epidural space, penetrates the dura and arachnoid mater of the spinal cord, and ultimately ends up in the subarachnoid space where CSF bathes and protects the cauda equina, spinal cord, and brain (Fig. 49.1).

The actual cause of PLPH is unknown, but it is hypothesized that there is a leakage of CSF through the hole caused by the needle puncture through the dura and arachnoid mater and into the epidural space. Symptoms arise when the leakage rate into the epidural space exceeds the production rate of new CSF by the choroid plexus. Once there is an overall net loss of CSF into

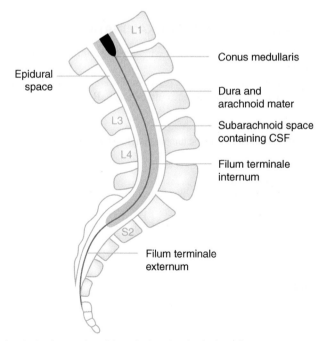

Fig. 49.1   Showing the lumbar portion of the spinal cord and spinal canal.

the epidural space, the support and cushioning provided by CSF is lost, which results in a stretch of the sensory part of the nerves resulting in pain. The intracranial pressure could also play a role because if the intracranial pressure drops because of increased CSF leakage, the venous vasculature dilates, which causes acute distention leading to pain.

The diagnosis of PLPH is dependent on the patient's history. The obvious clue to the correct diagnosis is having a lumbar puncture performed within the last seven days. Another big clue that points to PLPH is the positional nature of the headache. PLPH tends to resolve if the patient is completely supine and not moving. PLPH tends to acutely worsen with sitting, standing, or rapid body movements. There are three main severity classes of PLPH, which are discussed in Table 49.1.

The treatment of PLPH is dependent on the severity of symptoms. Treatment can be either symptomatic management with pain relief and antiemetics or curative with an epidural blood patch. The epidural blood patch is the definitive treatment for a patient with a PLPH. During an epidural blood patch, around 20 cc of the patient's whole blood is drawn. The blood is then injected into the epidural space. It is believed that the blood acts to help clot the CSF leak and acts to promote a healing inflammatory response. The increased pressure of the epidural space with the addition of the blood volume may also act to tamponade the CSF leak into the epidural space. After the blood patch has been performed, the patient must remain supine for the next 2 h to ensure that the patch has enough time to set. Anesthesia or interventional radiology typically performs the epidural blood patches depending on institutional policy.

Suggested Approach to a Patient With PLPH in a Rapid Response Event

For a patient with PLPH, the following approach can be used to evaluate and treat the acute event. See Fig. 49.2 for a flowchart of management of PLPH.

FOCUSED HISTORY AND PHYSICAL EXAMINATION

- The timing of onset and acuity of signs and symptoms, the timing and condition of patient's last known well state.
- A detailed history of the headache with a particular focus on the timing of the headache and the presence of any red flag symptoms should be taken. Red flags symptoms are discussed

TABLE 49.1 ■ Severity classification of post lumbar puncture headache

Severity of PLPH	Comments
Mild	Postural headache slightly restricting daily activities, the patient is not bedridden at any time of the day, and there are no associated symptoms
Moderate	The patient is bedridden for some part of the day because of postural symptoms that significantly restrict daily activities; associated symptoms may or may not be present
Severe	The patient might stay in bed the whole day because of severe postural symptoms; associated symptoms are almost always present

Associated symptoms:
Vestibular: Nausea, vomiting, and dizziness
Cochlear: Hearing loss, tinnitus, and hyperacusis
Musculoskeletal: Neck stiffness, scapular pain
Ocular: Photophobia, diplopia, difficulty in accommodation, and teichopsia

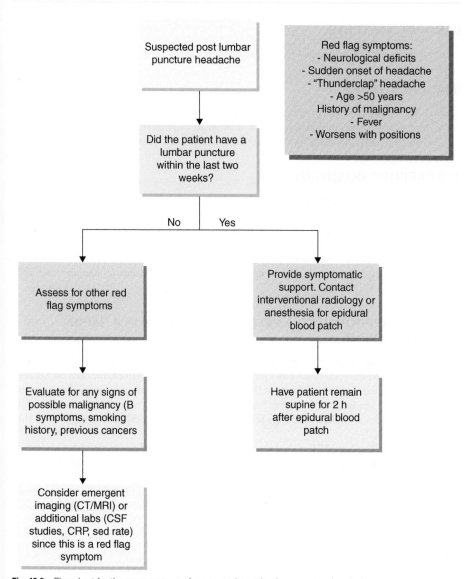

Fig. 49.2 Flowchart for the management of suspected post lumbar puncture headache.

in detail in Chapter 48. PLPH usually occurs within one week of having a lumbar puncture but has been reported to occur up to two weeks after the lumbar puncture. If the timeline does not match, re-evaluate the diagnosis.

- Past medical history, the reason for admission, hospital course, and baseline mental status.
- History of home medications and inpatient medications.
- Physical exam should begin with an assessment of airway, breathing, and circulation.
- A detailed neurological exam should be performed to evaluate for any deficits.

LABORATORY TESTS

- No emergent labs are needed for the diagnosis of PLPH.

IMAGING STUDIES

- A CT of the head or magnetic resonance imaging (MRI) of the brain can be obtained depending on the clinician's suspicion of an alternate or more sinister cause of the headache. Positional headaches are associated with raised intracranial pressure as well.

THERAPEUTIC INTERVENTIONS

As PLPH is a clinical diagnosis, an astute physician will rely heavily on focused history and physical exam to diagnose this condition during a rapid response event. As in any rapid response event, airway, breathing, and circulation should be secured per advanced cardiac life support guidelines. IV access is crucial for administering medications; therefore, two peripheral IV lines should be placed. The definitive treatment is an epidural blood patch which either the anesthesia or interventional radiology teams can do. Providing supportive care with analgesics and antiemetics is also appropriate.

STEPWISE APPROACH TO A PATIENT WITH A PLPH IN A RAPID RESPONSE EVENT

Step 1: Management should start with an assessment of airway, breathing, and circulation.

Step 2: Detailed neurological history and physical exam should be obtained, focusing on the history of prior headaches and similarity of the current episode to previous episodes. The temporal relationship of headache with lumbar puncture should be evaluated as PLPH occurs within seven days of the procedure. Red flags for more sinister neurological pathologies should also be assessed.

Step 3: CT of the head or MRI of the brain can be obtained depending on the clinician's suspicion of an alternate cause. Positional headaches are also associated with increased intracranial pressure.

Step 4: Anesthesiology or interventional radiology should be consulted for definitive management with an epidural blood patch. Symptomatic relief can be provided with non-steroidal anti-inflammatory drugs and antiemetic medications.

Suggested Reading

Ahmed SV, Jayawarna C, Jude E. Post lumbar puncture headache: diagnosis and management. *Postgrad Med J*. 2006;82(973):713–716. https://doi.org/10.1136/pgmj.2006.044792.

Alstadhaug KB, Odeh F, Baloch FK, Berg DH, Salvesen R. Post-lumbar puncture headache. *Tidsskr Nor Laegeforen*. 2012;132(7):818–821. https://doi.org/10.4045/tidsskr.11.0832.

Bateman BT, Cole N, Sun-Edelstein C, Lay CL. Post dural puncture headache. UpToDate.com. 2021. Available at: https://www.uptodate.com/contents/post-dural-puncture-headache

Kwak K-H. Postdural puncture headache. *Korean J Anesthesiol*. 2017;70(2):136–143. https://doi.org/10.4097/kjae.2017.70.2.136.

CHAPTER 50

Hyperthermia in a Patient on Polypharmacy

Melissa Chrites ▓ Mohammad Adrish

Case Study

A rapid response event was initiated by the bedside nurse for a patient who developed severe hyperthermia. Upon the arrival of the rapid response team (RRT), the patient was noted to be a 45-year-old male admitted to the hospital for severe depression. The bedside nurse informed the RRT that his temperature had been normal on morning vital signs. The patient had reported a racing heart to the nurse, who checked his vitals and found him to have elevated temperature. A review of his chart showed that he was taking sertraline for depressive disorder. Buspirone had been added to the patient's regimen that morning. He had also received his usual dose of trazodone the evening before, which he was taking for insomnia. The patient denied taking any illicit substances. He was not on any other prescription or over-the-counter medications or supplements.

VITAL SIGNS

Temperature: 105 °F, axillary
Blood Pressure: 180/90 mmHg
Heart Rate: 102 beats per min (bpm), sinus tachycardia on the monitor
Respiratory Rate: 22 breaths per min
Pulse Oximetry: 98% saturation on room air

FOCUSED PHYSICAL EXAMINATION

A quick exam revealed a middle-aged male, awake and alert, and answering questions. His face was flushed, and there was visible perspiration on his forehead. He appeared agitated. Visual tracking was intact without evidence of nystagmus. His cranial nerve exam was unremarkable. There was evidence of rigidity with passive movement of his extremities, and his patellar reflexes were noted to be 3+ bilaterally. A cardiac exam revealed tachycardia without evidence of murmurs. His lung exam was unremarkable, and his abdominal examination revealed hyperactive bowel sounds.

INTERVENTIONS

A cardiac monitor and pacer pads were attached to the patient immediately. Blood sample for stat laboratory tests was drawn, which included a complete blood count (CBC), comprehensive metabolic panel (CMP), creatine phosphokinase (CPK), lactate level, and blood cultures. A urine drug screen was also ordered. Then, 1 g of intravenous acetaminophen was administered immediately, which had no effect on the patient's temperature. Ice packs were placed along his neck, axilla, and groin. The patient's labs were later reported and showed elevated CPK level, elevated lactate level, and mild acute renal insufficiency. With relevant history and laboratory examination, a presumptive diagnosis of serotonin syndrome was made. Intravenous fluids were started, and the patient was immediately given 2 mg of IV lorazepam to induce mild sedation and decrease muscle activity. The orders for the patient's sertraline, buspirone, and trazodone were discontinued, and a consult was placed for psychiatry to evaluate the patient's medication regimen. The patient was transferred to the intensive care unit (ICU) for further management and possible need of further sedation, neuromuscular blockage, and mechanical ventilation.

FINAL DIAGNOSIS

Hyperthermia secondary to serotonin syndrome.

Severe Hyperthermia

Hyperthermia is the elevation of core body temperature above 38.5°C or 101.3°F. Severe hyperthermia is the elevation of core body temperature to greater than 40°C or 104°F. The various mechanisms underlying the development of hyperthermia are discussed in Table 50.1.

The underlying pathophysiology of hyperthermia is different from fever. Fever is mediated by the release of cytokines, whereas hyperthermia is mediated by a failure of thermoregulation. Clinical differences between fever and hyperthermia are discussed in Table 50.2.

TABLE 50.1 ■ Mechanisms of hyperthermia

Mechanism	Example
Increased environmental heat load	Heatwave Humidity
Increased heat production	Overexertion Thyroid storm Pheochromocytoma Malignant hyperthermia Neuroleptic malignant syndrome Serotonin syndrome Delirium tremens Illicit drugs such as MDMA Anticholinergic toxicity Hypothalamic dysfunction – hemorrhage or stroke
Decreased heat dissipation	Humidity Poor sweat production Anticholinergic toxicity

TABLE 50.2 ■ Clinical comparison of fever and hyperthermia

Fever	Hyperthermia
Temp generally lower than 104°F	Temp higher than 104°F
Improves with acetaminophen	Antipyretics have no effect
The patient may have rigors, no changes in muscle tone or reflexes	The patient may exhibit rigidity or clonus if hyperthermia is caused by medication side effect

As seen in Table 50.1, drug toxicities are one of the common causes of hyperthermia. A comparison of common hyperthermia syndromes associated with drug toxicities is discussed in Table 50.3.

Suggested Approach to a Patient With Severe Hyperthermia in a Rapid Response Event

We suggest the following approach to evaluate and treat the acute event for a patient with severe hyperthermia. This can be expanded and used as such in emergency room situations as well, as this protocol is based on guidelines for the management of severe hyperthermia. See Fig. 50.1 for a flowchart of evaluation and management of hyperthermia.

FOCUSED HISTORY AND PHYSICAL EXAMINATION

- Timing of onset and duration of symptoms.
- History of exposure to environmental triggers or drugs triggers listed in Table 50.1.
- Medication history.
- Family history of hyperthermia – malignant hyperthermia is a genetic disorder.
- Physical exam should begin with the assessment of airway, breathing, and circulation.

TABLE 50.3 ■ Features of common hyperthermia syndromes

Syndrome	Serotonin syndrome	Neuroleptic malignant syndrome	Malignant hyperthermia	Anticholinergic toxicity
Causative agent	Serotonin agonists such as selective serotonin reuptake inhibitors, monoamine oxidase inhibitors	Dopamine antagonists such as typical antipsychotics	Inhalational anesthetics such as enflurane and depolarizing neuromuscular blockers such as succinylcholine	Anticholinergic agents such as organophosphates, diphenhydramine
Resolution of symptoms	24 h after initiation of treatment	Within two weeks with treatment	24–48 h with treatment	Hours to days with treatment
Features	Altered mental status Muscle rigidity Hyperreflexia Increased bowel sounds Diaphoresis	Altered mental status Rigidity Hyporeflexia Dysautonomia	Increased end-tidal CO_2 Mottled kin Rigidity Hyporeflexia Dysautonomia	Altered mental status Urinary retention Decreased bowel sounds Normal muscle tone and reflexes
Treatment	Discontinuation of the offending agent Supportive care Intubation in patients with temp >41.1°C Benzodiazepines Cyproheptadine	Discontinuation of the offending agent Supportive care Benzodiazepines Dantrolene	Call for help Discontinuation of the offending agent Optimize oxygenation Dantrolene Calcium channel blockers are contraindicated	Discontinuation of the offending agent Decontamination if indicated Supportive care Sodium bicarbonate Benzodiazepines

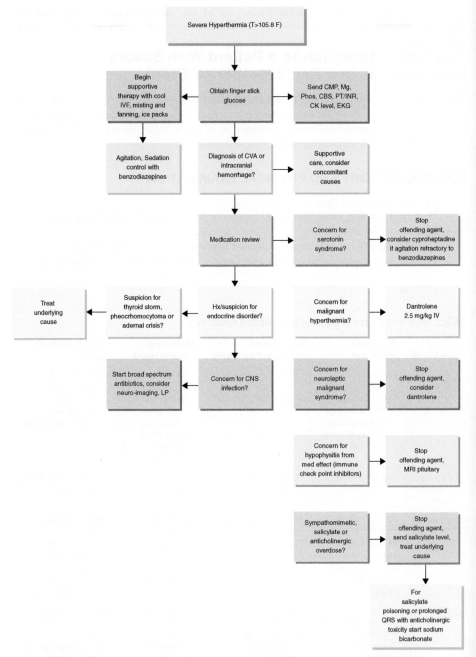

Fig. 50.1 Flowchart to guide the management of severe hyperthermia in a hospitalized patient.

- A detailed neurological exam should be done, including an assessment of muscle tone and reflexes.
- Although rare, sepsis and malignancies can also present with very high-grade fevers, and assessment should be made for these causes as well.

LABORATORY TESTS

- CBC – elevated white count can point toward an infection.
- CMP – to evaluate for change in renal or liver function, which can lead to decreased drug clearance and drug-drug interactions. Electrolyte abnormalities are seen with certain hyperthermia syndromes.
- CPK – to assess for rhabdomyolysis.
- Blood cultures – to assess for infection.
- Thyroid-stimulating hormone level, urine toxicology screen – can be obtained if suspicion of thyroid cause or drug abuse, respectively.

EKG

- Should be obtained in all patients to assess for QTc changes which are seen in many hyperthermia syndromes. EKG does not need to be obtained emergently.

IMAGING STUDIES

- CT head or MRI brain can be obtained if there is suspicion of acute hemorrhage or stroke in the hypothalamic region.

THERAPEUTIC INTERVENTIONS

Hyperthermia syndromes are medical emergencies and carry a high mortality rate. Management should begin with an assessment of airway, breathing, and circulation. Patients with hyperthermia because of serotonin syndrome should be intubated, paralyzed, and sedated to reduce muscle rigidity, which would bring down the temperature. Succinylcholine should not be used if malignant hyperthermia is suspected. Patients with arrhythmias should be treated according to the advanced cardiac life support protocol for the treatment of arrhythmias. Acetaminophen does not have a role in hyperthermia management. However, it is often used regardless, given the difficulty in pinpointing the exact diagnosis in a rapid response setting. General supportive measures including evaporative and convective cooling should be initiated. Benzodiazepines are used to reduce agitation, which can help reduce muscle activity and, subsequently, patient's temperature. Benzodiazepines also help reduce shivering. A brief overview of the treatment of specific hyperthermia syndromes is discussed in Table 50.3. Electrolyte abnormalities should be treated per protocol. Patients should be transferred to ICU for further care.

STEPWISE APPROACH TO THE MANAGEMENT OF A PATIENT WITH SEVERE HYPERTHERMIA IN HOSPITAL

Step 1: Assess airway, breathing, and circulation. Patients with serotonin syndrome require intubation to reduce muscle activity.

Step 2: Begin supportive care with cooling techniques and control of agitation and shivering with benzodiazepines.

Step 3: Investigation of underlying causes, including intracranial pathologic conditions (very recent cerebrovascular accident (CVA) or intracranial hemorrhage), review medication interactions and toxicities, consider endocrinopathies and infectious causes.

Step 4: Send labs to rule out complications secondary to severe hyperthermia, blood cultures to rule out infection/sepsis.

Step 5: Patients should be transferred to ICU for further care.

Suggested Readings

Caroff SN, Watson CB, Rosenberg H. Drug-induced hyperthermic syndromes in psychiatry. *Clin Psychopharmacol Neurosci Off Sci J Korean Coll Neuropsychopharmacol.* 2021;19(1):1–11. https://doi.org/10.9758/cpn.2021.19.1.1.

Mørch SS, Andersen JDH, Bestle MH. Treatment of hyperthermia. *Ugeskr Laeger.* 2017;179(30).

Rusyniak DE, Sprague JE. Toxin-induced hyperthermic syndromes. *Med Clin North Am.* 2005;89(6): 1277–1296. https://doi.org/10.1016/j.mcna.2005.06.002.

PART 4

Cases With Gastrointestinal Pathologies

CHAPTER 51

Hematemesis in a Patient With Alcohol Use Disorder

Abdelrhman M. Abo-zed ▦ Mohammad Adrish ▦ Syed Arsalan Akhter Zaidi

Case Study

A rapid response event was initiated by the bedside nurse after the patient had an episode of large volume, bloody vomiting. On prompt arrival of the rapid response team, it was noted that the patient was a 28-year-old male with a known history of alcohol use and IV drug abuse who was admitted earlier for alcohol withdrawal syndrome and two episodes of bloody vomiting. A quick review of his charts indicated that the patient's hemoglobin had been trending down.

VITAL SIGNS

Temperature: 98.2 °F, axillary
Blood Pressure: 100/54 mmHg
Pulse: 109 beats per min (bpm) – sinus rhythm on telemetry
Respiratory Rate: 28 breaths per min
Pulse Oximetry: 95% saturation on room air

FOCUSED PHYSICAL EXAMINATION

A quick exam showed a young, jaundiced male in moderate distress, with blood all over his hospital gown. The patient was using accessory muscles of respiration. He had evidence of fresh, bright red blood in his mouth as well. His lungs were clear on auscultation. His cardiac exam was significant for tachycardia but was otherwise unremarkable. His abdomen was distended with dullness to percussion in flanks. No tenderness on palpation was appreciated.

INTERVENTIONS

A cardiac monitor with pads was attached. Two large-bore IV lines were established. A stat order of a liter bolus of lactated ringers was administered. Stat labs were drawn, including a complete blood count (CBC), serum chemistry, liver tests, coagulation studies, and type and screen. Consent was obtained from the patient to allow for blood transfusion if required. Emergent placement of advanced airway was deferred at the time given stable oxygen saturation on room air and the ability of the patient to protect his airway. Pantoprazole (80 mg), ceftriaxone, and octreotide were ordered to be given intravenously. Stat consult was obtained from gastroenterology, and the patient was transferred to the intensive care unit (ICU), where he underwent elective intubation and upper GI endoscopy for suspected variceal banding.

FINAL DIAGNOSIS

Acute upper gastrointestinal (GI) bleeding.

Upper Gastrointestinal Bleeding

Bleeding from an upper GI source usually presents as hematemesis, coffee-ground emesis, or melena. Hematemesis, or frank bloody emesis, is indicative of moderate to severe active bleeding. Patients can also present with hematochezia in cases with very brisk bleeding (5%-10% cases of hematochezia). The common causes of upper GI bleed are discussed in Table 51.1.

The patient's history and physical exam are of paramount importance in upper GI bleeding. Certain symptoms can point toward specific causes. These symptoms and associations are discussed in Table 51.2.

It is often difficult to gauge the amount of bleeding in any episode. Clues such as resting tachycardia could represent less than 15% blood volume lost. If greater than 15% of blood volume is lost, orthostatic hypotension might be present. Supine hypotension is indicative of at least 40% blood volume loss. Fluid resuscitation should be initiated immediately in patients with an upper

TABLE 51.1 ■ Common causes of upper gastrointestinal bleed

Ulcerative	Vascular
• Peptic ulcer disease – most common cause • Esophagitis • Gastritis	• Angiodysplasia • Esophageal and gastric varices • Dieulafoy lesion • Gastric antral vascular atresia
Neoplastic	**Traumatic**
• Polyps • Carcinoma	• Malory Weiss tear • Boerhaave syndrome • Cameron lesions • Aorto-enteric fistula

TABLE 51.2 ■ History and physical exam findings of various causes of upper gastrointestinal bleed

Disease	History and physical findings
Peptic ulcer disease	Sharp or burning, epigastric or upper abdominal pain History of non-steroidal anti-inflammatory drugs use (most common culprit), selective serotonin reuptake inhibitors, calcium channel blockers, aldosterone antagonists
Esophagitis	Odynophagia, chest pain History of gastroesophageal reflux disease. Intake of bisphosphonates or doxycycline is associated with pill esophagitis
Mallory-Weiss tear	Chest pain History of emesis, retching, or violent coughing prior to hematemesis
Varices	Painless bleeding History of cirrhosis or portal hypertension
Malignancy	Painless bleeding History of dysphagia, involuntary weight loss, cachexia, early satiety

GI bleed. Blood products should be used in those with active bleeding or hemodynamic instability, regardless of the hemoglobin level. It should be kept in mind that a CBC obtained immediately after a large volume bleed might not be reflective of actual hemoglobin levels as whole blood is being lost.

Suggested Approach to the Patient With Upper GI Bleed in a Rapid Response Setting

For patients with acute upper GI bleed warranting a rapid response, the following approach can be used for rapid evaluation and management.

FOCUSED HISTORY AND PHYSICAL EXAMINATION

- Timing of onset and duration of symptoms. The volume of hematemesis.
- Prior history of hematemesis or melena; history of any of the causes mentioned in Table 51.1.
- History of coagulopathy or anticoagulation. If yes, the agent and last dose should be recorded.
- The presence of abdominal or chest symptoms mentioned in Table 51.2 could point toward a specific cause.
- Physical exam should begin with an evaluation of airway, breathing, and circulation. Patients with high volume hematemesis are at increased risk of airway compromise.
- Exam findings such as abdominal tenderness, distension can point toward different causes.

LABORATORY TESTS

- CBC – to evaluate the degree of anemia and for the presence of thrombocytopenia. As mentioned before, a CBC drawn immediately after large volume hematemesis might not be reflective of the true hemoglobin as whole blood is being lost.
- Coagulation profile – to assess for elevated international normalized ratio, which is of particular importance in patients on anticoagulation and those with cirrhosis.
- Blood type and screen – in anticipation of blood transfusion.
- Other labs such as comprehensive metabolic panel, troponin, and lactate levels are dependent on the clinical scenario and clinician judgment.

IMAGING STUDIES

- Unlike lower GI bleed, where imaging studies might be the first step in the evaluation of active bleeding, upper GI bleed is evaluated with endoscopy.

THERAPEUTIC INTERVENTIONS

A large volume upper GI bleed is a medical emergency. We recommend assessment of airway, breathing, and circulation in all patients. The airway should be secured in those with active large volume hematemesis, given the high risk for aspiration and in preparation for endoscopic evaluation. The patient should be made *nil per os*. Two large-bore IV lines should be placed. Fluid resuscitation should be started immediately. Packed red cells should be transfused immediately in those with hemodynamic instability or those with active hematemesis regardless of blood hemoglobin levels. In stable patients, packed red cells should be transfused to a goal hemoglobin greater than 7 gm/dL. In patients with deranged coagulation profile, fresh frozen plasma, vitamin K, or prothrombin complex concentrate can be used as appropriate (see Chapter 8). Patients should be started on intravenous proton pump inhibitors, e.g., pantoprazole, at a loading dose of 80 mg followed by 40 mg IV BID. Patients with cirrhosis should be initiated on octreotide (to reduce splanchnic pressures) and ceftriaxone (for prophylaxis of spontaneous bacterial peritonitis). Stat consult should be obtained from gastroenterology for upper GI endoscopy. Patients with large volume hematemesis should be monitored in an ICU setting regardless of the hemodynamic status, given the potential for rapid deterioration.

STEPWISE APPROACH TO THE MANAGEMENT OF A PATIENT WITH LARGE VOLUME HEMATEMESIS

Step 1: The patient should be assessed for airway, breathing, and circulation. The airway should be secured in those with active large volume hematemesis, given the potential for aspiration.
Step 2: Two large-bore IVs should be established. Fluid resuscitation should be initiated.
Step 3: Labs including CBC, coagulation profile, and blood type and screen should be drawn.
Step 4: Packed red cells should be transfused to those with active bleeding or hemodynamic instability regardless of hemoglobin level. Stable patients should be transfused to goal hemoglobin >7 gm/dL. IV PPI, octreotide, and ceftriaxone should be used in appropriate clinical scenarios.
Step 5: Stat consult should be called to GI, and the patient should be transferred to ICU for close monitoring.

Suggested Reading

Saleem S, Thomas AL. Management of upper gastrointestinal bleeding by an internist. *Cureus*. 2018;10(6): e2878-e2878. https://doi.org/10.7759/cureus.2878.
Wilkins T, Wheeler B, Carpenter M. Upper gastrointestinal bleeding in adults: evaluation and management. *Am Fam Physician*. 2020;101(5):294–300.

CHAPTER 52

Hematochezia in a Patient With Diverticulosis

Abdelrhman M. Abo-zed   Syed Arsalan Akhter Zaidi   Firas Abdulmajeed

Case Study

A rapid response event was initiated by the bedside nurse after the patient had a large bloody bowel movement. On prompt arrival of the rapid response team, it was noted that the patient was a 72-year-old male with a known history of atrial fibrillation, for which he was anticoagulated with rivaroxaban. He had a history of diverticulosis as well. The patient was admitted to the hospital earlier in the day for evaluation of one episode of bright blood per rectum. At that time, he was found to have a hemoglobin of 6.7 gm/dL and had received one unit of packed red blood cells with an appropriate hematological response. Anticoagulation was held upon admission. A quick review of his chart indicated that the patient's blood pressure had been slowly trending down, and per the registered nurse, the patient was starting to get more lethargic.

VITAL SIGNS

Temperature: 98.2 °F, axillary
Blood Pressure: 86/50 mmHg
Pulse: 132 beats per min (bpm) – sinus rhythm on telemetry
Respiratory Rate: 22 breaths per min
Pulse Oximetry: 96% saturation on room air

FOCUSED PHYSICAL EXAMINATION

A quick exam revealed an elderly Caucasian male who appeared pale and lethargic but could respond to questions appropriately. He had one 18 gauge peripheral IV line in his left antecubital fossa. He was cold to touch. His abdomen was soft, non-distended, and bowel sounds were hyperactive. The patient's underpants were soaked in bright red blood. His pulmonary and cardiac examination was unremarkable.

INTERVENTIONS

A cardiac monitor and pacer pads were attached to the patient. In addition, 1 L bolus of Ringer lactate was started immediately. Labs were drawn, including complete blood count (CBC), serum chemistries, liver tests, and coagulation studies. Two units of packed red cells were ordered stat. The patient's blood pressure failed to improve with the first fluid bolus. Another 16-gauge IV line was placed, and the patient was given one unit of blood through a pressure bag, which improved systolic blood pressure to 90 s. Stat consult was obtained from gastroenterology, and a computed tomography (CT) angiogram of the abdomen was obtained. The patient was transferred to the intensive care unit (ICU) for further resuscitation, GI evaluation, and possible interventional radiology consultation.

FINAL DIAGNOSIS

Acute frank lower gastrointestinal (GI) bleeding.

Acute Lower GI Bleed

Twenty percent of all cases of GI bleeding originate in the colon or rectum. Patients with a lower GI bleed usually present with sudden onset of hematochezia (maroon or red blood per rectum). Rarely, bleeding from the right side of the colon can present with melena. About 15% of the patients with presumed lower GI bleeding are bleeding from an upper GI source. Literature suggests that hematochezia associated with hemodynamic instability, orthostasis, and an elevated BUN/Cr ratio may indicate an upper GI bleeding source and warrant an upper GI endoscopy. The common causes of lower GI bleed are discussed in Table 52.1.

More than 80% of cases of lower GI bleed stop spontaneously; the rest require intervention. Higher morbidity and mortality are seen in older patients and those with comorbid conditions. Risk stratification based on clinical parameters should be performed to help distinguish patients at high- and low-risk of adverse outcomes. These risk factors are outlined in Table 52.2.

A decision regarding discontinuation of anticoagulation and antiplatelet agents and reversal of coagulopathy should be weighed carefully. Anticoagulation should be withheld in patients with active bleeding. Vitamin K, fresh frozen plasma, and prothrombin complex concentrate can be used to reverse anticoagulation in patients with an international normalized ratio (INR) >2.5.

TABLE 52.1 ■ Common causes of lower gastrointestinal (GI) bleeds

Anatomic causes	Vascular causes
• Diverticulosis – the most common cause of lower GI bleeding. It also carries a high recurrence rate	• Hemorrhoids • Ischemia • Angiodysplasia • Post-polypectomy • Radiation-induced telangiectasia
Inflammatory causes	**Neoplastic causes**
• Inflammatory bowel disease • Infections • Ulcers – non-steroidal anti-inflammatory drugs enteropathy • Radiation-induced inflammation	• Polyps • Cancers

TABLE 52.2 ■ Risk factors associated with poor outcomes in lower gastrointestinal bleeds

High-risk features	Low-risk features
• Tachycardia (heart rate >100) • Hypotension (systolic blood pressure <100) • Syncope • Gross blood on digital rectal exam • Recurrent hematochezia • Age >60 years • History of diverticulosis or angioectasia • Creatinine >1.5 • Initial hematocrit <35	• Hemodynamic stability • Age <60 years • No signs of recurrent bleeding • Hematocrit >35 and creatinine <1.5

Aspirin that is being administered for secondary prophylaxis should be continued as its discontinuation in GI bleed has been associated with increased all-cause mortality. In patients with a recent cardiovascular procedure (coronary stent placement, bypass graft, vascular grafts), dual antiplatelet therapy should be discontinued only in consultation with cardiology or vascular surgery.

Suggested Approach to a Patient With Lower GI Bleed in a Rapid Response Setting

The following approach can be used for evaluation and management for patients with an acute lower GI bleed. This approach can be utilized in the emergency department, and this management is universal.

FOCUSED HISTORY AND PHYSICAL EXAMINATION

- Timing of onset and duration of symptoms.
- Presence or absence of abdominal pain.
- Prior history of upper or lower GI bleed.
- History of any of the causes mentioned in Table 52.1, which are the common culprits in lower GI bleeding.
- History of use of anticoagulation or antiplatelet agents. If yes, the last dose should be documented.
- Cardiac history – in case of ongoing cardiac ischemia, the hemoglobin goal should be increased to a Hb level of >9 gm/dL instead of the usual 7 gm/dL.
- Physical exam should begin with the assessment of airway, breathing, and circulation.
- An abdominal exam should be done to identify any tenderness. Pain out of proportion to the exam can point toward ischemia. A palpable mass could point toward malignancy.

LABORATORY TESTS

- CBC – to assess the degree of anemia. In acute large volume bleed, the change in hemoglobin might not be reflected in the CBC right away.
- Electrolyte panel – elevated BUN/creatinine ratio could point toward an upper GI source in large volume bleed.
- Coagulation profile – to assess for the requirement of reversal agents.
- Lactate – would be elevated in shock and ischemic bowel.
- Blood type and screen – in anticipation of blood transfusion.

IMAGING STUDIES

- The decision to pursue imaging would depend on the patient's stability and suspected underlying cause of the bleed
  - CT angiogram of the abdomen can be obtained if there is suspicion of ongoing ischemia. It can also help localize the site of a bleeding vessel in patients with active, rapid bleeding.
  - CT of the abdomen and pelvis with contrast can be obtained to look for malignancies, radiation-associated colitis, and inflammatory bowel disease.

THERAPEUTIC INTERVENTIONS

Management should start with an assessment of the airway, breathing, and circulation. An advanced airway should be placed in patients who cannot protect the airway or those with concomitant large volume hematemesis. Large bore IVs should be placed in all patients. IV fluid boluses should be initiated in hypotensive patients. A drop in hemoglobin level is occasionally not seen on CBC immediately after a large volume bleed. Type and screen should be obtained regardless, and packed red blood cells should be reserved for stable patients. Stable patients with hemoglobin <7 gm/dL should be transfused with packed red blood cells. Unstable patients or those with active bleeding should be transfused regardless of the hemoglobin level. Platelets should be transfused for a platelet count <50,000. For patients on anticoagulation, the reversal should be done if they have active bleeding and hemodynamic instability (see Chapter 8). IV vitamin K and prothrombin complex concentrate should be utilized. Fresh frozen plasma can be used if prothrombin complex concentrate is not available. Reversal of direct oral anticoagulants (DOACs) with drug-specific antidotes should be done only with expert consultation and per institutional guidelines. It is generally safe to continue aspirin. In patients with a recent cardiac procedure, antiplatelet agents should be discontinued only after consultation with cardiology. Stopping the antiplatelet agents is generally outside the scope of a rapid response event. A stat consult should be obtained from gastroenterology. Large volume active lower GI bleeds generally require arterial embolization through interventional radiology rather than colonoscopic treatment. This should be discussed with the gastroenterology. Patients should be monitored in an ICU setting given a high probability of decompensation.

STEPWISE APPROACH TO PATIENTS WITH ACUTE LOWER GI BLEED

Step 1: Assessment of airway, breathing, and circulation should be done. The airway should be secured.

Step 2: Two large bore IVs should be placed, and fluid resuscitation should be initiated in patients with hypotension.

Step 3: Baseline labs including CBC, BMP, coagulation profile, and type and screen should be obtained in all patients.

Step 4: Transfuse hemodynamically stable patients to Hb >7. Unstable patients and those with active bleeding should be transfused regardless of Hb levels.

Step 5: IV vitamin K and prothrombin complex concentrate should be used to reverse INR in unstable patients. Fresh frozen plasma can be used if the prothrombin complex concentrate is not available.

Step 6: Stat consultation should be obtained from gastroenterology.

Step 7: CT angiogram vs. plain CT abdomen pelvis can be obtained in stable patients depending on clinical suspicion of the underlying cause.

Suggested Readings

Aoki T, Hirata Y, Yamada A, Koike K. Initial management for acute lower gastrointestinal bleeding. *World J Gastroenterol.* 2019;25(1):69–84. https://doi.org/10.3748/wjg.v25.i1.69.

Moss AJ, Tuffaha H, Malik A. Lower GI bleeding: a review of current management, controversies and advances. *Int J Colorectal Dis.* 2016;31(2):175–188. https://doi.org/10.1007/s00384-015-2400-x.

CHAPTER 53

Acute Abdominal Pain in a Patient on High Dose Steroids

Abdelrhman M. Abo-zed ▓ Syed Arsalan Akhter Zaidi ▓ Firas Abdulmajeed

Case Study

A rapid response event was activated for a patient for acute onset abdominal pain and hypotension. On arrival of rapid response (RRT) personnel, the patient was a 65-year-old male with a known history of chronic obstructive pulmonary disease (COPD), active smoking, and chronic back pain for which he was taking ibuprofen daily. The patient was admitted two days before for a COPD exacerbation and was receiving prednisone 60 mg daily. He had received a dose of 125 mg of IV methylprednisolone at the time of admission.

VITAL SIGNS

Temperature: 98 °F, axillary
Blood Pressure: 80/55 mmHg
Heart Rate: 135 beats per min (bpm)
Respiratory Rate: 25 breaths per min
Pulse Oximetry: 97% on 2 L nasal cannula

FOCUSED PHYSICAL EXAMINATION

A quick exam showed a severely distressed man who appeared tachypneic and was attempting to lay in bed motionless. His abdominal exam showed diffuse guarding and rigidity. Significant tenderness was noted on palpation of all quadrants. Bowel sounds were hyperactive. Lungs had mild expiratory wheezing. His cardiac exam was unremarkable.

INTERVENTIONS

A cardiac monitor and pads were attached immediately. A 16-G intravenous (IV) access was established, and a 1 L IV fluid bolus was started. In addition, 1 mg IV hydromorphone was administered for pain. A stat lactate level, troponin level, complete metabolic panel, complete blood count (CBC), and lipase level were ordered. Electrocardiogram (EKG) was obtained, which showed sinus tachycardia; no acute ST changes were seen. An upright abdominal X-ray was ordered but could not be completed given the patient's severe distress. Blood pressure showed improvement with the fluid bolus, and emergent computed tomography (CT) scan of the abdomen was obtained (Fig. 53.1). Findings were consistent with acute duodenal perforation. Based on the patient's clinical history, a perforated duodenal ulcer seemed like the most probable cause. The patient was immediately given a dose of IV pantoprazole, and a stat consult was placed for surgery. The patient was transferred to the intensive care unit for further management and treatment planning.

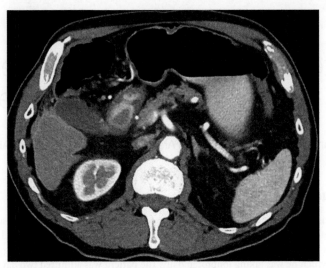

Fig. 53.1   CT abdomen without contrast showing free air in the abdomen (pneumoperitoneum)

FINAL DIAGNOSIS

Duodenal perforation from peptic ulcer disease (PUD).

Gastric/Duodenal Perforation

Perforation of an abdominal viscus requires full-thickness injury to the wall leading to the expulsion of the contents into the peritoneal cavity. This leads to irritation of the peritoneum and presents as severe acute abdominal pain. As peritoneal inflammation worsens, it leads to the development of severe abdominal tenderness, guarding, and rigidity.

The most common cause of gastric and duodenal perforation is PUD and is seen in about 3-6.5 per 100,000 individuals suffering from the disorder. Despite the widespread use of aggressive acid-lowering therapies such as proton pump inhibitors, the incidence of peptic ulcer perforation has remained the same over the years. Perforated peptic ulcers carry a high mortality rate (10%–40%), and most of these patients require surgical intervention.

Helicobacter pylori infections and non-steroidal anti-inflammatory drugs (NSAIDs) (especially in combination with medications like steroids) are most commonly associated with the development of complications related to PUD (see Table 53.1 for the risk factors of PUD. Table 53.2 describes other causes of gastric and duodenal perforation.

Suggested Approach to a Patient With Suspicion of Perforated Gastric/Duodenal Ulcer

The following approach can be used when dealing with a patient suspected of having gastric or duodenal ulcer perforation in a rapid response setting. This approach can also be used when other etiologies of gastric/duodenal perforation are suspected.

TABLE 53.1 ■ **Risk factors associated with the development of peptic ulcer disease (PUD)**

- Infections
  - *Helicobacter pylori*
  - Herpes simplex
  - Cytomegalovirus
  - Tuberculosis, syphilis
- Medications
  - NSAIDs
  - Glucocorticoids
  - Bisphosphonates
  - Clopidogrel
  - Potassium chloride
- Lifestyle factors
  - Smoking
  - Alcohol
  - Caffeinated beverages
  - Physiological/psychological stress
- Hypersecretory states
  - Zollinger-Ellison syndrome
- Radiation therapy
- Systemic disease
  - Sarcoidosis
  - Crohn disease

TABLE 53.2 ■ **Non-peptic ulcer disease-related causes of gastric and duodenal perforation**

Mechanism	Examples
Iatrogenic trauma	• Upper endoscopy • Enteral stent placement • Nasogastric intubation • Surgery
Non-iatrogenic trauma	• Blunt or penetrating abdominal trauma • Foreign body ingestion
Ischemia	• Shock state • Vasopressor use • Recreational drugs like crack cocaine
Other	• Neoplasms, especially during chemotherapy • Cardiopulmonary resuscitation

FOCUSED HISTORY AND PHYSICAL EXAMINATION

- The acuity of signs and symptoms.
- History of PUD.
- History of NSAID use, corticosteroid use, and other risk factors, including recent instrumentation. Proton pump inhibitor use does not rule out ulcer perforation.
- Physical exam should begin with an assessment of airway, breathing, and circulation.
- An abdominal exam should be done with a special focus on evaluating for signs of peritonitis.

LABORATORY TESTS

- CBC to evaluate for sepsis and acute hemorrhage.
- Electrolyte panel to assess for any electrolyte derangements as a consequence of peritonitis.
- Lactate level to evaluate for ischemia.
- Troponin and lipase levels to rule out differentials of acute abdominal pain such as cardiac ischemia and severe pancreatitis.
- Coagulation profile and type and screen can be obtained in anticipation of emergent surgery.
- C-reactive protein can be considered in patients with recent surgery as its elevation can be an indicator of anastomotic leak.

EKG

- It can be done to rule out cardiac ischemia in ambiguous cases.

IMAGING STUDIES

- Upright radiograph of the chest and abdomen can serve as a good screening tool for perforated viscus. Supine and lateral decubitus films can be obtained in patients who cannot sit or stand; negative imaging cannot rule out a perforation because of low sensitivity.
- CT abdomen and pelvis should be obtained emergently and will help determine the site of perforation. Oral barium contrast should not be used if perforation is suspected.
- Concomitant CT chest can be considered in ambiguous cases to evaluate for esophageal rupture in the appropriate setting.

THERAPEUTIC INTERVENTIONS

A perforated viscus is a medical and surgical emergency. We recommend that all patients be assessed for airway, breathing, and circulation. Hypotension should be corrected with IV fluids and pressors as indicated. Broad-spectrum antibiotics should be initiated empirically if suspicion of sepsis and shock. Pain control should be instituted to allow for detailed exams and investigations. IV proton pump inhibitors should be given based on institutional protocol. All offending medications should be stopped. The patient should be made *nil per os*. Emergent abdominal imaging should be obtained; CT abdomen and pelvis can identify the site of perforation. Emergent surgical consultation should be obtained for surgical evaluation and possible early repair of perforation.

STEPWISE APPROACH TO PATIENTS WITH SUSPECTED PERFORATED VISCUS

Step 1: Assessment of airway, breathing, and circulation should be done. The airway should be secured and hemodynamics stabilized.

Step 2: Two large bore IVs should be placed, and fluid resuscitation should be initiated in patients with hypotension (+/− vasopressor support).

Step 3: Baseline labs including CBC, BMP, coagulation profile, and type and screen should be obtained in all patients.

Step 4: Stat abdominal imaging should be obtained. Abdominal flat film (X-ray) vs. CT abdomen and pelvis can be obtained in appropriate clinical scenarios.

Step 5: If viscus rupture is confirmed, a stat consult to surgery should be placed for emergent surgical evaluation.

Step 6: The patient should be kept *nil per os* and started on broad-spectrum antibiotics as soon as possible for impending sepsis/peritonitis.

Step 7: The patient should be monitored in an ICU.

Suggested Reading

Freeman HJ. Spontaneous free perforation of the small intestine in adults. *World J Gastroenterol.* 2014;20(29):9990–9997. https://doi.org/10.3748/wjg.v20.i29.9990.

Langell JT, Mulvihill SJ. Gastrointestinal perforation and the acute abdomen. *Med Clin North Am.* 2008;92(3):599–625. https://doi.org/10.1016/j.mcna.2007.12.004. viii-ix.

Narum S, Westergren T, Klemp M. Corticosteroids and risk of gastrointestinal bleeding: a systematic review and meta-analysis. *BMJ Open.* 2014;4(5):e004587. https://doi.org/10.1136/bmjopen-2013-004587.

Sigmon DF, Tuma F, Kamel BG, et al. Gastric Perforation. [Updated 2021 Jul 1]. In: StatPearls [Internet]. Treasure Island (FL): StatPearls Publishing; 2022 Jan-. https://www.ncbi.nlm.nih.gov/books/NBK519554/.

CHAPTER 54

Acute Abdominal Pain in a Patient With Atrial Fibrillation

Abdelrhman M. Abo-zed   ■   Syed Arsalan Akhter Zaidi   ■   Firas Abdulmajeed

Case Study

The bedside nurse initiated a rapid response event after the patient had an abrupt onset of severe abdominal pain while sitting calmly watching television. On prompt arrival of the rapid response team, the patient started to have severe nausea and vomiting. It was noted that the patient was a 70-year-old female with a known history of persistent atrial fibrillation, coronary artery disease with coronary stent placement a month before. She was admitted to the hospital for evaluation after a mechanical fall at home. Her apixaban was currently being held while the safety of restarting anticoagulation in the patient was being determined.

VITAL SIGNS

Temperature: 98.2 °F, axillary
Blood Pressure: 130/85 mmHg
Pulse: 120 beats per min – irregular rhythm with rapid ventricular rate on telemetry
Respiratory Rate: 25 breaths per min
Pulse Oximetry: 97% on room air

FOCUSED PHYSICAL EXAMINATION

A quick exam showed an elderly African American female in significant distress. Her abdominal exam showed a soft, non-tender, non-distended abdomen without peritoneal signs indicating pain out of proportion to the exam. A cardiovascular exam showed an irregular rhythm with no abnormal heart sounds. The pulmonary exam was benign.

INTERVENTIONS

A cardiac monitor with pacer pads was attached. The patient was immediately given 2 mg intravenous (IV) morphine with some improvement in pain. 4 mg IV ondansetron was administered for nausea. A stat abdominal X-ray was unremarkable. Lab workup, including a complete blood count, comprehensive metabolic panel, lactic acid level, and lipase level, were sent. Fluid resuscitation was provided after the laboratory results showed increased hematocrit with concerns for hemoconcentration and metabolic derangements. Because of the pain out of proportion of abdominal exam and history of atrial fibrillation, there was a high suspicion of mesenteric ischemia; thus, a stat mesenteric angiography was ordered. Computed tomography (CT) angiography showed a complete lack of visualization of the superior mesenteric artery (SMA) origin. Stat general surgery consult was placed, the patient was started on therapeutic heparin infusion, and was transferred to the intensive care unit for further care.

FINAL DIAGNOSIS

Acute mesenteric ischemic secondary to arterial embolism.

Acute Mesenteric Ischemia

The gastrointestinal (GI) tract has a rich blood supply which aids in the absorption of nutrients in the gut. The intestines derive a significant portion of their blood flow through direct branches of the aorta: celiac trunk, SMA, and inferior mesenteric artery (Table 54.1). The venous circulation parallels the arterial circulation. The presence of significant collateral circulation between the branches of these three major vessels protects the gut from ischemia. This collateral blood flow allows the intestine to tolerate up to 12 h of reduced blood flow without significant damage. However, some "watershed" areas of the colon (splenic flexure and rectosigmoid junction) are not as richly supplied by collateral circulation and are more prone to develop ischemia in the setting of reduced blood flow.

DEFINITION AND DIAGNOSIS

Acute mesenteric ischemia (AMI) generally refers to ischemia of the small bowel in contrast to acute colonic ischemia (or ischemic colitis), which refers to ischemia of the large bowel. AMI is a life-threatening vascular emergency requiring early diagnosis and intervention to adequately restore mesenteric blood flow and prevent bowel necrosis and patient death.

AMI remains a diagnostic challenge for clinicians, and the delay in diagnosis contributes to the continued high mortality rate (Table 54.2 for common differential diagnosis of AMI). Early diagnosis and prompt, effective treatment are essential to improve the clinical outcome. The classic presentation of AMI remains "pain out of proportion to the exam." Involvement of proximal small bowel can also produce signs and symptoms such as nausea and vomiting. AMI has often been classified into four distinct types (Table 54.3).

TABLE 54.1 ■ **Blood supply of gastrointestinal tract**

Artery	Supply
Celiac artery	Distal esophagus, stomach, liver, spleen, pancreas, proximal duodenum
Superior mesenteric artery	Duodenum, pancreas, small intestine, cecum, ascending colon, proximal two-third of the transverse colon
Inferior mesenteric artery	Distal one-third of transverse colon, descending colon, sigmoid colon, rectum

TABLE 54.2 ■ **Differentials of acute mesenteric ischemia**

Causes of acute, diffuse abdominal pain	
Acute gastroenteritis	Inflammatory bowel disease flare
Abdominal aortic aneurysm	Porphyria
Appendicitis – early stage	Pancreatitis
Perforation of the gastrointestinal tract	Peritonitis
Diabetic ketoacidosis	Abdominal compartment syndrome

Suggested Approach to a Patient With Suspected AMI

We suggest the following approach based on a thorough literature search and updated guidelines for inpatient scenarios where AMI is being considered. This can be applied to emergency room scenarios as well, as the management is universal.

FOCUSED HISTORY AND PHYSICAL EXAM

- The acuity of signs and symptoms.
- History of thromboembolism, atherosclerotic vascular disease, and use of antiplatelet and anticoagulation agents.
- History of alternate causes of abdominal pain.
- Assess for signs of shock and decreased end-organ perfusion.
- Physical exam should begin with the assessment of airway, breathing, and circulation.
- An abdominal exam should be done to identify any tenderness. Pain out of proportion to the exam can point toward ischemia. A palpable mass could point toward malignancy.

LABORATORY WORKUP

- Complete blood count to evaluate for leukocytosis and hemoconcentration.
- Comprehensive metabolic panel to assess for metabolic acidosis, glucose level.
- Lipase level to evaluate for pancreatitis.

TABLE 54.3 ■ Classification of acute mesenteric ischemia

Subtype	Features
Arterial embolism	Sudden onset, severe occlusion Embolus originates from a cardiac or aortic source Most frequent cause of AMI (~40%-50% of cases) Superior mesenteric artery (SMA) is affected more commonly than other splanchnic arteries
Arterial thrombosis	"Acute on chronic ischemia" – superimposed thrombosis in patients with chronic atherosclerotic splanchnic vasculature Accounts for 25%-30% of all ischemic events Involves celiac trunk and SMA. Involvement of both is usually required to produce symptoms given the acute on chronic nature and presence of collaterals
Non-occlusive mesenteric ischemia	Produced by a low output state associated with diffuse mesenteric vasoconstriction Accounts for 5%-15% of patients with AMI Predisposing factors include heart failure, cardiogenic shock, aortic insufficiency, septic shock, use of vasoconstrictive medications, cardiopulmonary bypass, severe burns Carries high mortality given the difficulty and delay in diagnosis as the precipitating cause usually overshadows this disease
Mesenteric venous thrombosis	Produced by primary causes such as hypercoagulable disorders vs. secondary causes such as abdominal surgery, pancreatitis Accounts for 10% of patients with AMI The superior mesenteric vein is the most common site of involvement Abdominal pain is usually less severe than arterial occlusion and leads to delay in presentation and diagnosis

- Lactate level with or without arterial blood gas to evaluate for the degree of ischemia and acidosis.
- A coagulation profile can be obtained in anticipation of any further interventions.

IMAGING

- A bedside abdominal radiograph can be obtained while waiting for more clinical data. It is a non-specific study but can be used to rule out certain differentials like high-grade small bowel obstruction and viscus perforation.
- CT angiography of the abdomen should be obtained as soon as possible.

THERAPEUTIC INTERVENTIONS

AMI is a medical and surgical emergency. We recommend that all patients be assessed for airway, breathing, and circulation. Hemodynamic stability should be ensured as a priority. IV fluids should be used as indicated with pressor support to ensure adequate end-organ perfusion if a low output state or shock is suspected. It should be kept in mind that pressors can exacerbate splanchnic vasoconstriction. Judicious use of IV opioids should be used for pain control. Therapeutic anticoagulation and broad-spectrum antibiotics should be initiated immediately. Some studies have shown the benefit of early IV glucagon infusion in reducing splanchnic vasoconstriction. Stat consultation should be obtained from general surgery and vascular surgery teams for further therapeutic interventions.

SUMMARY OF STEPWISE APPROACH IN PATIENTS WITH SUSPECTED AMI

Step 1: A focused history and physical exam. Is the pain out of proportion to the exam?
Step 2: Ensure hemodynamic stability and secure the airway.
Step 3: Obtain laboratory data for sepsis, electrolyte derangements, acidosis, and alternate differentials.
Step 4: Obtain a CT angiogram of the abdomen as soon as possible. Consider empiric therapeutic anticoagulation based on the clinical judgment if there is a delay in obtaining a CT angiogram.
Step 5: Initiate broad-spectrum antibiotics.
Step 6: Obtain stat general surgery and vascular surgery consults.

Suggested Readings

Bala M, Kashuk J, Moore EE, et al. Acute mesenteric ischemia: guidelines of the world society of emergency surgery. *World J Emerg Surg.* 2017;12:38. https://doi.org/10.1186/s13017-017-0150-5.

Gnanapandithan K, Feuerstadt P. Review article: mesenteric ischemia. *Curr Gastroenterol Rep.* 2020;22(4):17. https://doi.org/10.1007/s11894-020-0754-x.

Mastoraki A, Mastoraki S, Tziava E, et al. Mesenteric ischemia: pathogenesis and challenging diagnostic and therapeutic modalities. *World J Gastrointest Pathophysiol.* 2016;7(1):125–130. https://doi.org/10.4291/wjgp.v7.i1.125.

CHAPTER 55

Foreign Body Ingestion

Abdelrhman M. Abo-zed ▪ Kainat Saleem ▪ Syed Arsalan Akhter Zaidi

Case Study

A rapid response event was initiated by the bedside nurse after the patient threatened to kill himself and swallowed a needle with no visualization in the oropharynx. Upon the prompt arrival of the rapid response team, it was noted that the patient was a 35-year-old male with a known history of prior severe suicidal ideation, bipolar disorder, alcohol use disorder, and recent imprisonment who was admitted earlier to the psychiatric ward because of suicidal plans and thoughts. The patient had attempted to swallow other foreign bodies in the past, and after one of the prior episodes, he had an endoscopy done for concerns of esophageal perforation.

VITAL SIGNS

Temperature: 98.2 °F, axillary
Blood Pressure: 160/92 mmHg
Pulse: 88 beats per min (bpm) – sinus rhythm on telemetry
Respiratory Rate: 22 breaths per min
Pulse Oximetry: 94% saturation on room air

FOCUSED PHYSICAL EXAMINATION

A quick exam showed an anxious appearing young male in mild distress. Exam of the oropharynx showed erythema and hypersalivation. He had mild tenderness along the left submandibular area. No subcutaneous crepitus was palpated. No foreign objects were visualized in the oropharynx. Pulmonary, cardiac, and abdominal exams were unremarkable.

INTERVENTIONS

A cardiac monitor and pads were attached. Airway, breathing, and circulation were assessed and secured. A stat chest X-ray was obtained at the bedside, which showed a metallic object in the esophagus. Stat consult was called to ear, nose, and throat (ENT) given submandibular tenderness and hypersalivation. Mild erythema was seen in the posterior oropharynx and laryngopharynx on flexible bedside laryngoscopy. No obvious evidence of perforation was seen. Once it was ensured that there was no airway compromise, a stat consult was called to gastroenterology, and the patient was transferred to the gastrointestinal (GI) lab for emergent endoscopy.

FINAL DIAGNOSIS

Foreign body ingestion.

Foreign Body Ingestion

Foreign body ingestion is more commonly seen in children than adults. In the adult population, it is more frequently seen in older patients, in individuals with underlying psychiatric diseases or alcohol intoxication, in prison inmates, and for the purpose of drug trafficking. The esophagus is the most common site of obstruction in the GI tract, and this chapter will focus on esophageal symptomatology and management. Physiologic narrowing of the esophagus occurs at three sites: at the upper esophageal sphincter, at the level of the aortic arch, and the diaphragmatic hiatus. These sites are the most common spots of foreign body lodgment.

The most common symptom of foreign body ingestion is dysphagia. It can be caused by both a retained foreign body and by the trauma left by the uncomplicated passage of the foreign body through the esophagus. Symptoms such as odynophagia, hypersalivation, blood-tinged saliva, drooling, and inability to swallow can be indicative of complications. Most ingested foreign bodies pass without the need for intervention. Endoscopic intervention is required in 10%-20% of patients, and surgical intervention is needed in less than 1% of cases. Foreign body ingestions are associated with complications such as perforation, obstruction, aorto-esophageal fistula formation, and tracheoesophageal fistula formation; the presentation of these complications is discussed in Table 55.1.

Imaging is obtained for all patients and is dependent on the type of object ingested. An anteroposterior (AP) view chest X-ray is the first investigation and can show most objects located in the esophagus. Tracheal foreign bodies can align in the sagittal plane and require a lateral view X-ray. Neck imaging should be obtained in patients where the site of lodgment is higher up. Computed tomography (CT) of the neck and chest can provide a more detailed view of the object and its complications but should be pursued after consultation with ENT or GI, depending on the clinical scenario. The management of ingested foreign bodies depends on the type of object ingested. The management of objects that require endoscopic removal is described in Table 55.2.

Suggested Approach to a Patient With Suspected Foreign Body Ingestion

We suggest the following approach based on a thorough literature review for a patient with suspected foreign body ingestion. This approach can be used in the emergency department as well.

HISTORY AND PHYSICAL EXAMINATION

- The acuity of signs and symptoms.
- Type of foreign body ingested and time since ingestion.
- Presence of red flags that indicate the development of a complication, as described in Table 55.2.

TABLE 55.1 ■ Signs and symptoms of esophageal complications from foreign body ingestion

Complication	Signs and symptoms
Obstruction	Dysphagia, odynophagia, choking, chest pain, drooling
Perforation	Fever, tachycardia, tachypnea, neck pain in case of cervical perforation, chest pain in case of thoracic perforation, blood-tinged saliva, subcutaneous emphysema
Tracheoesophageal fistula	Coughing, purulent sputum, pulmonary infiltrates because of aspiration, hypoxia

TABLE 55.2 ■ **Endoscopic management of ingested foreign bodies**

Type of object	Management
Food bolus	Emergent removal is indicated if associated with signs of complete obstruction Removed via grasp devices or endoscopy gently
Blunt objects	The removal technique is based on the shape of the object Coins are removed via foreign body forceps Smooth objects are removed by retrieval net or basket
Long objects	Urgent removal indicated (within 24 h) – unless the object is sharp Objects >5 cm in length are less likely to pass duodenal sweep and are unlikely to pass without intervention Removal is done via snare or basket
Sharp pointed objects	Emergent removal indicated If ingestion was <24 h ago and no complication (abscess or perforation), endoscopic removal is pursued If ingestion was >24 h ago or complication seen (abscess, esophageal perforation), then surgical treatment is required
Disk batteries	Emergent removal is indicated The poles of the battery conduct electricity and cause liquefication necrosis and perforation Removal done via retrievable basket or net
Magnets	Urgent removal is indicated The attractive force between magnets or a metal object can trap a portion of the bowel wall and cause necrosis Endoscopic retrieval should be done as soon as possible

- Physical exam should begin with an assessment of airway, breathing, and circulation.
- Assessment should be done to determine accidental vs. deliberate ingestion, suicidal intent, or intent to harm self.

LABORATORY TESTS

- Lab testing is not required for the diagnosis of foreign body ingestion.
- A complete blood count, basic metabolic panel, and venous blood gas can be obtained in appropriate clinical scenarios to assess the severity of complications if there are red flags indicating the presence of a complication.

IMAGING STUDIES

A chest X-ray should be pursued in all stable patients. CT of the chest can be done to look for complications, as discussed in the review section of this chapter.

THERAPEUTIC INTERVENTIONS

All patients should be assessed for airway, breathing, and circulation per the advanced cardiac life support algorithm. The scene should also be secured, and it should be ensured that the patient is not an active threat to himself or others. After determining the type of object ingested and time since ingestion, imaging should be pursued in stable patients to locate the object and assess for complications. In unstable patients, imaging should be skipped, and stat consult should be called to ENT vs. GI for further interventions.

STEPWISE APPROACH TO A PATIENT SUSPECTED OF FOREIGN BODY INGESTION

Step 1: Airway, breathing, and circulation should be assessed and secured.

Step 2: The type of object ingested should be determined along with the time since ingestion.

Step 3: Deliberate vs. accidental ingestion should be determined. Suicidality or intent to harm self should be assessed.

Step 4: Imaging should be obtained in stable patients to assess the foreign body's location and assess for associated complications.

Step 5: Stat consult should be called to ENT or GI for unstable patients or objects requiring urgent or emergent removal.

Suggested Readings

Chirica M, Kelly MD, Siboni S, et al. Esophageal emergencies: WSES guidelines. *World J Emerg Surg.* 2019;14(1):1–15. https://doi.org/10.1186/s13017-019-0245-2.

Libânio D, Garrido M, Jácome F, Dinis-Ribeiro M, Pedroto I, Marcos-Pinto R. Foreign body ingestion and food impaction in adults: better to scope than to wait. *United Eur Gastroenterol J.* 2018;6(7):974–980. https://doi.org/10.1177/2050640618765804.

Cases With Endocrinological Pathologies

CHAPTER 56

Hypotension in a Patient With Adrenal Insufficiency

Melissa Chrites ▪ Mohammad Adrish ▪ Kainat Saleem

Case Study

A rapid response code was called for a patient because of new-onset hypotension. The patient was a 52-year-old male with a known history of adrenal insufficiency and asthma admitted one day prior because of pneumonia and was being treated with ceftriaxone and azithromycin. He was chronically on prednisone 5 mg daily as outpatient for primary adrenal insufficiency. Per the bedside nurse (RN), the patient appeared lethargic compared to when he was admitted to the hospital.

VITAL SIGNS

Temperature: 102.0 °F, oral
Blood Pressure: 85/60 mmHg
Heart Rate: 110 beats per min, sinus tachycardia with peaked T waves on telemetry (Fig. 56.1)
Respiratory Rate: 20 breaths per min
Pulse Oximetry: 92% on 4 L O$_2$ via nasal cannula

FOCUSED PHYSICAL EXAMINATION

A quick exam revealed a middle-aged male in no apparent distress. He was awake but appeared lethargic, with slow but appropriate responses to questions. During the exam, it was noted that he was becoming more somnolent, and beads of sweat were starting to form over his forehead. He stated that he felt sick to his stomach and started to dry heave. A cardiac exam showed tachycardia with regular heart sounds. There were rhonchi noted over the left posterior lung fields on the lung exam. The neurological exam was non-focal.

INTERVENTIONS

A cardiac monitor and pads were attached to the patient. Two large-bore IVs were established, and a 1 L bolus of Ringer's lactate was started. Point-of-care-test (POCT) blood glucose level was checked, which was noted to be 60 mg/dL. He was administered 25 g of dextrose 50% IV. A stat EKG was negative for any acute ischemic changes; however, it showed peaked T waves in most leads. Stat blood tests were drawn. Complete blood count (CBC) and troponin tests were unremarkable. A comprehensive metabolic panel was concerning for a mild acute kidney injury and potassium level of 5.5 mEq/dL. Lactate was elevated at 4 mmol/L. His blood pressure failed to improve midway through the 1 L fluid bolus, and his clinical condition, especially his mental status, started deteriorating. Due to worsening hemodynamics, vasopressor support with norepinephrine was initiated. 100 mg IV hydrocortisone was administered for the suspicion of

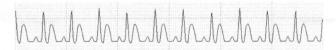

Fig. 56.1　Telemetry strip showing sinus tachycardia at 110 bpm with peaked T waves

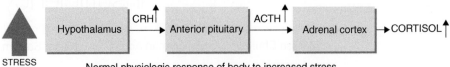

Normal physiologic response of body to increased stress
This response is unable to be mounted in states of adrenal
insufficiency, and enough cortisol is not produced

Fig. 56.2　Schematic representation of the hypothalamic-pituitary-adrenal axis

adrenal crisis in the setting of sepsis. Blood cultures were obtained, broad-spectrum antibiotics were ordered, and the patient was transferred to the intensive care unit (ICU) for further care.

FINAL DIAGNOSIS

Adrenal crisis in the setting of sepsis.

Adrenal Crisis

Adrenal glands are a vital part of the human stress response system. Adrenal glands are the effector organ in the hypothalamic-pituitary-adrenal (HPA) axis, essential for the successful adaptive response to stress. The HPA axis is shown in Figure. 56.2. Adrenal insufficiency can arise from defects at any level along the HPA axis. These causes are discussed in Table 56.1.

Adrenal crisis is a state of shock caused by acute or acute on chronic adrenal insufficiency. Hypotension, which is usually refractory to intravenous fluids or vasopressors, is the primary presenting feature. Other symptoms include nausea, vomiting, abdominal pain, or fever. Adrenal crisis can be precipitated in the following scenarios:

1. Adrenal crisis can be the presenting feature in a patient with undiagnosed adrenal insufficiency.
2. In patients with an established diagnosis, inability to escalate glucocorticoid and/or mineralocorticoid replacement in the setting of acute stressors.
3. Abrupt withdrawal of glucocorticoids in patients who have been on supraphysiologic doses of steroids.
4. Acute destruction of the adrenal glands, such as in bilateral adrenal hemorrhage or infarct.
5. Acute destruction of the pituitary gland as in pituitary infarct.
6. Initiation of thyroid replacement in a patient with severe hypothyroidism without concomitant adrenal replacement.

Adrenal crisis can occur from a deficiency of either mineralocorticoid or glucocorticoid hormones, and thus, it is important that if this condition is suspected, both components are replaced. Lab work is extremely helpful in the diagnosis of this condition. Electrolyte abnormalities may occur from lack of mineralocorticoid activity, including hyponatremia and hyperkalemia from lack of aldosterone. This will lead to vascular depletion and hypotension. Hypoglycemia will occur because of a lack of glucocorticoids.

TABLE 56.1 ■ Causes and types of adrenal insufficiency

Adrenal insufficiency	Level of defect	Hormone deficiency	Exam findings	Labs
Primary	Adrenal gland	Glucocorticoid + Mineralocorticoid	Hypotension	Hypoglycemia Hyperkalemia Hyponatremia
Secondary	Pituitary	Adrenocorticotropic hormone	Hypotension	Hypoglycemia Hyperkalemia may not be seen acutely
Tertiary	Hypothalamus	Corticotrophin-releasing hormone	Hypotension	Hypoglycemia Hyperkalemia may not be seen acutely

Suggested Approach to a Patient With an Adrenal Crisis in a Rapid Response Event

For a patient with an inpatient adrenal crisis, we suggest the following approach to evaluate and treat the acute event. This can be expanded and used as such in emergency room situations. See Figure. 56.3 for a flowchart of the management of an adrenal crisis. The usual sequence of history taking, physical exam, investigations, and resuscitative interventions is often not followed during a rapid response; these measures often run parallel to each other in a code situation. The following components of the rapid response are discussed in the traditional sequence only to ease understanding.

FOCUSED HISTORY AND PHYSICAL EXAMINATION

- The acuity of signs and symptoms.
- Past medical history, the reason for admission, hospital course, and baseline mental status.
- History of adrenal insufficiency or chronic steroid use.
- Complaints of dizziness, nausea, vomiting, abdominal pain.
- Vital signs, with attention to BP as there may be a need to initiate vasopressors.
- Physical exam should begin with an assessment of airway, breathing, and circulation.
- Mental status alteration because of decreased perfusion or hypoglycemia.

LABORATORY TESTS

- CBC to evaluate for leukocytosis in the setting of suspected infection.
- Basic metabolic panel (BMP) to evaluate for hyponatremia, hyperkalemia, and hypoglycemia.
- Lactate level and blood cultures to evaluate for infection as an underlying cause.
- Cortisol level needs to be drawn as a timed lab which is usually not possible during the rapid response event.

EKG

- Evaluation for the presence of arrhythmias and T wave changes because of increased risk for hyperkalemia. QTc interval shortening may be seen initially, and then PR interval lengthening and increased QRS duration, which predisposes to ventricular arrhythmia.

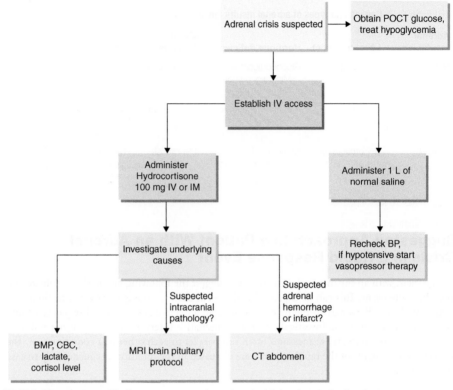

Fig. 56.3   Flowchart to guide the management of an adrenal crisis in a hospitalized patient.

IMAGING STUDIES

- Radiographic imaging of the brain may be required if pituitary involvement is suspected. A computed tomography (CT) scan of the head is not as sensitive as brain magnetic resonance imaging (MRI) for detecting pituitary abnormalities. If adrenal hemorrhage is suspected, a CT of the head without contrast may be obtained. MRI is the most sensitive modality for diagnosing adrenal hemorrhage but will not be feasible in the emergency setting.

THERAPEUTIC INTERVENTIONS

Adrenal crisis is a medical emergency. Management should begin with the assessment of the airway, breathing, and circulation. Maintaining an appropriate airway is the first step. IV access is crucial for administering medications. If there is suspicion of adrenal crisis, treatment should not be delayed while obtaining lab work or imaging. A bolus of hydrocortisone 100 mg IM/IO/ IV should be administered as the first step. After that, dosing should be continued with hydrocortisone 50 mg every 6 h. Hydrocortisone has both glucocorticoid and mineralocorticoid properties. Aggressive IV fluid hydration will be required, and the patient may require vasopressor use. Hypoglycemia should be corrected with IV dextrose. Hyperkalemia should be treated per institutional guidelines. Broad-spectrum antibiotics can be initiated until a definitive cause of hypotension is identified as sepsis is the top differential. Patients in adrenal crisis should be transferred to an ICU for closer monitoring. An endocrinologist should be consulted for assistance with management.

SUMMARY OF STEPS TO MANAGE ADRENAL CRISIS IN HOSPITAL

Step 1: Airway, breathing, and circulation should be assessed – because of concomitant hypotension and hypoglycemia, the patient may be unable to protect his airway. Advance airway would be indicated in that scenario.

Step 2: IV access should be established, and IV hydrocortisone 100 mg bolus should be administered.

Step 3: Lab work should be obtained, including CBC and blood cultures, to evaluate for sepsis which is the top differential, BMP, and lactate, which would show any electrolyte abnormalities present.

Step 4: Treatment of concomitant hypoglycemia with IV dextrose, hyponatremia with IV saline for adequate sodium replacement, and treatment of hyperkalemia should be initiated if appropriate.

Step 5: Broad-spectrum antibiotics should be initiated until a definitive cause of shock is identified

Step 4: Emergent consult with endocrinology should be obtained, and the patient should be transferred to ICU for further care.

Suggested Readings

Amrein K, Martucci G, Hahner S. Understanding adrenal crisis. *Intensive Care Med.* 2018;44(5):652–655. https://doi.org/10.1007/s00134-017-4954-2.

Harward M, Joyce C, Li Q, et al. Adjunctive glucocorticoid therapy in patients with septic shock. *NEJM.* 2018:797–808. https://doi.org/10.1056/NEJMoa1705835.

CHAPTER 57

Altered Mental Status in a Patient With Insulin-Dependent Diabetes

Melissa Chrites ▨ Kainat Saleem ▨ Syed Arsalan Akhter Zaidi

Case Study

A rapid response event was initiated for a patient with a blood glucose reading by finger stick of <10 mg/dL. On arrival of the rapid response team, the patient was somnolent but arousable to tactile stimuli. Nursing staff reported that the patient was a 75-year-old male with a history of end-stage renal disease on hemodialysis, type 2 diabetes mellitus, and congestive heart failure, who was admitted to the hospital for management of volume overload in the setting of missed dialysis. The patient had a malfunctioning atrioventricular (AV) fistula and was scheduled for fistula repair. He had been made *nil per os* (NPO) the night prior. It was noted that he received two-thirds of his usual dose of long-acting subcutaneous insulin and three units of short-acting insulin with a bedtime snack last evening. The patient's nurse noted that the patient has mentioned that his diabetes was difficult to control, and he often experienced wide fluctuations in his blood glucose.

VITAL SIGNS

Temperature: 98.9 °F, axillary
Blood Pressure: 105/85 mmHg
Heart Rate: 110 beats per min (bpm) – sinus tachycardia on telemetry
Respiratory Rate: 12 breaths per min
Pulse Oximetry: 98% oxygen saturation on room air

FOCUSED PHYSICAL EXAMINATION

A quick exam showed a frail elderly gentleman lying in bed with his eyes closed. He was arousable to medium pressure sternal rub, was protecting his airway, and was able to answer simple yes/no questions. However, he would quickly return to his somnolent state once the verbal and tactile stimulation was withdrawn. His pupils were equal and reactive to light. He moved all his extremities spontaneously but was unable to follow complex commands. His skin was clammy to touch, and his heart sounds revealed tachycardia and a flow murmur because of AV fistula. His chest was clear bilaterally.

INTERVENTIONS

A cardiac monitor and pacer pads were attached to the patient immediately. One ampule of intravenous 50% dextrose was ordered. However, the patient was noted to lack adequate IV access. One dose of intramuscular glucagon was administered while awaiting placement of IV line. Once the IV line was established, the ampule of dextrose was administered. Repeat blood glucose check after 1 min was 80 mg/dL. The patient was initiated on 10% intravenous dextrose infusion given concern for worsening volume overload with the 5% solution. He was retained on the medical floor with frequent glucose checks till his procedure.

FINAL DIAGNOSIS

Altered mental status secondary to hypoglycemia.

Hypoglycemia

Hypoglycemia is a common occurrence on medical floors, with an estimated prevalence of 3.5% in a non-ICU setting. Various factors contribute to the increased risk of deranged blood glucose control during hospitalization, namely, change in diet because of illness, dietary restrictions placed during hospitalization or dislike of hospital food, any discrepancy between insulin administration and meals, inadequate adjustment to insulin dose upon hospitalization, concomitant use of medications such as steroids, prolonged periods without meals such as during NPO while awaiting procedures, and changes in renal function which can lead to decreased insulin clearance. Other risk factors associated with the development of hypoglycemia are discussed in Table 57.1.

There are various degrees of hypoglycemia based on the severity of symptoms, as discussed in Table 57.2.

Suggested Approach to a Patient With Hypoglycemia in a Rapid Response Event

For a patient with an inpatient hypoglycemic event, we suggest the following approach to evaluate and treat the acute event. This can be expanded and used as such in emergency room situations, as this protocol is based on guidelines for the management of hypoglycemia. See Fig. 57.1 for a flowchart of evaluation and management of a hypoglycemic patient.

FOCUSED HISTORY AND PHYSICAL EXAMINATION

- Timing of onset and severity of symptoms.
- Prior history of hypoglycemic events.
- Diabetes history with particular focus on any recent change in diabetes medications, especially insulin.
- Inpatient medication administration history – high risk of recurrent or persistent hypoglycemia with long-acting insulin.

TABLE 57.1 ■ Risk factors associated with the development of hypoglycemia

Risk factors for hypoglycemia	
• Advanced age	• Tight glycemic control in older patients with diabetes
• Concomitant use of more than one hypoglycemic agent	• Recent or excessive alcohol intake
• Pharmacokinetic or pharmacodynamic drug interactions	• Increased carbohydrate utilization or reduced glycogen stores
• Inappropriate dose or misuse of the offending drug	• History of hypoglycemia
• Hepatic dysfunction	• Recent hospitalization

TABLE 57.2 ■ Overview of the degree of severity of hypoglycemia

Level of hypoglycemia	Blood glucose level (mg/dL)	Symptoms	Management
Level 1 Mild	≤54 to <70	Can be asymptomatic	Oral – 15-20 g of fast-acting carbo-hydrate load in the form of: three or four glucose tabs/1 tube glucose gel OR half a cup of juice or soda OR four or five saltine crackers
Level 2 Moderate	≤54	Possible presence of neurogenic symptoms – tremors, palpitations, anxiety/arousal sweating, hunger, and paresthesia	Oral – 30-40 mg of fast-acting carbo-hydrate load in the form of: two tubes glucose gel OR one cup of juice + four saltine crackers If unable to take PO: IV: 25 g 50% dextrose OR IM: glucagon 1 mg IM (nasal formula-tion can also be used)
Level 3 Severe	<40	Neuroglycopenic symptoms – dizziness, weakness, drowsiness, delirium, confusion, seizure, and coma	IV: 25 g of dextrose 50% solution +/– IM: glucagon 1 mg IM (nasal formula-tion can also be used)

- Symptoms pointing toward other causes of altered mental status (please refer to Chapter 39 for a detailed review of altered mental status).
- Physical exam should begin with the assessment of airway, breathing, and circulation.
- A detailed neurological exam should be done to evaluate for other causes of acute change in mental status.
- Assessment of ability to take per oral intake.

LABORATORY STUDIES

- Point-of-care capillary glucose testing should be done in all patients. Testing should be repeated every 15 min after interventions until blood glucose level is >70 mg/dL. The frequency of testing after hypoglycemia resolves is dependent on clinician judgment.
- Basal metabolic panel (BMP) can be obtained to assess for a venous blood glucose level. Any changes in renal function would also reflect in the BMP.

EKG AND IMAGING STUDIES

EKG and imaging studies are not needed to evaluate or manage an acute hypoglycemic event.

THERAPEUTIC INTERVENTIONS

Management should begin with an assessment of airway, breathing, and circulation. Severe hypoglycemia can lead to severe neuroglycopenic symptoms such as seizures and coma. Patients

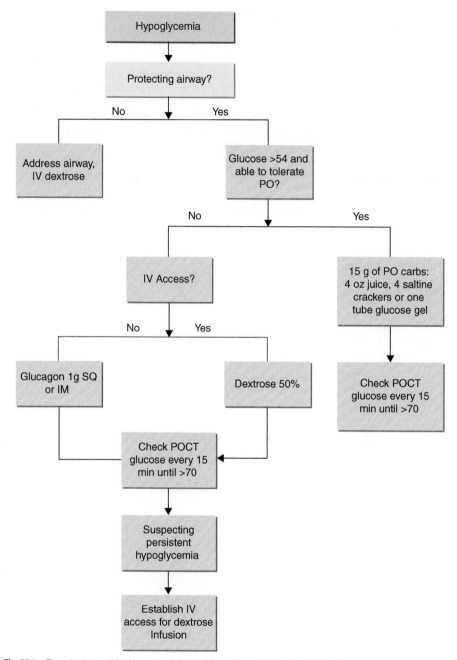

Fig. 57.1   Flowchart to guide the management of hypoglycemia in a hospitalized patient

with concern for airway protection should have the airway secured as a priority. Hypoxia and hypotension should be corrected. In patients with mild symptoms, oral interventions discussed in Table 57.1 should be initiated. Patients with moderate to severe symptoms should have their blood glucose repleted with IV 50% dextrose. The IV push of 50% dextrose can be followed by initiating dextrose infusion if prolonged or recurrent hypoglycemia is anticipated, per clinician judgment. Intramuscular (IM) or subcutaneous (SQ) glucagon can be administered as a bridge in patients with poor IV access. The IM/SQ dose can be repeated every 15 min. As mentioned above, blood glucose should be checked every 15 min till levels are greater than 70 mg/dL. The frequency of blood glucose checks after that is dependent on clinician judgment. Please refer to Fig. 57.1 for an algorithm for the management of hypoglycemia.

Suggested Readings

Evans Kreider K, Pereira K, Padilla BI. Practical approaches to diagnosing, treating and preventing hypoglycemia in diabetes. *Diabetes Ther.* 2017;8(6):1427–1435. https://doi.org/10.1007/s13300-017-0325-9.

CHAPTER 58

Hypotension in a Patient With Progressive Neurological Decline

Melissa Chrites ▪ Kainat Saleem

Case Study

A rapid response was called for a patient because of new-onset hypothermia and hypotension. Upon the rapid response team's arrival, the patient was noted to be a 78-year-old female with a known history of hypertension treated with amlodipine and osteoporosis. She was admitted earlier in the day as a direct admission from the clinic for failure to thrive. Her daughter had found her unable to care for herself at home because of progressive fatigue, lethargy, somnolence, and dyspnea on exertion. She had also been unsteady on her feet and had had a few near falls.

VITAL SIGNS

Temperature: 93.7 °F, rectal
Blood Pressure: 80/62 mmHg
Heart Rate: 48 beats per min (bpm), sinus bradycardia on telemetry (Fig. 58.1)
Respiratory Rate: 8 breaths per min
Pulse Oximetry: 97% on room air

FOCUSED PHYSICAL EXAMINATION

A quick exam revealed a somnolent older woman in no apparent distress. She was opening her eyes only to painful stimuli and was responding in a garbled voice. Her responses were incomprehensible. She could move all limbs spontaneously but could not follow simple commands. Cardiac and pulmonary exams were unremarkable. The abdomen was benign.

INTERVENTIONS

A cardiac monitor and pacer pads were attached to the patient's chest. A 1 L bolus of normal saline was ordered stat. Point-of-care glucose level was checked and noted to be 65 mg/dL. Then, 25 g of 50% IV dextrose was administered, which improved the blood glucose but had no effect on the patient's mental status. Stat complete blood count (CBC), comprehensive metabolic panel (CMP), arterial blood gas (ABG), and lactate were obtained, which came back unremarkable except for mild hyponatremia of 131. Blood cultures were drawn, and broad-spectrum antibiotics were initiated. A review of labs from admission showed a thyroid-stimulating hormone (TSH) of 125 mIU/L. Free T4 was undetectable. The patient was given 100 mg IV hydrocortisone. Stat consult was called to endocrinology, who recommended 200 mcg IV levothyroxine which was initiated. Given worsening altered mentation, there was a concern for the protection of the airway. The patient was intubated and transferred to the intensive care unit for further care.

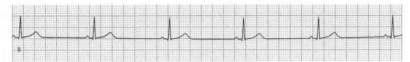

Fig. 58.1   Telemetry strip showing sinus bradycardia with a heart rate of 48 bpm.

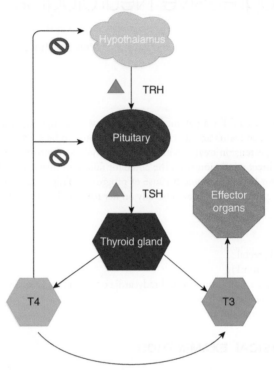

Fig. 58.2   Schematic of the hypothalamic-pituitary-thyroid axis.

FINAL DIAGNOSIS

Myxedema coma.

Myxedema Coma

The thyroid hormone is one of the primary regulators of metabolism in the human body. The thyroid hormone production is regulated by a negative feedback loop in the hypothalamic-pituitary-thyroid (HPT) axis. Reduction in circulating levels of thyroid hormone or increase in the body's demand for thyroid hormone leads to a fall in blood levels, which then leads to increased production of thyrotropin-releasing hormone from the hypothalamus, which in turn stimulates the production of TSH from the pituitary gland, which leads to increased production of T4 and T3 (Fig. 58.2). The reverse occurs when there is excess thyroid hormone (T4 and T3) in the blood.

Myxedema coma is a severe, life-threatening endocrinopathy caused by a severe deficiency of thyroid hormone. The mortality rate approaches 30%-50%. The dysfunction of thyroid hormone production can occur at any level of the HPT axis. It is usually seen in patients with uncontrolled hypothyroidism when they face a precipitating event. See Table 58.1 for classification of hypothyroidism.

Patients with myxedema coma usually present with depressed mental status, although frank coma is rare. Other findings include hypothermia, bradycardia, hyponatremia, hypoglycemia, hypotension, hypoventilation. Generalized non-pitting edema (myxedema) is often seen. Myxedema coma can be precipitated by any number of causes (Table 58.2).

Treatment for myxedema coma should be initiated immediately, given the high mortality associated with this disease. The turnaround time for the testing of TSH levels is quick. However, empiric treatment with IV levothyroxine should be initiated empirically in consultation with endocrinology if delays are expected. IV liothyronine supplementation should be done only with expert consultation. Administration of glucocorticoids before initiation of IV levothyroxine replacement is essential as hypothyroidism can mask adrenal insufficiency. Thyroid replacement in such patients can rapidly precipitate an adrenal crisis. Severe hypothyroidism is associated with a reduced cardiac reserve from a decrease in cardiac myocyte activity. Active rewarming of hypothermic patients should be avoided as it can lead to peripheral vasodilation and shock because of inadequate cardiac compensatory mechanisms.

TABLE 58.1 ■ Classification of hypothyroidism

	Primary hypothyroidism	Central hypothyroidism	
		Secondary	Tertiary
Mechanism	Defect at the level of the thyroid gland	Defect at the level of the pituitary gland	Defect at the level of the hypothalamus
Examples	Hashimoto thyroiditis	Pituitary macroadenoma	Stroke affecting hypothalamus
Lab features	Increased thyrotropin-releasing hormone (TRH), thyroid-stimulating hormone (TSH) Decreased T4, T3	Increased TRH Decreased TSH, T4, T3	Decreased TRH, TSH, T4, T3

TABLE 58.2 ■ Common causes associated with precipitation of myxedema coma

Precipitating causes of myxedema coma

- Infections
- Drugs
  - Amiodarone, lithium, propylthiouracil, methimazole
- Medication non-adherence
- Burns
- Hypothermia
- Trauma
- Acute cardiovascular conditions
  - Myocardial infarction, congestive heart failure, pulmonary embolism
- Infiltrative diseases
  - Hemochromatosis, amyloidosis
- Acute pituitary or hypothalamic diseases
  - Stroke

Suggested Approach to a Patient With Myxedema Coma in a Rapid Response Event

We suggest the following approach to evaluate and treat the acute event for a patient with suspected myxedema coma (see Fig. 58.3 for a flowchart of its management). This approach can also be used in the emergency room setting.

FOCUSED HISTORY AND PHYSICAL EXAMINATION

- Timing of onset and duration of symptoms.
- History of hypothyroidism and compliance to medications.
- History of precipitants associated with acute decompensation as listed in Table 58.2.
- Most recent thyroid hormone levels, if available.
- Physical exam should begin with an assessment of airway, breathing, and circulation.
- Assess for signs of infection, as sepsis is one of the differentials of thyroid dysfunction.
- Assess for focal neurological deficits which can point toward acute CVA.

LABORATORY TESTS

- Point-of-care blood glucose testing – hypoglycemia is a common feature of myxedema coma and also a differential.
- CBC – to assess for signs of infection.

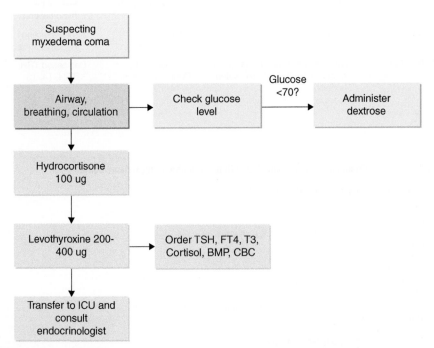

Fig. 58.3 Flowchart to guide the management of myxedema coma in a hospitalized patient.

- CMP – to assess for hyponatremia which is commonly seen with myxedema coma. Also, to evaluate for any other causes of encephalopathy.
- TSH level – screening test with a rapid turnaround time.
- Free T4, T3 level – can be sent off during a rapid response, however unlikely to affect management in the acute setting.
- Blood cultures – to assess for concomitant infection, which is a common trigger of myxedema coma and a top differential.
- ABG – should be obtained in the appropriate setting where hypoxia or CO_2 narcosis is considered a differential.

EKG

- Should be done in all patients with bradycardia. Heart block is not common.

IMAGING STUDIES

- Imaging studies are not required for the diagnosis of myxedema coma. However, imaging studies such as computed tomography (CT) of the head can be done to rule out other causes of altered mental status.

THERAPEUTIC INTERVENTIONS

Myxedema coma is a life-threatening emergency. All patients should be assessed for airway, breathing, and circulation. The airway should be secured in patients who cannot protect the airway because of obtundation. Hypotension should be treated with IV fluids. Pressors can be utilized for severe refractory hypotension with evidence of end-organ damage. However, the definitive treatment remains thyroid hormone replacement. Hypoglycemia should be treated with intravenous dextrose. Expert consultation with endocrinology should be obtained immediately, and intravenous thyroid replacement (T4 +/– T3 replacement) should be initiated. Stress dose glucocorticoids should be administered prior to initiating thyroid replacement to prevent precipitation of an adrenal crisis. Broad-spectrum antibiotics should be considered per the clinician's judgment, given the similarity of signs between severe hypothyroidism and sepsis.

SUMMARY OF THE STEPS FOR THE MANAGEMENT OF SUSPECTED MYXEDEMA COMA IN A RAPID RESPONSE SETTING

Step 1: Assess the patient for airway, breathing, and circulation.
Step 2: Secure airway in patients with poor neurological status. IV fluids should be initiated in patients with hypotension.
Step 3: Assess for hypoglycemia and correct with IV dextrose.
Step 4: Obtain appropriate labs, including CBC, CMP, ABG, and TSH. Treatment should not wait for lab results unless an alternate cause is strongly suspected.
Step 5: Before considering IV thyroid replacement, IV stress dose glucocorticoids should be initiated.
Step 6: Emergent consultation should be obtained from endocrinology, and the patient should be initiated on intravenous thyroid replacement. If there is a delay in obtaining an endocrinology consult, empiric IV levothyroxine should be initiated.
Step 7: CT of the head can be considered in stable patients where an alternative diagnosis is more likely.

Step 8: Broad-spectrum antibiotics should be considered per clinician judgment as sepsis is a trigger as well as a differential.

Step 9: Patients should be managed in a high acuity unit per institutional protocol.

Suggested Reading

Acharya R, Cheng C, Bourgeois M, Masoud J, McCray E. Myxedema coma: a forgotten medical emergency with a precipitous onset. *Cureus*. 2020;12(9). https://doi.org/10.7759/cureus.10478. e10478–e10478.

Wall CR. Myxedema coma: diagnosis and treatment. *Am Fam Physician*. 2000;62(11):2485–2490.

CHAPTER 59

Tachycardia in a Patient on Amiodarone

Melissa Chrites ▪ Kainat Saleem ▪ Syed Arsalan Akhter Zaidi

Case Study

A rapid response event was initiated for a patient who complained of worsening shortness of breath and was found to be tachycardic. Upon the arrival of the rapid response team, the patient was found to be a 65-year-old female with a history of atrial fibrillation, ischemic cardiomyopathy (the last known left ventricular ejection fraction was 40%), and chronic kidney disease. She was admitted to the hospital with complaints of generalized weakness, shortness of breath, and increased lower extremity edema over the prior few weeks. She had received one dose of 40 mg IV furosemide for acute exacerbation of congestive heart failure. Since admission, she had become progressively more tachycardic, with her heart rate increasing from 100 beats per min (bpm) to 140 bpm. Her home medications included furosemide 20 mg oral daily, carvedilol 25 mg oral BID, lisinopril 20 mg oral daily, amiodarone 200 mg oral daily, apixaban 5 mg oral BID, and atorvastatin 80 mg oral daily.

VITAL SIGNS

Temperature: 102.2 °F, oral
Blood Pressure: 110/80 mmHg
Heart Rate: 140 bpm, irregular rhythm on telemetry (Fig. 59.1)
Respiratory Rate: 25 breaths per min
Pulse Oximetry: 99% saturation on 2 L oxygen via nasal cannula (NC)

FOCUSED PHYSICAL EXAMINATION

A quick exam revealed a cachectic female who appeared older than her stated age. The patient was diaphoretic and tachypneic. She also seemed to be jittery and anxious. The pulmonary exam showed clear lungs, no crackles or wheezes. The cardiac exam showed an irregularly, irregular rhythm, normal heart sounds, no murmur. She had 2+ to 3+ bilateral lower extremity pitting edema. The rest of the exam was benign.

INTERVENTIONS

A cardiac monitor and pads were attached to the patient immediately. A point of care blood glucose level was checked and found to be 80 mg/dL. Stat EKG was obtained, which showed atrial fibrillation with a rapid ventricular response. The patient was given 1 g acetaminophen for fever and 5 mg IV metoprolol for tachycardia. These interventions brought down her heart rate to 120 bpm. Stat labs including complete blood count (CBC), basal metabolic panel (BMP),

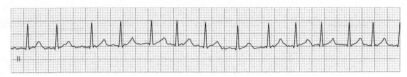

Fig. 59.1 Telemetry strip showing irregularly irregular rhythm with a ventricular rate of 140 bpm.

TABLE 59.1 ■ **Causes and associations of thyrotoxicosis**

Systemic causes	Medications	Other
Stroke	Amiodarone	Labor
Myocardial infarction	Lithium	Iodinated contrast
Pulmonary embolus	Checkpoint inhibitors	dye
Sepsis	Non-compliance with anti-thyroid	Thyroid/neck
Cerebrovascular accident	medications	surgery
Graves disease	Iatrogenic	
Thyroid carcinoma		
Diabetic ketoacidosis		

magnesium, troponin, arterial blood gas, and thyroid-stimulating hormone (TSH) were drawn. All labs came back unremarkable except TSH, which was undetectable. The patient was immediately given 100 mg IV hydrocortisone, and urgent consultation was obtained from endocrinology and cardiology. The patient was transferred to the stepdown unit for close monitoring.

FINAL DIAGNOSIS

Amiodarone-induced thyrotoxicosis (AIT).

Thyrotoxicosis

Thyrotoxicosis is a hypermetabolic state caused by excess thyroid hormone in the presence or even the absence of excess thyroid hormone production. As thyroid hormone receptors are expressed widely throughout the body, excess stimulation leads to a wide variety of signs and symptoms, including:

- General symptoms – fever, diaphoresis, tremors, increased appetite.
- Central nervous system symptoms – anxiety, agitation, delirium, psychosis, seizures, coma.
- Cardiovascular system (CVS) symptoms – elevated blood pressure, tachycardia, palpitations, arrhythmias (especially atrial fibrillation), heart failure.
- Respiratory symptoms – tachypnea (because of increased ventilation).
- Gastrointestinal (GI) symptoms – diarrhea, hyperphagia.
- Genitourinary (GU) symptoms – urinary frequency and nocturia.

Given the multi-organ system involvement, thyrotoxicosis can often be confused with other diseases with similar signs and symptoms, such as sepsis and heart failure. Table 59.1 lists some common causes of thyrotoxicosis.

"Thyroid storm" is a life-threatening form of thyrotoxicosis that is associated with severe signs and symptoms such as hyperpyrexia, altered mentation, and cardiovascular collapse. The Burch-Wartofsky scoring system can be used to determine the likelihood of impending storm (score 25-44) and established thyroid storm (score ≥ 45).

TABLE 59.2 ■ **Alternatives to beta-blockers for rate control in thyrotoxicosis associated atrial fibrillation**

Alternative agents for rate control

- Calcium channel blockers – diltiazem, verapamil
- Amiodarone – should be given concomitantly with anti-thyroid drugs
- Digoxin

Prompt identification of thyrotoxicosis and thyroid storm is necessary. General management is supportive care and blockade of stimulating effects of thyroid hormone. Non-selective beta-blockers such as propranolol are preferred because of their effect on the peripheral conversion of T4 to T3 (Table 59.2). Corticosteroids and anti-thyroid drugs can also be considered. Lugol's iodine can saturate the iodine receptors and block the release of thyroid hormone.

Amiodarone has been associated with both hypo- and hyperthyroid states. Discontinuation of amiodarone therapy should be done in consultation with cardiology and endocrinology. The long half-life of this drug makes discontinuation unlikely to have an immediate effect. Two types of AIT have been identified.

- Type I AIT
  - Caused by increased synthesis of T4 and T3 because of increased iodine availability.
  - Seen in patients with pre-existing multi-nodular goiter or latent Graves disease.
  - Treated with anti-thyroid drugs. Surgery is done in refractory cases.
- Type II AIT
  - Caused by the destruction of thyroid follicular cells and release of excess T4 and T3.
  - The hyperthyroid phase is followed by a subsequent hypothyroid phase.
  - Treated with glucocorticoids. Surgery is done in refractory cases.

Suggested Approach to a Patient With Suspected Thyrotoxicosis

For inpatient scenarios of suspected thyrotoxicosis, we suggest the following approach to evaluate and treat the acute event (Fig. 59.2). This approach can be expanded and used in emergency room situations, as the management is universal.

FOCUSED HISTORY AND PHYSICAL EXAMINATION

- Time of onset and duration of signs and symptoms.
- History of thyroid disease, especially multi-nodular goiter, or Graves disease.
- History of thyroid hormone use, access to thyroid hormone, and use of other medications associated with hyperthyroidism are mentioned in Table 59.1.
- History of other precipitants such as trauma or surgery to the neck.
- History of infectious signs and symptoms.
- Physical exam should begin with an assessment of airway, breathing, and circulation.
- Cardiovascular collapse is a common side effect of thyrotoxicosis.

LABORATORY TESTS

- CBC – can be done to look for signs of infection as sepsis is in differential.
- BMP and magnesium – should be done to evaluate for electrolyte abnormalities that can precipitate atrial fibrillation.

- TSH – should be done as the screening test for thyroid dysfunction.
- Free T4 and T3 levels – should be obtained if there is a high suspicion of thyrotoxicosis in the setting of normal TSH. It can take some time for TSH to get deranged.
- Blood cultures – should be obtained as infection/sepsis is in the differential.

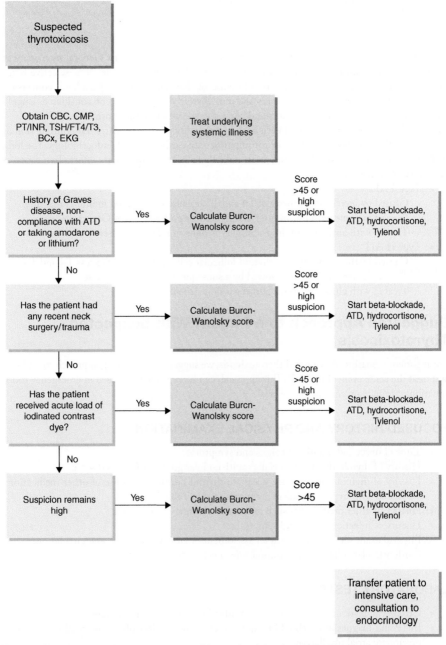

Fig. 59.2 Flowchart to guide the management of thyrotoxicosis in a hospitalized patient.

EKG

- It should be done in all patients with tachycardia, as atrial fibrillation commonly accompanies thyrotoxicosis.

IMAGING STUDIES

- No imaging studies are required for the diagnosis of thyrotoxicosis in the setting of rapid response. A chest X-ray can be considered if there is hypoxia and concomitant heart failure.

THERAPEUTIC INTERVENTIONS

A cardiac monitor and pacer pads should be attached to the patient immediately. Assessment of airway, breathing, and circulation should be done. Rapid assessment should also be made for the presence of thyroid storm; evaluate for hemodynamic instability, altered mental status, and hyperpyrexia. Airway and hemodynamics should be secured. Thyrotoxicosis and thyroid storm are associated with high output cardiac failure. IV fluids and pressors should be used judiciously. Beta-blockers should be used to control heart rate. Non-selective agents such as propranolol have the added benefit of halting the conversion of T4 into T3. However, in a rapid response setting, any fast-acting beta-blocker is reasonable. IV steroids can be considered, which also block the peripheral conversion of T4 into T3. Acetaminophen should be administered for fever. Aspirin should not be used as it releases thyroid hormones from protein bindings sites. Broad-spectrum antibiotics can be initiated per clinician judgment as it is often difficult to differentiate between thyrotoxicosis and sepsis initially. Urgent endocrine consult should be obtained for further guidance regarding therapy. Patients should be monitored closely in a high acuity unit.

SUMMARY OF STEPS FOR THE MANAGEMENT OF THYROTOXICOSIS IN A RAPID RESPONSE SETTING

Step 1: Assess airway, breathing, and circulation. Assess for the presence of thyroid storm, which would present as hemodynamic instability, altered mental status, and hyperpyrexia.
Step 2: Secure hemodynamics.
Step 3: Obtain EKG and treat atrial fibrillation with beta-blockers.
Step 4: Evaluate for precipitants, including factitious use of exogenous thyroid hormone.
Step 5: Obtain labs including CBC, CMP, troponin, TSH, and free T4 and T3 levels. Blood cultures can be obtained per the clinician's judgment, as sepsis is one of the differentials.
Step 6: Initiate steroids based on clinical judgment and in consultation with endocrinology.
Step 7: Transfer patient to a high acuity unit.

Suggested Reading

De Leo S, Lee SY, Braverman LE. Hyperthyroidism. *Lancet.*. 2016;388(10047):906–918. https://doi.org/10.1016/S0140-6736(16)00278-6.

Doubleday AR, Sippel RS. Hyperthyroidism. *Gland Surg.* 2020;9(1):124–135. https://doi.org/10.21037/gs.2019.11.01.

Gilbert J. Thyrotoxicosis – investigation and management. *Clin Med.* 2017;17(3):274–277. https://doi.org/10.7861/clinmedicine.17-3-274.

CHAPTER 60

Muscle Spasms in a Patient With a History of Thyroidectomy

Melissa Chrites ▪ Kainat Saleem ▪ Syed Arsalan Akhter Zaidi

Case Study

A rapid response was initiated by the bedside registered nurse for uncontrollable spasms in the hands and feet. Upon the arrival of the rapid response team, the patient was a 72-year-old gentleman with a known history of coronary artery disease, diabetes, hypothyroidism, and morbid obesity. The patient had been admitted earlier for viral gastroenteritis associated with intractable nausea and vomiting. The patient had been experiencing a "Charlie horse" in his left leg for at least 1 h. He had tried stretching his leg and foot, which had been ineffective in relieving the spasm. Eventually, the spasm resolved. However, 5 min before the rapid response event, the patient experienced another severe spasm in his left leg. An attempt by the nurse to check blood pressure had resulted in a spasm of his left arm and hand as well.

VITAL SIGNS

Temperature: 98.6 °F, oral
Blood Pressure: not available – had been within normal limits on last vitals check
Heart Rate: 130 beats per min (bpm), sinus tachycardia on telemetry (Fig. 60.1)
Respiratory Rate: 30 breaths per min
Pulse Oximetry: 90% on 3 L O_2

FOCUSED PHYSICAL EXAMINATION

A quick exam revealed an obese gentleman sitting at the edge of the bed in moderate to severe distress. Appropriate personal protective equipment was established, and the patient was examined. He was holding his left wrist with his right hand. The left wrist was flexed, with the thumb adducted and flexed into the crease between the index and middle fingers. Other fingers of the left hand were in full extension at the interphalangeal joints. When trying to pull back on his thumb, there was resistance. Left lower extremity exam showed the foot in dorsiflexion at the ankle and toes in plantarflexion. The exam was unremarkable otherwise. A surgical scar was noted on his throat, which he stated was from a thyroidectomy three years ago.

INTERVENTIONS

The patient was immediately given 2 mg IV morphine for pain relief. Stat labs, including comprehensive metabolic panel (CMP), ionized calcium, magnesium, lactate, and creatine phosphokinase (CPK) level, were drawn. The patient was given 1 g IV calcium gluconate while awaiting lab results. The patient's pain and muscle spasms improved with the administration of morphine and IV calcium. Labs showed an adjusted calcium level of 5.8 mg/dL, ionized calcium 0.6 mmol/L,

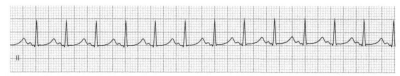

Fig. 60.1 Telemetry strip showing sinus tachycardia with a ventricular rate of 130 bpm and prolonged QT interval.

TABLE 60.1 ■ **Hypocalcemia causes and associations**

Causes of hypocalcemia		
Hypoparathyroidism	Anticonvulsants	Chemotherapy (cisplatin, 5-FU)
Vitamin D deficiency	Loop diuretics	Antibiotics (isoniazid, rifampin, pentamidine, aminoglycosides, amphotericin)
Osteoblastic metastases	Bisphosphonates, denosumab	Inflammation (pancreatitis, sepsis, burns)
Massive transfusion	Plasmapheresis/leukapheresis	Renal replacement therapy
Hypo-/ hypermagnesemia	Hyperphosphatemia	Alkalosis

magnesium 0.8 mg/dL. Lactate, CPK, and CMP were unremarkable otherwise. A stat EKG was obtained given these findings, which showed a prolonged QTc of 620 ms. The patient was started on a 4g IV magnesium infusion, and an urgent consult was obtained from endocrinology. The patient was also started on a continuous calcium infusion per endocrinology recommendations and transferred to the stepdown unit for closer monitoring.

FINAL DIAGNOSIS

Tetany secondary to severe hypocalcemia in the setting of inadequate dietary calcium intake and undiagnosed hypoparathyroidism

Hypocalcemia

Hypocalcemia is defined as a corrected calcium level <8.5 or ionized calcium <1.1. Table 60.1 lists the common causes of hypocalcemia. Calcium is mainly found bound to albumin in the plasma, and a low albumin level would result in a falsely low measured calcium level. The corrected calcium can be calculated by using the formula:

Corrected calcium = calcium (mg/dL) + 0.8 (4.0-serum albumin mg/dL)

The symptoms of hypocalcemia can range from asymptomatic hypocalcemia to life-threatening seizures and heart failure. Mild symptoms include paresthesia (peri-oral numbness), abdominal pain, and generalized weakness. Severe hypocalcemia has been associated with seizures, spasms, tetany, and arrhythmias.

The neuromuscular manifestations of hypocalcemia are produced by the loss of the "calming" effect of calcium on the nerve and muscle action potential. This leads to increased neuromuscular irritability, which produces spasms and tetany (Table 60.2). The cardiac manifestations of hypocalcemia are produced by the prolongation of phase II of the cardiac conduction cycle, which is

TABLE 60.2 ■ Evaluation of latent tetany

Trousseau sign	Chvostek sign
Induction of carpal spasm by inflation of a blood pressure cuff above the systolic blood pressure for 3 min or greater	Induction of contraction/spasm of ipsilateral facial muscles by tapping the facial nerve anterior to the ear

TABLE 60.3 ■ Calcium repletion for hypocalcemia

Degree of hypocalcemia	Ionized calcium level	Calcium dose
Mild hypocalcemia	1-1.2 mmol/L	Calcium gluconate 1 to 2 g IV over 2 h
Moderate to severe asymptomatic hypocalcemia (no seizures or tetany)	<1 mmol/L	Calcium gluconate 4 g IV over 4 h
Severe symptomatic hypocalcemia (presence of seizures or tetany)	Irrespective of levels	Intermittent dosing: Calcium gluconate 1-2 g IV over 10 min; repeat every 60 min until symptoms resolve
		Continuous infusion: Calcium gluconate 5-20 mg/kg/h

Recheck calcium every 4-6 h for severe or symptomatic hypocalcemia

mediated by extracellular calcium. This results in prolongation of the QT interval and can trigger arrhythmias such as Torsades de pointes. Heart block is a less common manifestation of hypocalcemia. Rapid onset hypocalcemia such as that seen with massive transfusions can cause heart failure because of reduced myocyte function and contractility.

Patients with symptomatic hypocalcemia should be treated with intravenous calcium supplementation. Chronic or asymptomatic hypocalcemia can be treated with oral calcium. However, the patients who develop hypocalcemia acutely (e.g., after massive transfusion) or those with serum ionized calcium below 0.8 mmol/L are at a high risk of developing complications. These patients should be treated with intravenous calcium (Table 60.3).

Suggested Approach to a Patient With Hypocalcemia

We recommend the following approach for evaluation and treatment for patients with neuromuscular or cardiological signs suspected to be secondary to hypocalcemia. This approach can also be utilized in the emergency department. Fig. 60.2 provides a simple flowchart for evaluating and managing hypocalcemia in a rapid response setting.

FOCUSED HISTORY AND PHYSICAL EXAMINATION

- Timing of onset and duration of symptoms.
- Prior history of similar symptoms.
- History of precipitatory causes, especially recent thyroid or neck surgery, massive transfusion, loop diuretics, and other causes mentioned in Table 60.1.

- History of renal dysfunction.
- Physical exam should begin with an assessment of airway, breathing, and circulation. Severe hypocalcemia can be associated with laryngeal muscle spasms, which can compromise the airway.
- The degree of symptoms should be assessed, mild vs. moderate vs. severe symptoms.

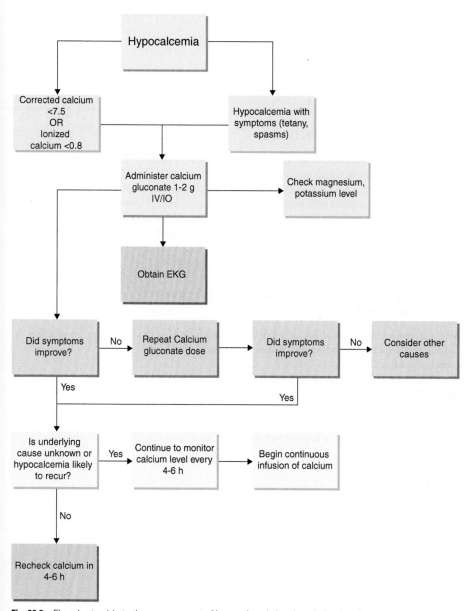

Fig. 60.2   Flowchart guide to the management of hypocalcemia in a hospitalized patient.

LABORATORY TESTS

- CMP – to calculate adjusted calcium level based on albumin level. The levels should be rechecked every 4-6 h in severe cases.
- Ionized calcium level.
- Magnesium level – hypomagnesemia can precipitate hypocalcemia through its effect on parathyroid hormone (PTH) production.
- PTH level – not required in rapid response setting, but a baseline level can help plan future interventions.

EKG

- EKG should be obtained in all patients with moderate to severe hypocalcemia to assess the degree of QT prolongation.

THERAPEUTIC INTERVENTIONS

All patients should be assessed for airway, breathing, and circulation. Hypocalcemia can cause laryngeal muscle spasms, which can compromise the airway which should be evaluated. IV access should be established if not present. IV calcium can be administered empirically after blood levels have been drawn in patients with normal renal function. Calcium gluconate is preferred over calcium chloride in this setting as there is less risk of tissue necrosis from extravasation. Concomitant hypomagnesemia should be corrected. Endocrine or renal consult should be obtained depending on the suspected underlying cause. The decision for continuous calcium infusion should be made with expert consultation. Cardiac monitoring should be instituted.

STEPWISE APPROACH TO A PATIENT WITH SYMPTOMATIC HYPOCALCEMIA

Step 1: Confirm true hypocalcemia (either by calculating corrected calcium level for albumin or by an ionized calcium level can be obtained on arterial blood gas).
Step 2: Establish IV access.
Step 3: Obtain an EKG to assess QTc interval and place the patient on telemetry.
Step 4: Provide calcium gluconate 1-2 g in D5W or normal saline over 10-20 min.
Step 5: Treat any concomitant hypomagnesemia.
Step 6: Recheck calcium level within 4-6 h (or earlier if indicated).
Step 7: Obtain expert consultation from endocrine or renal regarding continuous calcium infusion in appropriate cases.

Suggested Reading

Gafni RI, Collins MT. Hypoparathyroidism. *N Engl J Med.* 2019;380(18):1738–1747. https://doi.org/10.1056/NEJMcp1800213.
Pepe J, Colangelo L, Biamonte F, et al. Diagnosis and management of hypocalcemia. *Endocrine.* 2020;69(3):485–495. https://doi.org/10.1007/s12020-020-02324-2.

Cases With Musculoskeletal Pathologies

CHAPTER 61

Acute Foot Discoloration in a Patient With Peripheral Vascular Disease

Abdelrhman M. Abo-zed ▪ Syed Arsalan Akhter Zaidi ▪ Firas Abdulmajeed

Case Study

A rapid response event was initiated by the bedside nurse after the patient had symptoms of sudden pain in his left foot. Prior to calling the condition, the nurse assessed the patient's pulse in the affected foot, and she did not feel it. On prompt arrival of the rapid response team, a quick chart review suggested that the patient was a 55-year-old male with a known history of persistent atrial fibrillation and peripheral vascular disease. He was admitted earlier for a traumatic left lower extremity injury at the job when a cement block fell on his extremity. The nurse had responded initially to the patient's screaming and yelling that this was the worst pain he had ever felt and called the rapid response code after she was unable to locate patient's dorsalis pedis or posterior tibial pulse. Patient also described pins and needles in his foot.

VITAL SIGNS

Temperature: 99 °F, axillary
Blood Pressure: 170/95 mmHg
Pulse Rate: 125 beats per min (bpm) – irregular rhythm
Respiratory Rate: 22 breaths per min
Pulse Oximetry: 97% saturation on room air

FOCUSED PHYSICAL EXAMINATION

A quick exam showed a middle-aged male in severe distress. His left foot had a shiny appearance with a bluish coloration, and the foot was cool to the touch. Pulses were checked and were not palpable at the dorsalis pedis and posterior tibial level on the affected side; these pulses were inaudible on bedside Doppler ultrasound as well. Pulses were present and 1+ in the femoral arteries bilaterally. Muscle strength and neurologic examination were difficult to be assessed in the left foot because of pain but were diminished compared to the right.

INTERVENTIONS

The patient was given 4 mg intravenous (IV) morphine for pain. A dose of 5 mg IV metoprolol was given with improvement in his heart rate. Stat consult was called to vascular surgery for evaluation. IV unfractionated heparin was started, and stat arterial Doppler of lower extremities were ordered. The patient was transferred to the vascular surgery service for evaluation for revascularization vs. open embolectomy.

FINAL DIAGNOSIS

Acute limb ischemia in the setting of atrial fibrillation with a rapid ventricular response.

Acute Limb Ischemia

Acute lower extremity ischemia is generally related to arterial occlusion, although there are occasional cases where severe venous occlusion can also cause ischemia (phlegmasia cerulea dolens). The most common underlying mechanism of acute limb ischemia is thromboembolism. The thrombi typically form at, and the emboli typically lodge at sites of arterial narrowing, such as in places with an atherosclerotic plaque or at a vessel branch point (see Table 61.1 for the causes of acute limb ischemia). The classic presentation is characterized by the "6 Ps": paresthesia, pain, pallor, pulselessness, poikilothermic (coolness), and paralysis (late sign). Acute limb ischemia is typically categorized into three classes of severity, described in detail in Table 61.2. Early diagnosis and initiation of therapy (medical vs. surgical) are critical to prevent limb loss. Despite all efforts for early attempts for reversal of ischemia, the morbidity and mortality from acute lower extremity ischemia remain high.

Blue toe Syndrome is a syndrome of small vessel occlusion typically caused by embolic occlusion of small vessels of the toes with atherothrombotic material from proximal arterial sources. Compared to thromboemboli, atheroemboli are less likely to produce acute limb ischemia (Table 61.3).

Suggested Approach to a Patient With Suspected Acute Limb Ischemia

We suggest the following approach to a patient with suspected acute limb ischemia based on an extensive literature review. This approach can also be used in emergency departments as the management is universal.

TABLE 61.1 ■ Causes of acute limb ischemia

Mechanism	Associations

Native arterial thrombus	• Generally stems from pre-existing plaques
	• Other causes include:
	  • Aneurysm thrombosis
	  • Arterial dissection
	  • Arterial entrapment/compression
	  • Thrombophilia – malignancy, disseminated intravascular coagulation, heparin-induced thrombocytopenia
	  • Low flow state – shock

Injury	• Iatrogenic (interventional procedures, closure device, device embolization) • Trauma
Iatrogenic/idiopathic thrombosis	• Vein bypass graft • Prosthetic bypass graft • Angioplasty site • Stent placement
Embolism	• Cardiac (atrial fibrillation, myocardial infarction, endocarditis, valvular disease, atrial myxoma, prosthetic valve) • Aneurysm (atherosclerotic plaque) • Paradoxical embolus
Peripheral vasospasm	• Raynaud phenomenon, shock (meningococcal sepsis, cardiogenic shock)

TABLE 61.2 ■ **Classification of the severity of acute limb ischemia**

Category	Features
Class I – Viable	• Mild pain; intact capillary refill • No sensory or motor deficits • Arterial and venous Doppler audible
Class IIa – Marginally threatened	• Moderate pain; delayed capillary refill • Mild to no sensory deficits (usually in toes only); no motor deficits • Arterial Doppler inaudible; venous audible
Class IIb – Immediately threatened	• Severe pain; delayed capillary refill • Major sensory deficits (involving more than toes); mild to moderate motor deficits • Arterial Doppler inaudible; venous Doppler audible
Class III – Non-viable	• Variable pain, can have complete anesthesia; absent capillary refill • Complete sensory deficit (anesthesia) and motor deficit (paralysis) • Inaudible arterial and venous Doppler

TABLE 61.3 ■ **Clinical presentation of thrombotic vs. embolic arterial occlusion**

Thrombosis	Embolism
• Typically occurs in patients with underlying peripheral vascular disease. Patients might have a history of claudication or be on antiplatelet agents. Exceptions include patients with severe hypercoagulable states and low flow states as above	• It can occur in patients with underlying peripheral vascular disease and those with normal vasculature
• The presence of collaterals might lead to the slow development of symptoms over hours to days	• The suddenness of occlusion and absence of collaterals would lead to the development of symptoms acutely
• Signs and symptoms are usually focal unless a major artery is thrombosed that supplied multiple organs	• Other organs can be affected in case of a shower of emboli

FOCUSED HISTORY AND PHYSICAL EXAMINATION

- The timing of onset and acuity of signs and symptoms.
- History of atherosclerotic vascular disease, recent limb injury, hypercoagulable conditions, recent vascular instrumentation.
- History of use of antiplatelet agents and anticoagulants.
- Physical exam should assess for airway, breathing, and circulation. Assess for hypotension.
- A limb exam should be done to evaluate for 6 Ps. Bedside Doppler should be used to evaluate pulses, especially if the patient is morbidly obese.

LABORATORY TESTS

- Lab tests are not required for the diagnosis of acute limb ischemia. Ancillary testing can be done to guide further therapy and can include:
  - Complete blood count to assess hemoglobin and platelet count in anticipation of thrombectomy and anticoagulation and evaluate for causes like heparin-induced thrombocytopenia (HIT).

- Renal function panel to assess for acid-base (acidosis) and electrolyte disturbances (hyperkalemia).
- Lactate level to assess the degree of ischemia (normal levels do not rule limb ischemia).
- Coagulation profile including fibrinogen levels to help guide anticoagulation and to rule out disseminated intravascular coagulation.

EKG

- EKG is not required for the diagnosis of acute limb ischemia and should not delay other limb-saving investigations and interventions.
- It can be obtained to evaluate for cardiac arrhythmias like atrial fibrillation, which can cause emboli.

IMAGING STUDIES

- Imaging studies should not delay initiation of anticoagulation if there is a high clinical suspicion of acute limb ischemia, based on institutional guidelines. The following studies can be obtained:
  - Emergent arterial and venous Doppler should be obtained to evaluate the degree of arterial and venous compromise.
  - If emergent Doppler are not available, a computed tomography (CT) angiogram of the limb should be considered, which can assess for complete arterial occlusion.

THERAPEUTIC INTERVENTIONS

Acute limb ischemia is a limb-threatening and potentially life-threatening emergency. We recommend that all patients be assessed for airway, breathing, and circulation. Hemodynamics should be evaluated, and hypotension should be corrected to improve blood flow to the affected limb. Vasopressors should be used for shock states as indicated and per institutional guidelines. Pain control should be considered early. Anticoagulation should be initiated as soon as possible while considering differentials like HIT. An emergent arterial Doppler or CT angiogram should be obtained after emergent consultation with vascular surgery. Anticoagulation should not be delayed while waiting for imaging if clinical suspicion of acute limb ischemia is high. Stat consultation should be obtained from vascular surgery or interventional radiology for catheter-directed thrombectomy vs. open embolectomy.

STEPWISE APPROACH TO THE MANAGEMENT OF SUSPECTED ACUTE LIMB ISCHEMIA

Step 1: Assess airway, breathing, and circulation—correct hypotension.

Step 2: Assess for the acuity of signs and symptoms.

Step 3: Evaluate for underlying causes of ischemia, prior use of antiplatelet and anticoagulant agents.

Step 4: Initiate anticoagulation as soon as possible, choice of agent depending on the suspected underlying cause (special case: HIT).

Step 5: Emergent arterial and venous Doppler should be obtained. CT angiogram can be considered as an alternative. Therapeutic anticoagulation should not wait for imaging studies if suspicion for acute limb ischemia is high.

Step 6: Emergent surgical +/− interventional radiology consultation should be obtained for further therapeutic options.

Suggested Reading

McNally MM, Univers J. Acute limb ischemia. *Surg Clin North Am*. 2018;98(5):1081–1096. https://doi. org/10.1016/j.suc.2018.05.002.

Obara H, Matsubara K, Kitagawa Y. Acute limb ischemia. *Ann Vasc Dis*. 2018;11(4):443–448. https://doi. org/10.3400/avd.ra.18-00074.

Olinic D-M, Stanek A, Tătaru D-A, Homorodean C, Olinic M. Acute limb ischemia: an update on diagnosis and management. *J Clin Med*. 2019;8(8):1215. https://doi.org/10.3390/jcm8081215.

CHAPTER 62

Acute Leg Pain in a Patient With Cellulitis

Melissa Chrites ■ Syed Arsalan Akhter Zaidi ■ Kainat Saleem

Case Study

A rapid response was initiated by the bedside nurse (RN) for a patient with severe leg pain. Upon the arrival of the rapid response team, the patient was a 48-year-old male with a known history of type 2 diabetes mellitus with insulin dependence, stage III chronic kidney disease, and chronic hypertension. The patient had been admitted two days earlier for lower extremity cellulitis, for which he was receiving broad-spectrum antibiotics. He had been experiencing increasing pain in his affected extremity over the past few hours before the rapid response event was initiated. He reported new numbness of 15 min duration to the code team.

VITAL SIGNS

Temperature: 100.2 °F, oral
Blood Pressure: 125/70 mmHg
Heart Rate: 125 beats per min (bpm), sinus tachycardia on telemetry
Respiratory Rate: 35 breaths per min
Pulse Oximetry: 99% saturation on room air

FOCUSED PHYSICAL EXAMINATION

A quick exam revealed an overweight male lying in bed in severe distress. The lower extremity exam showed erythema and swelling of the left leg. The erythema had spread beyond the margins of the border that was drawn earlier in the day. There was no evidence of pallor or cyanosis of the toes, feet, or leg. The range of movements was intact at the left knee, as was plantarflexion. The patient was unable to dorsiflex his left ankle. The extremity was warm to touch, and the calf was extremely tender to palpation. Posterior tibial and dorsalis pedis were not palpable. However, the bedside RN could locate the posterior tibial pulse in the affected extremity with Doppler.

INTERVENTIONS

The patient was immediately given 2 mg IV morphine for pain relief. Stat consult was called to orthopedic surgery for evaluation of the patient's lower extremity. Bedside manometry was done by the surgical team, which showed a pressure of 35 mmHg in the anterior compartment. The patient was taken immediately to the operating room for emergent fasciotomy.

FINAL DIAGNOSIS

Acute compartment syndrome in a patient with cellulitis.

Acute Compartment Syndrome

Human limbs are organized into groups of muscles divided by thick fascial membranes. These sections or compartments are limited-space areas with neurovascular bundles traversing the space to supply distal parts of the body. Any increase in the volume of this closed compartment would lead to compression of the blood vessels and nerves, which is the basic underlying pathophysiology of acute compartment syndrome. Table 62.1 lists some common traumatic and non-traumatic causes of acute compartment syndrome.

The normal pressure within a musculoskeletal compartment ranges between 0 and 8 mmHg. Pain occurs when pressure increases to 20 mmHg. An increase in pressure to 25 mmHg or greater leads to compromised capillary blood flow. When the intracompartmental pressure reaches diastolic blood pressure, ischemia ensues.

Acute compartment syndrome is a time-sensitive, life-threatening emergency. Failure to recognize the syndrome within 4 h can lead to irreversible neurovascular damage and myocyte death. Clinical features of acute compartment syndrome are pain, pallor, pulselessness, paralysis, and paresthesia, similar to the five Ps of critical limb ischemia (Table 62.2). Other common causes of acute limb pain should be ruled out (Table 62.3). Definitive diagnosis is made by direct measurement of compartment pressure using a hand-held manometer. A delta pressure is obtained by calculating the difference between the diastolic blood pressure and the measured compartment pressure. A delta pressure <20-30 mmHg is an indication of urgent fasciotomy. Surgical consultation should be obtained as soon as acute compartment syndrome is being suspected.

Suggested Approach to a Patient With Acute Compartment Syndrome

For inpatient scenarios where acute compartment syndrome is suspected, we suggest the following approach to evaluate and treat the acute event. This approach can be expanded and used in emergency room situations as well, as this protocol is based on guidelines for the management of compartment syndrome (Fig. 62.1).

FOCUSED HISTORY AND PHYSICAL EXAMINATION

- Timing of onset of signs and symptoms.
- History of trauma, burns, recent procedure (especially vascular procedures), or infection.
- History of anticoagulation – deep vein thrombosis prophylaxis post-orthopedic surgery.

TABLE 62.1 ■ Common causes of acute compartment syndrome

Traumatic	Non-traumatic

• Fractures – open or closed (~75% of cases)
  • Tibia fractures – most common
  • Supracondylar humeral fractures
• Crush injuries
• Severe thermal burns
• Constrictive circumferential bandages, casts, or splints
• High-pressure injections
• Vascular injury
• Animal bites
	• Reperfusion injury – post-embolectomy, thrombolysis, or bypass
	• Hemorrhage
	• Thrombosis
	• Anticoagulation
	• Injections of illicit drugs
	• Extravasation of fluids
	• Prolonged compression of the limb
	• Infection of musculature
	• Rhabdomyolysis

TABLE 62.2 ■ **Signs and symptoms of compartment syndrome (notice similarity to signs of limb ischemia)**

5 Ps of compartment syndrome
Pain (especially with passive stretch)
Pallor
Pulselessness
Paralysis
Paresthesia

TABLE 62.3 ■ **Differential diagnosis of acute compartment syndrome**

Differentials of acute compartment syndrome	
Cellulitis	Stress fracture
Deep venous thrombosis	Rhabdomyolysis
Necrotizing soft tissue infection	Hemorrhage

- Physical exam would show tense and tenderly affected compartment, severe pain on a passive stretch of the muscles within the compartment.
- Pulses would be diminished or absent in severe elevation of compartment pressure and prolonged cases.

LABORATORY TESTS

- Lab testing is not required for the diagnosis of compartment syndrome. Ancillary testing can be obtained to evaluate for concomitant issues.
  - Creatine phosphokinase level (CPK) – to evaluate for rhabdomyolysis.
  - Electrolytes – to evaluate for hyperkalemia and hyperphosphatemia, which are seen with muscle damage.
  - Coagulation profile – to evaluate for bleeding diathesis in the appropriate setting
  - Lactate level – can be obtained to evaluate for the degree of hypoperfusion.

IMAGING STUDIES

- Acute compartment syndrome is a clinical diagnosis, and imaging studies are not required. Imaging can lead to a delay in diagnosis and should be considered only if there is a strong suspicion of an alternate diagnosis.

THERAPEUTIC INTERVENTIONS

Acute compartment syndrome is a surgical emergency. Airway, breathing, and circulation should be assessed, and the airway should be secured. Hypoxia should be corrected with oxygen supplementation. To reduce hypoperfusion to the affected limb, hypotension should be corrected with IV fluids. Pain control should be instituted with intravenous opioids. The limb should be

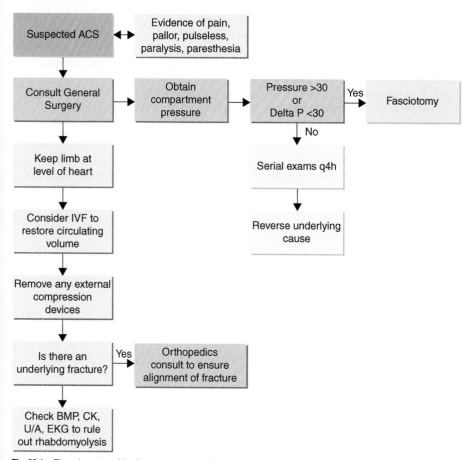

Fig. 62.1   Flowchart to guide the management of acute compartment syndrome in a hospitalized patient

positioned at the level of the heart. Elevating the limb would lead to decreased perfusion while putting the limb in a dependent position increases the risk of edema and increased compartment pressures. An emergent consult should be obtained from orthopedic surgery or general surgery to evaluate the compartment and further management. Any tight bandages, casts, or splints should be removed after consultation with surgical teams. Measurement of compartment pressure is not required for making a diagnosis of acute compartment syndrome. If an emergent in-house surgical consultation cannot be obtained, the patient should be transferred emergently to a facility with in-house surgery and the capability of conducting fasciotomy.

STEPWISE APPROACH TO THE MANAGEMENT OF SUSPECTED ACUTE COMPARTMENT SYNDROME

Step 1: Assess the limb for the cause of acute pain. Rule out differentials such as acute limb ischemia by ensuring the presence of distal pulses.

Step 2: Emergent surgical consultation should be obtained to evaluate the compartments.

Step 3: Ensure adequate perfusion to the limb. The limb should be positioned at the level of the heart;
avoid elevation or dependent positioning. IV fluids should be used to ensure adequate perfusion.

Step 4: For patients with known fractures or limb injuries, any immobilizing devices such as plaster casts should be removed after consultation with the surgical team.

Step 5: Adequate analgesia should be instituted.

Step 6: Ancillary lab work can be obtained to evaluate for complications from myocyte injury such as hyperkalemia and acidosis.

Step 7: If in-house surgical services are not present, the patient should be transferred immediately to a center where an emergent surgical evaluation and intervention can be done.

Suggested Reading

Guo J, Yin Y, Jin L, Zhang R, Hou Z, Zhang Y. Acute compartment syndrome: cause, diagnosis, and new viewpoint. *Medicine (Baltimore)*. 2019;98(27):e16260. https://doi.org/10.1097/MD.0000000000016260.

Page numbers followed by '*f*' indicate figures, '*t*' indicate tables.

ClinicalKey®

Confidence
is ClinicalKey

Evidence-based answers,
continually updated

The latest answers, always at your fingertips

A subscription to ClinicalKey draws content from
countless procedural videos, peer-reviewed journals,
patient education materials, and books authored by
the most respected names in medicine.

Your patients trust you. You can trust ClinicalKey.

Equip yourself with trusted, current content that provides you with
the clinical knowledge to improve patient outcomes.

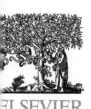

Printed and bound by CPI Group (UK) Ltd, Croydon, CR0 4YY

08/05/2025

01864764-0001